Minimally Invasive Surgery of the Lumbar Spine

Pier Paolo Maria Menchetti

Editor

Minimally Invasive Surgery of the Lumbar Spine

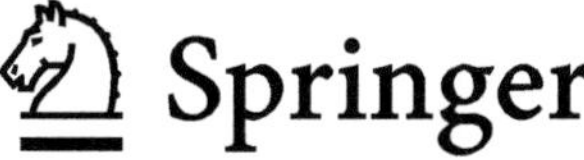 Springer

Editor
Pier Paolo Maria Menchetti, MD, FRCS (US)
Florence University
Florence
Italy

Department of Orthopaedics
Rome American Hospital
Rome
Italy

ISBN 978-1-4471-5279-8   ISBN 978-1-4471-5280-4   (eBook)
DOI 10.1007/978-1-4471-5280-4
Springer London Heidelberg New York Dordrecht

Library of Congress Control Number: 2013950486

*To the dear memory of my mother.
To my father.*

Preface

The growing interest in minimally invasive lumbar spinal surgery (lumbar MISS) with the actual possibility to perform different lumbar spinal surgical procedures was the motivation behind gathering the contributions and editing a book on this innovative topic. Because of the multidisciplinary nature of MISS, professionals including orthopedic surgeons, neurosurgeons, radiologists, anesthesiologists, and pain management specialists have been involved in order to create a handbook in which all the aspects of lumbar MISS are treated.

Lumbar back and/or radicular pain is encountered at least once in their lifetimes by 80 % of the adult population. When conservative treatment fails, before undertaking standard open surgery, lumbar MISS can offer to the patient a panel of surgical procedures with a low rate of morbidity and complications, permitting a fast return to daily activities.

This handbook on the current status on lumbar MISS may be useful both to expert surgeons and to young surgeons or clinicians with little or no experience in this field of surgery. Because of the involvement of different and highly trained specialists from all over the world, the aim of this handbook is to satisfy the requirements for knowing the most advanced surgical techniques and their application.

A chapter is presented on new anesthesiology methods applied in the minimally invasive field, as general anesthesia is usually not required; in fact, mild sedation allows safe operations for patients with cardiopulmonary diseases or compromised general conditions. A section dedicated to lumbar pain management using a percutaneous approach with radiofrequency has been widely investigated, before introducing percutaneous lumbar disc herniation treatments and degenerated intervertebral disc treatments.

Most of the chapters concern the osteodiscoarthrosic pathology, mainly responsible for chronic lumbar and/or radicular pain in the fourth to sixth decade of life, with step-by-step presentation of either the most advanced MISS (endoscopically placed cage) or the standard procedures such as interspinous devices, minimally invasive dynamic stabilization systems designed to restore the physiological intervertebral motion, and interlaminar lumbar interbody systems of fusion. Looking to the future, a chapter about robotic assistance in lumbar spine surgery is also presented.

I would like to thank all the authors for the high scientific value of their contribution. The handbook is foreworded by ISLASS (International Society Laser and Percutaneous Procedures in Spinal Surgery), a multidisciplinary society devoted to the standard and the most innovative procedures in spinal surgery.

Florence, Italy   Pier Paolo Maria Menchetti, MD, FRCS (US)

Contents

Contributors

Massimo Balsano, MD Department of Orthopaedic, Regional Spinal Department, Santorso Hospital, Santorso, Vicenza, Italy

Rapahel Bartalesi, PhD Department of Bioengineering, University of Pisa, Pisa, Italy

Yair Barzilay, MD Spine Unit, Department of Orthopedic Surgery, Hadassah-Hebrew University Medical Center, Jerusalem, Israel

Lorin Michael Benneker, MD Department of Orthopaedic Surgery, Inselspital Bern, Bern, Switzerland

Walter Bini, MD, FRCS Department of Neurosurgery, The City Hospital, Dubai, UAE

Francesco Cacciola, MD Department of Neurosurgery, Siena University, Siena, Italy

Giuseppe Calvosa, MD Department of Orthopaedics and Traumatology, Santa Maria Maddalena Hospital, Volterra, Italy

Angelo Chierichini, MD Department of Anesthesiology and Intensive Care, Catholic University School of Medicine, Rome, Italy

Riccardo Ciarpaglini, MD Department of Orthopaedic Surgery, Hospital Cantonal Fribourg, Fribourg, Switzerland

Gianluca Cinotti, MD Orthopedic Department, University Sapienza, Rome, Italy

Cesare Colosimo, MD Department of Bioimaging and Radiological Sciences, Institute of Radiology, Catholic University, Rome, Italy

Alessandro Maria Costantini, MD Department of Bioimaging and Radiological Sciences, Institute of Radiology, Catholic University, Rome, Italy

Giuseppe Costanzo, MD Department of Orthopedic Surgery,
Polo Pontino, University of Rome Sapienza, Rome, Italy

Roberto Delfini, MD Division of Neurosurgery, Department of Neurology
and Psychiatry, University of Rome Sapienza, Rome, Italy

Nicola Di Lorenzo, MD Department of Neurosurgery, Florence University,
Florence, Italy

Maurizio Domenicucci, MD Division of Neurosurgery,
Department of Neurology and Psychiatry, University of Rome Sapienza,
Rome, Italy

Carlo Doria, MD U.O.C. Orthopedics and Traumatology,
San Martino Hospital, Oristano, Italy

Luciano Frassanito, MD Department of Anesthesiology and Intensive Care,
Catholic University School of Medicine, Rome, Italy

Matteo Galgani, MD Department of Orthopaedics and Traumatology,
Santa Maria Maddalena Hospital, Volterra, Italy

Charles A. Gauci, MD, KHS, FRCA, FIPP, FFPMRCA Department of Pain
Management, Whipps Cross University Hospital, London, UK

Christian Giannetti, MD Department of Orthopaedics and Traumatology,
Santa Maria Maddalena Hospital, Volterra, Italy

Eyal Itshayek, MD Department of Neurosurgery, Hadassah-Hebrew
University Medical Center, Jerusalem, Israel

Leon Kaplan, MD Spine Unit, Department of Orthopedic Surgery,
Hadassah-Hebrew University Medical Center, Jerusalem, Israel

Alessandro Landi, MD, PhD Division of Neurosurgery, Department
of Neurology and Psychiatry, University of Rome Sapienza, Rome, Italy

Wanda Lattanzi, MD Department of Anatomy and Cell Biology,
Università Cattolica del Sacro Cuore, Rome, Italy

Meir Liebergall, MD Spine Unit, Department of Orthopedic Surgery,
Hadassah-Hebrew University Medical Center, Jerusalem, Israel

Giandomenico Logroscino, MD Department of Orthopaedics
and Traumatology, Università Cattolica del Sacro Cuore, Rome, Italy

Gianluca Maestretti, MD Department of Orthopaedic Surgery,
Hospital Cantonal Fribourg, Fribourg, Switzerland

Pier Paolo Maria Menchetti, MD, FRCS (US) Florence University,
Florence, Italy
Department of Orthopaedics, Rome American Hospital, Rome, Italy

Etienne Monnard, MD Department of Radiology, Hospital Cantonal Fribourg, Fribourg, Switzerland

Christian Morgenstern, MD, PhD Centrum für Muskuloskeletale Chirurgie, Charité Universitätsmedizin Berlin, Berlin, Germany

Centrum für Muskuloskeletale Chirurgie, Charitè Hospital, Berlin, Germany

Rudolf Morgenstern, MD, PhD Orthopedic Spine Surgery Unit, Centro Médico Teknon, Barcelona, Spain

Francesco Muresu, MD Department of Orthopedics, University of Sassari, Sassari, Italy

Alessandro Pedicelli, MD Department of Bioimaging and Radiological Sciences, Institute of Radiology, Catholic University, Rome, Italy

Germano Perotti, MD Department of Bioimaging and Radiological Sciences, Nuclear Medicine Institute, Catholic University, Rome, Italy

Department of Bio-Imaging, Radiology/Neuroradiology Institute – Nuclear Medicine Institute, Catholic University of Sacred Heart, Polyclinic A Gemelli, School of Medicine, Rome, Italy

Marco Pileggi, MD Department of Bioimaging and Radiological Sciences, Institute of Radiology, Catholic University, Rome, Italy

Roberto Postacchini, MD Italian University of Sport and Movement (IUSM), Rome, Italy

Israelitic Hospital Rome, Rome, Italy

Alessandro Ramieri, MD, PhD Division of Orthopedic, Don Gnocchi Foundation, Milan, Italy

Stefano Santoprete, MD Department of Anesthesiology and Intensive Care, Catholic University School of Medicine, Rome, Italy

Josh E. Schroeder, MD Spine Unit, Department of Orthopedic Surgery, Hadassah-Hebrew University Medical Center, Jerusalem, Israel

Bengt Sturesson, MD Department of Orthopedics, Ängelholm County Hospital, Ängelholm, Sweden

Miria Tenucci, MD Department of Orthopaedics and Traumatology, Santa Maria Maddalena Hospital, Volterra, Italy

Anton A. Thompkins, MD Department of Orthopaedic, Lakeshore Bone and Joint Institute, Chesterton, IN, USA

Paolo Tranquilli Leali, MD Department of Orthopedics, University of Sassari, Sassari, Italy

Chapter 1
Anesthesia and Perioperative Care in MISS

Angelo Chierichini, Stefano Santoprete, and Luciano Frassanito

General Considerations

The work of the anesthesiologist in MISS ranges widely, from mild to deep sedation and Monitored Anesthesia Care (MAC) to general anesthesia, in some cases with single-lung ventilation and/or invasive systemic blood pressure or central venous pressure monitoring. There is also great variability in surgical techniques, ranging from percutaneous or mini-open posterior approaches to laparo- or thoracoscopic anterior procedures. The choice of the anesthetic technique, drugs, and the appropriate treatment setting is made by considering both the planned surgical procedure and the patient's preoperative conditions [1]. Especially in the elderly, coexisting diseases are frequent and often chronic therapies can often interfere with anesthetics or increase the rate of some surgical or anesthesiological complications.

Population aging is a well-known phenomenon, leading to various social and economic problems. As a consequence, we have an increase in healthcare demand while, on the other hand, worldwide economic difficulties are increasing, especially in the last few years.

In the future, we will probably be driven to expand the indications for outpatient (OP) or day-surgery (DS) treatments, enrolling not only low-risk patients [2].

Obviously, the aim of the anesthesiologist in MISS has to be oriented towards a fast-track protocol, allowing the return of the patient to their normal activity as soon as possible (Fig. 1.1).

In some cases, this can be a challenge.

The availability of modern drugs, characterized by a rapid and full recovery, and the improvement in the cardiorespiratory monitoring in the operating room has even

A. Chierichini, MD (✉) • S. Santoprete, MD • L. Frassanito, MD
Department of Anesthesiology and Intensive Care, Catholic University School of Medicine,
Largo Agostino Gemelli 8, Rome 00168, Italy
e-mail: angelo.chierichini@rm.unicatt.it, achierichini@gmail.com

P.P.M. Menchetti (ed.), *Minimally Invasive Surgery of the Lumbar Spine*,
DOI 10.1007/978-1-4471-5280-4_1, © Springer-Verlag London 2014

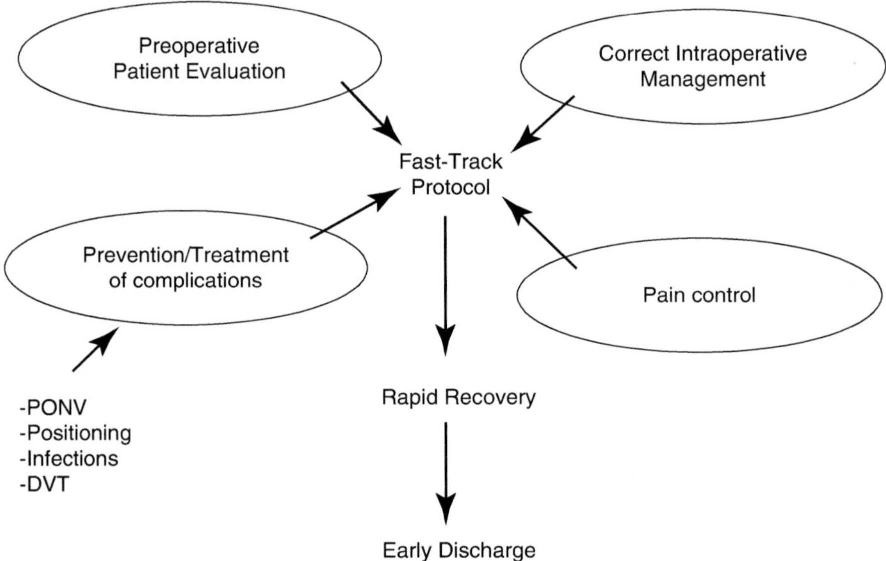

Fig. 1.1 The fast-track treatment in MISS

made possible the administering of general anesthesia to many patients in OP or DS setting.

The preoperative patient assessment is crucial, determining most of the subsequent clinical decisions and therapeutic choices. Moreover, most of the postoperative complications can be minimized or avoided if some preoperative situations are correctly pondered. The prevention of post operative nausea and vomiting (PONV) and post discharge nausea and vomiting (PDNV) could have better results if risk factors are previously detected, influencing the drug choice and, in some cases, the anesthetic technique. The incidence of deep venous thrombosis (DVT) after spine surgery is not negligible [3]. Despite the lack of data concerning MISS in the literature, the potential risk of devastating outcomes deserves particular care. The preoperative evaluation of thromboembolic risk is mandatory in order to decide whether or not to apply some kind of prophylaxis.

Preventing infections is important in spine surgery. In fact, the treatment of established infections is slow and difficult and the outcome is not always good [4, 5].

Indeed, the real secret of success of fast-track treatment in MISS is a good team; surgeons, anesthesiologists, nurses, and physiotherapists, as well as other specialists, can achieve good results only by working together and sharing information [6, 7].

Preoperative Patient Assessment

In order to establish the proper treatment setting for every patient, multiple aspects must be considered. Some factors are patient related, such as age, comorbidities, and grade of autonomy.

Every patient scheduled for surgery should be studied in order to customize the treatment. The assessment of the patient-related risk, together with the consideration of the surgical procedure and the most appropriate anesthetic technique, lead to proper clinical decisions.

Today, there is great interest in the new trends for preoperative risk assessment in DS. The subject is really too wide to be treated deeply in this chapter. We will only try to provide here some simple indications emerging from recent experiences.

The simplest approach to risk assessment is the stratification according to the American Society of Anesthesiologists Physical Status Classification System (ASA class). For years, patients exceeding ASA I-II have been considered not suitable to be treated in an OP or DS setting. More recent studies evidenced that patients in ASA III can be treated as OPs without significant increase in perioperative complications [2, 8]. ASA IV patients are generally addressed for an inpatient treatment.

Most authors are now focusing their attention on the single comorbidities rather than on the ASA class, and particularly on their grade of stabilization. Older patients especially are often affected by one or more chronic diseases, leading to possible perioperative complications. Mainly, patients suffering from diabetes, cardiovascular diseases, and/or chronic obstructive pulmonary disease (COPD) need a careful evaluation. In addition, especially if a fast-track treatment is proposed, patients with already-diagnosed or suspected obstructive sleep apnea (OSA) deserve special attention. Untreated or poorly stabilized situations should suggest delaying surgery or deciding on an inpatient protocol [9].

For diabetic patients, it is strongly advised to assess the level of control of the disease, based on the history, the number of previous hospital admissions for hypo- or hyperglycemia, and so on. It is also important to assess the level of compliance of the patient with their disease. Commonly, a good compliance consists of the ability to perform blood glucose tests by oneself and to detect the early symptoms of hypoglycemia.

Oral antidiabetics should not be taken on the day of surgery, and are to be avoided until normal alimentation is resumed.

Patients on insulin often take a combined therapy consisting of a basal component, a single dose of long-acting insulin, and a postprandial correction with a short-acting insulin. Usually, if the patient has not experienced preprandial hypoglycemia in the last months, it is safe and advisable to administer 75–100 % of basal-dose long-acting insulin the morning of surgery. However, the main objective is to avoid hypoglycemia, so it is advisable to keep blood glucose levels under control and to be ready to administer 5–10 % glucose solutions IV perioperatively.

High levels of glycosylated hemoglobin A1c (HbA1c) can help to detect patients with poor control of the disease. Levels of HbA1c lower than 7 %, representing the ideal therapeutic target according to the American Diabetes Association Guidelines [10], were found to be associated with a significantly lower rate of postoperative infections [11].

Patients affected by coronary artery disease (CAD) should be carefully investigated. They can be enrolled for a fast-track treatment only if a good coronary functional reserve is documented, but they should be excluded in case of instability or recent modifications in the appearance of symptoms [8].

Recent works suggest that congestive heart failure (CHF) is actually the most important risk factor for perioperative morbidity and mortality [12]. CHF leading to a NYHA (New York Heart Association) class higher than II suggests an inpatient treatment.

With cardiac patients there is general agreement to continue chronic medications until the morning of surgery, with a few exceptions. Recent reviews suggest a short preoperative suspension of all renin-angiotensin-aldosterone system antagonists. According to their results, these drugs increased the rate of significant hypotension episodes after the induction of anesthesia, or during neuraxial blocks, and the incidence of postoperative acute renal failure [13].

The perioperative continuation of antiplatelet drugs should be carefully considered. While it is commonly accepted, in the presence of a bleeding risk, to suspend the therapy in primary prevention, many reports suggest that the antiplatelet withdrawal during secondary prevention for ischemic diseases may lead to serious complications [14]. When a double antiplatelet therapy is administered, elective surgery should be postponed. Moreover, when surgery is performed in closed spaces, such as the spinal canal, the risk of bleeding should be carefully evaluated. The average increase in bleeding risk in non-cardiac surgery is about 20 % with aspirin or clopidogrel alone [15, 16]. The risk rises to 50 % above the basic risk when aspirin and clopidogrel are used in combination [17]. In such situations, a multidisciplinary approach involving surgeon, anesthesiologist, and cardiologist or neurologist is advisable to optimize a case-by-case clinical decision [18, 19].

COPD is a frequent condition among the older patients and is often associated with obesity. The increase in the rate of postoperative bronchopulmonary complications is well known, despite the lack of large clinical studies in minimally invasive surgery [20, 21]. If general anesthesia or deep sedation are needed, a severe or poorly compensated COPD with increased bronchial secretions and clinically relevant bronchial reactivity suggests treatment in an inpatient setting. Prophylactic antibiotic therapy is advised. In the compliant patient, banning smoking at least 6–8 weeks before surgery has significantly lowered the rate of bronchopulmonary complications and improved surgical wound healing [22]. If possible, local anesthesia and monitored anesthesia care should be preferred. However, if tracheal intubation is mandatory, the early weaning from invasive ventilation helps prevent complications [23].

Particularly in the elderly, smokers, and obese patients, OSA is not uncommon and is often underdiagnosed. The frequent association of anatomical abnormalities in the upper airways suggests a careful evaluation for suspected difficult intubation and the availability of all emergency airway equipment [24]. In recent years, simple questionnaires to detect patients with suspected OSA have been proposed, compared with others, and validated [25].

Patients with already diagnosed and treated OSA can be managed in OP or DS settings if they are able and skilled in the use of a continuous positive air pressure (CPAP) device (a device they may possibly already use at home) in the postoperative period. Patients with suspected OSA and without comorbidities, with a low risk emerging from clinical evaluation and from the questionnaire results, can be treated in OP or DS settings only if the postoperative pain can be easily controlled without opioids. In cases with high risk for suspected OSA or with comorbidities, or when postoperative opioid use is mandatory, it is more prudent to opt for an inpatient treatment [26].

Postoperative Pain Control

Pain after spine surgery is often more intense than in other surgical settings. Skin incision involves more frequently multiple adjacent dermatomes, and painful anatomical structures are often involved, such as periosteum, ligaments, facet joints, and muscular fascial tissue. In particular, periosteum seems to be one of the most painful tissues, having the lowest pain threshold nerve fibers among the deep somatic structures [27]. Complex mechanisms of peripheral and central sensitization of pain receptors and spinal cord pathways are also involved in explaining the resistance to treatment and the tendency to persist even after days. In addition, patients scheduled for spine surgery are often under preoperative chronic pain therapy. In some patients, a heavy use of opioids in the preoperative period creates serious therapeutic challenges postoperatively, making pain less responsive to incremental doses of opioids [28].

MISS techniques are already helpful in and of themselves in reducing postoperative pain, thanks to the generally small skin incisions and the reduced damage to muscles and deep tissues. However, pain represents, among the postoperative "side effects" of surgery, one of the most common causes of hospital re-admission or delayed discharge in an OP or DS setting. Currently, the multimodal approach to pain therapy is considered the best treatment model, as it reduces the doses of the single drugs used and minimizes the potential side effects. The multimodal or balanced treatment consists of combining, starting in the preoperative period, opioid and non-opioid analgesics that have additive or synergistic actions [29].

Other techniques can be adopted, together with drug therapy, to help decrease postoperative pain. Skin and tissue infiltration with a long-acting local anesthetic along with epinephrine before the surgical incision is a common practice, reducing intraoperative bleeding and requirement for analgesics, at least in the earlier postoperative period. Continuous postoperative wound infiltration with local anesthetics through microcatheters of various length is also available, but not so widely used, even though the efficacy and the slow rate of complications have been demonstrated [30, 31].

Because of its large margin of safety and the rarity of complications, acetaminophen deserves a special place in the management of pain after MISS, as in every other minimally invasive surgery. Acetaminophen alone or in combination with other NSAIDs or mild opiates, can efficiently control pain or significantly reduce the consumption of other analgesics in the postoperative period. The availability of oral and intravenous (IV) preparations makes it suitable both for perioperative and postoperative use, and also allows continuation of the therapy easy after the patient's discharge [29].

Non-steroidal anti-inflammatory drugs (NSAIDs) and cyclooxygenase-2 inhibitors (COX-2) lead to increased risk of nonunion after spine fusion surgery, but this adverse effect seems limited to a prolonged use (>14 days) or high doses. The use of more than 120 mg/day of ketorolac, even for few days, or the use of more than 300 mg of diclofenac in total significantly affect the risk of nonunion [32]. When used at lower doses and for fewer days, these drugs help in postoperative pain treatment.

Opioids still have an important role in the treatment of moderate-to-severe postoperative pain, but because of the important side effects, especially in a fast-track approach, it is advisable to avoid their use if possible, or at least to reduce the doses in a multimodal protocol. The association of NSAIDs or celecoxib with a slow-release oxycodone, starting during the preoperative period, when compared with intravenous morphine, improved outcome in spine surgery, providing earlier recovery of the bowel function [33]. Patients treated preoperatively with opiates for chronic back pain could need higher doses of opiates in the perioperative period. The use of intraoperative ketamine infusion in these patients has significantly lowered opiate consumption in the postoperative period and even for 6 weeks after surgery, but the clinical benefits in terms of reduction in opiate-related side-effects has been minimal [34].

The gabapentinoids (gabapentin, pregabalin) have also been used in association with other drugs for multimodal postoperative pain treatment, but their role remains uncertain as some studies failed to demonstrate a reduced opioids consumption. Furthermore, the frequent side effects, such as somnolence and sedation, dizziness, and ataxia, could slow the physical and psychological recovery, especially in older patients [29].

Prophylaxis of Infections

Infection is a serious complication in spine surgery, with an incidence varying from 0.4 to 3.5 %, and it deserves great attention in its prevention and treatment [4, 5]. Despite many attempts to extract valid meta-analysis from the literature data, the lack of randomized controlled studies and the presence of many confounding factors made researchers' efforts in vain [35].

The best approach to the problem is to establish the most context-sensitive protocol of treatment possible. It would be advisable to work in a multidisciplinary way, involving in the decisions an infectious diseases specialist and considering local epidemiological data regarding both the bacteria involved and the resistances detected [36, 37].

However, in most cases, a prophylaxis with a low-cost first-generation cephalosporin should be adopted. Cefazolin 2 g IV immediately before surgery is the most common prophylaxis as first choice, with a good activity against staphylococci, streptococci, and other Gram-positive bacteria, and also against common and dangerous Gram-negative bacteria as *Escherichia coli, Klebsiella pneumoniae,* and *Proteus mirabilis.* In case of allergy to penicillin or cephalosporins, a slow IV administration of vancomycin 1 g is normally recommended. In any case, the administration should be completed within 1 h before the beginning of surgery. There are not clear indications in the literature about the cost or effectiveness of the continuation of the antibiotic therapy in the postoperative period [4, 38].

Obviously, prevention of infection should go beyond antibiotic therapy and should involve the efforts of the entire surgical team, meaning the surgeon, the nurses, and also the anesthesiologist. Particular care is needed in establishing procedures for preoperative hygienic preparation of the patient, in adopting behavioral rules against contamination in the operating room, and so on. Furthermore, special attention is necessary with diabetic patients; metabolic control in the perioperative period is crucial for the reduction of bacterial colonization of the surgical site [4].

Thromboprophylaxis

This is a perfect example of a matter in which the level of understanding and good teamwork between the surgeon and the anesthesiologist is crucial. The decision about the adoption of a possible pharmacological and/or mechanical prophylaxis of the deep venous thrombosis (DVT) should follow a careful evaluation of the risk factors, both patient and procedure related [39, 40]. Nevertheless, other drugs, such as NSAIDs and antiplatelet agents, could interfere with surgical hemostasis, particularly if used in association with low-molecular-weight heparin (LMWH) or other anticoagulants.

There is lack of data about the incidence of DVT and pulmonary embolism (PE) in MISS, but it can probably be assumed that it should be lower than the rates observed for spine surgery in general. In a recent large review, observing more than 100,000 procedures from 2004 to 2007, the incidence of thromboembolic events (pulmonary embolism) in spine surgery varied widely from 0.47 per 1,000 cases for first-time lumbar microdiscectomy to 12.4 per 1,000 cases for metastatic tumor [41]. Probably, the risk of DVT and PE in MISS should not always be considered negligible; often the procedures are really mini-invasive, but sometimes this can be counterbalanced by an increase in patient-related risk factors, such as age, obesity, and comorbidities.

Among the surgical procedures considered in MISS, percutaneous vertebroplasty (PVP) deserves a special consideration for thromboembolic complications due to the possible leakage of cement in the veins of the vertebral bone. In a recent study, among 78 patients treated with PVP, 18 (23 %) showed CT-scan evidence of cement lung embolization [42]. Fortunately, most episodes remain asymptomatic or evolve in mild and reversible dyspnea. Rarely, however, fatal episodes have been reported [43, 44]. The presence of cement in a vein could even lead to late embolic complications, with symptoms occurring even after years [45]. Less rarely, the beginning of the symptoms is at the end of surgery or in the following few days. In these cases, clinical observation of patients and the execution of a thoracic CT scan is advisable [42]. In the asymptomatic patients with peripheral embolisms incidentally revealed with CT scan, no treatment is recommended, but a frequent follow-up is advisable. Symptomatic patients should be treated according to the guidelines for the treatment of thrombotic pulmonary embolisms, in order to avoid the progression of occlusion. Initial treatment with LMWH, followed by 6 months of therapy with oral anticoagulants to avoid additional thrombosis, ensures the endothelialization of the cement embolus and therefore the end of its thrombogenic risk [46].

It is unclear whether it is advisable to start a prophylaxis with LMWH in patients undergoing PVP. There are no specific guidelines for DVT prophylaxis about PVP.

The new ninth ACCP's guidelines suggest mechanical prophylaxis preferably with intermittent pneumatic compression in patients undergoing spinal surgery; in patients at high risk for VTE (including those with malignant disease and those undergoing surgery with a combined anterior-posterior approach), it is suggested to add pharmacologic prophylaxis to the mechanical prophylaxis once adequate hemostasis is established and the risk of bleeding has decreased [40].

PONV and PDNV Prevention and Treatment

After postoperative pain, nausea and vomiting are the second most common cause of hospital readmission or delayed discharge after ambulatory or 1 day surgery and affect heavily the grade of patient's satisfaction. Furthermore, vomiting can cause other severe complications such as pulmonary aspiration. Several studies have been dedicated to the problem, and guidelines have been established to help physicians in clinical decisions [47].

Detecting risk factors preoperatively is crucial to providing a correct PONV prevention in each patient. A simple way to assess the risk of PONV after general anesthesia has been proposed; it is based on the detection of only four characteristics: female gender, history of motion sickness or PONV, non-smoking status, need for postoperative opioids [48]. When none of the above is present, no prophylaxis is recommended. Higher risk scores deserve prophylaxis with one or more drugs, and/ or the adoption of specific anesthetic techniques. Regional or local anesthesia and, when general anesthesia is needed, totally intravenous anesthesia (TIVA) are associated with lower PONV incidence than inhalational anesthesia, especially in the first hours after surgery [49, 50].

The protective effects of adequate preoperative and intraoperative hydration against PONV, drowsiness, and dizziness, if not contraindicated, are well known [51]. For the same reason, allowing oral intake of clear fluids until 3 h before surgery helps prevent postoperative nausea and is considered safe as far as inhalation is concerned [7].

Dexamethasone is a long-acting glucocorticoid with a largely demonstrated efficacy in reducing PONV and PDNV [52]. The mechanism of action, probably multifactorial, is still unclear. When administered intravenously during anesthesia induction at a dose ranging from 0.05 to 0.1 mg/kg, it significantly lowers the rate of PONV in various surgical settings and is considered safe in terms of side effects [53]. Although many authors suggest that rescue medication should not involve dexamethasone, when added to ondansetron and droperidol, it has been associated with a significant reduction in established PONV [54].

5-Hydroxytryptamine-3 (5-HT3) receptor antagonists are widely used in common practice for the prevention of PONV and of the side effects of chemotherapy. Ondansetron is the most famous drug of the family, normally used at a dose of 4 mg IV at the end of surgery. Palonosetron, a 5-HT3 antagonist with a longer half-life and a higher receptorial affinity, seems promising, especially for the prevention of PDNV. Even if more effective and safer than ondansetron (no action on QT interval), the use of palonosetron is still limited [53, 55].

Transdermal scopolamine is effective and the side effects are quite frequent, although generally mild and well tolerated [56]. In the elderly, however, the occurrence of confusion or an excessive sedation could be observed, suggesting the removal of the patch. The patch is applied the evening before surgery or at least 2 h before the induction of anesthesia, because the onset of the effect is about 2–4 h.

Droperidol is very effective in the prevention of PONV with a number needed to treat (NNT) of five, and is highly effective in the prevention of nausea during patient-controlled analgesia with opiates (NNT = 3). In the last years, however, the use of droperidol has been greatly limited after the black box warning issued from the Foods and Drug Administration in the USA in 2001. Droperidol has been associated with adverse cardiac events such as prolongation of QT interval and *torsades de pointes*. Although several authors have suggested a revision of that decision, the warning is still active, restricting the use of droperidol to the treatment of patients who fail to show an acceptable response to other adequate treatments [47, 50, 57].

More recent drugs, the neurokinin-1 receptor antagonists, appear to be of interest in the prevention of PONV. Aprepitant, casopitant, and rolapitant showed better results when compared in clinical trial to ondansetron in patients at high risk for PONV, even though the reduction in vomiting is more evident than the reduction of nausea. Especially rolapitant, for its long half-life, could represent the best choice in the future, especially if it is mandatory to avoid vomiting [53, 58].

Intraoperative Management

Spinal anesthesia has been proposed and used for lumbar procedures such as microdiscectomy [59], and could be adopted for minimally invasive lumbar arthrodesis. The assessment of motion recovery and preoperative symptoms relief has to be delayed until the reversal of the block. Also, the psychological compliance of the patient has to be carefully evaluated [1].

With few exceptions, MISS procedures can be performed under MAC, that is, local anesthesia administered together with conscious sedation and analgesia, or general anesthesia. An accurate evaluation of the preoperative patient's status together with the considerations regarding the planned surgical procedure is mandatory. All the features and implications should be considered in order to establish the most suitable clinical decision.

It is important to understand that MAC is not always safer than general anesthesia. Analyzing the trends of the last 30 years in the American Society of Anesthesiologists Closed Claims Database, even in absence of a denominator consisting of the total of the anesthetics performed, the results are quite impressive. MAC-related claims increased from only 2 % of total claims for injuries in the 1980s, to 5 % in the 1990s and 10 % after 2000, while claims deriving from general anesthesia slightly decreased in the same period. Furthermore, death was significantly the most frequent outcome in claims associated with MAC than in claims associated with general or regional anesthesia, and the most frequent damaging mechanism was respiratory depression resulting from oversedation [60, 61].

MISS procedures are often performed in aged patients, with various comorbidities, in the prone position. The increased sensitivity to sedative and opioid drugs and the difficult management of the airways because of the position could generate potentially harmful situations and should be carefully considered [61, 62].

MAC can be performed combining liberal infiltration of the surgical site with a mixture of local anesthetics such as lidocaine or mepivacaine and bupivacaine or ropivacaine to achieve a rapid onset and a long-lasting effect and intravenous sedoanalgesia. Drugs more commonly used for sedation are midazolam, from 0.5 mcg/kg in the elderly to higher doses in the younger patients, and propofol infusion, 25 mcg/kg/min or more, titrating the doses to achieve the control of anxiety while maintaining the ability to respond to verbal stimuli and the control of the airways. Remifentanil infusion at 0.025 mcg/kg/min or more is often added to improve analgesia [7]. Accurate monitoring of the vital signs is mandatory: basic monitoring, that is, continuous ECG, pulse oximetry, respiratory rate, and noninvasive intermittent blood pressure measurement. The assessment of the level of sedation through frequent clinical evaluations or instrumental methods, especially considering electroencephalographic bispectral index [62, 63], is also advisable. When supplemental oxygen is administered, the measurement of end tidal CO_2 obtained through a nasal cannula or simply leaving the probe near the external airways (Fig. 1.2), even if not reliable in the absolute value and with an irregularly shaped wave (Fig. 1.3), can help detect a respiratory depression earlier than pulse oximetry [64]. During a MAC procedure the continuous presence of a qualified and skilled anesthesiologist is crucial, and this is particularly true during procedures performed in the prone position, in which in case of oversedation and prolonged apnea the control of the airways could be very difficult. Laryngeal masks of different sizes and all other devices designed for airways management should always be quickly available, because difficult airways can become a problem throughout anesthesia care, not just during induction of anesthesia [61].

When general anesthesia is indicated, tracheal intubation is the usual technique used to secure the airways, inasmuch as MISS is normally performed with the patient in the prone position. In the last few years, some authors have used and validated the laryngeal masks in prone patients, also studying the differences between the various version of these supraglottic airway devices [65–67]. The results are encouraging, but they seem to depend too much on the skill of the operator. Certainly, the preoperative detection of a "difficult airway" is crucial.

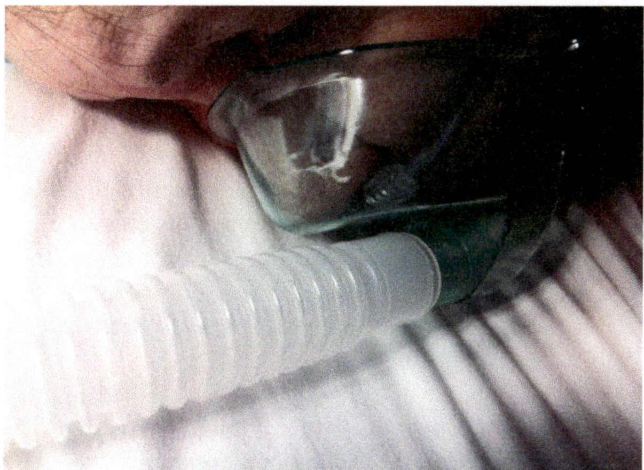

Fig. 1.2 A sampling probe near the external airways during a MAC procedure

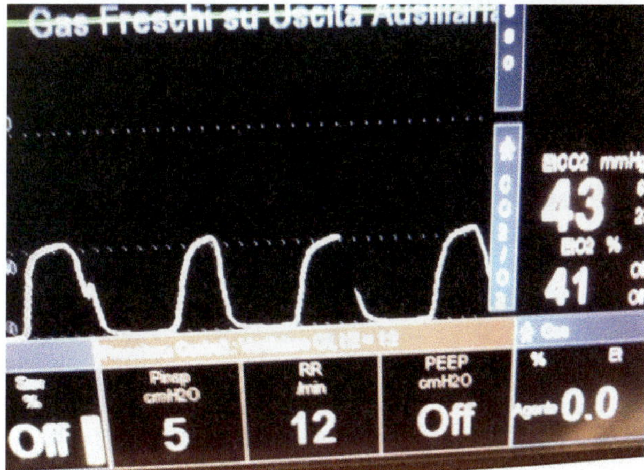

Fig. 1.3 The capnogram during MAC shows a regular spontaneous breathing

Propofol is the induction agent of choice, for its well-known pharmacodynamic and pharmacokinetic properties [68], supported by little doses of a medium-acting opioid such as fentanyl (0.5–2 mcg/kg) and/or by the starting of remifentanil infusion (0.05–0.2 mcg/kg/min) with or without an initial remifentanil bolus (0.1–0.5 mcg/kg) [7].

The choice of an eventual myorelaxant agent to facilitate intubation deserves some consideration. Normally, the neuromuscular block is not necessary for MISS; on the other hand, it could be undesirable if an intraoperative neuromuscular monitoring of lower limbs is planned. Some authors described techniques for performing tracheal intubation without the use of myorelaxant drugs, based on the use of propofol-opioid induction and topical anesthesia [69–71]. However, clinical experience and the literature data suggest that the use of a myorelaxant agent facilitates intubation and decreases the rate of some complications such as postoperative sore throat, hoarseness, and vocal cord injury [72]. In conclusion, the clinical decision about myorelaxation should be made case-by-case in order to minimize the technical difficulties in the airway management, shorten the postoperative recovery time, and avoid or minimize the interference with intraoperative electromyographic monitoring. When a nondepolarizing agent is chosen, the adoption of intraoperative train of four (TOF) monitoring, in addition to the clinical observation, helps in reducing the complications of postoperative residual curarization. A TOF ratio >0.9 is considered safe for the discharge of the patient, while the classical clinical test of the ability to lift the head for more than 5 s allows only a TOF ratio >0.5. Moreover, recent studies have focused on the importance of the use of reversal agents, even if associated with an increase in PONV [72].

Maintenance of anesthesia can be obtained mainly with a balanced technique based on inhalational agents and opioids or with a TIVA. The use of volatile anesthetics has increased the incidence of PONV, when compared with TIVA, especially in the first hours after surgery [49, 50]. Especially in the elderly, the choice of a TIVA could also help prevent postoperative agitation and confusion. In addition, in the wide and fascinating research field of the more subtle and sneaky postoperative cognitive dysfunction, animal and clinical studies seem to indicate a protective role of intravenous anesthesia when compared with inhalational anesthesia [73]. On the other hand, the recent less-soluble volatile agents sevoflurane and desflurane showed some advantages over propofol, facilitating the early discharge from the postoperative care unit [74, 75], especially when PONV prevention was administered.

Special considerations are needed when monitoring of somatosensory-evoked potentials (SSEP) and/or motor-evoked potentials (MEP) is planned, in order to detect intraoperative functional impairment of the spinal pathways. Anesthetic agents can heavily influence the quality of the monitoring, particularly for cortical MEPs (CMEPs). Generally, the first choice should be a TIVA, because of the impact of inhalational anesthetics on evoked potentials, even at low concentrations [76, 77]. Also, intravenous drugs should be chosen carefully: benzodiazepines and barbiturates produce CMEP depression at lower doses than the ones that alter SSEPs and their effect lasts for several minutes. Recently it has been noted that remifentanil, when used at higher doses, also can affect SSEPs monitoring, acting particularly on the amplitude of signals [78]. Spinal MEPs (stimulating cranially to the level of surgery) or pedicle screw testing during spinal instrumentation (EMG recording) are virtually insensitive to anesthetic agents, while they could be impaired from myorelaxant drugs. In any case, because of the complex pattern of interference between anesthesia and intraoperative neurophysiologic monitoring, a continuous exchange of information among all the specialists involved can improve the interpretation of data and the outcome of the patient [76].

Particularly when general anesthesia is performed, great care in patient positioning is needed. In the prone patient, the position of the head, neck, and arms should be carefully checked in order to minimize the rate of certain complications.

One of the most devastating complications in nonocular surgery is perioperative visual loss (POVL). POVL is rare if considered in the whole population of surgical patients, ranging from 1:60,000 to 1:125,000, but is more frequent in cardiac surgery (8.64:10,000), followed by spine surgery (3.09:10,000). The causes of POVL are mainly two: central retinal artery occlusion (CRAO) and ischemic optic nerve neuropathy (ION). The CRAO leads to the ischemia of the entire retina, while the less severe obstruction of a branch of the artery (BRAO) leads to impaired function only in a visual sector. While during cardiac surgery the more common mechanism involved is the arterial microembolism, during spine surgery the complication derives mainly from an improper head position, leading to mono or bilateral ocular compression [79]. Recently, a task force of the ASA has proposed some practical advice for POVL prevention in spine surgery. For the prevention of CRAO and other ocular damage, direct pressure on the eye should be avoided, and the eyes of prone-positioned patients should be assessed regularly and documented [80]. The mechanisms underlying the development of ION are not completely known, but the pathogenesis seems to be multifactorial [79]. Fortunately, the occurrence of ION after spine surgery of short duration, which is a characteristic of MISS procedures, is rare. In a survey of 83 ION after spine surgery, the majority of cases (94 %) occurred for 6 h anesthetic duration or longer, while only one case was associated with surgery lasting less than 4 h [81].

Other complications deriving from improper positioning should be prevented using gel or foam-made dedicated devices (Fig. 1.4) or even normal pillows put together with the active contribution of the surgeons, the nurses, and the anesthesiologist. The final result must ensure the distribution of pressure over larger extensions of tissues, avoiding excessive and localized compressions, and excessive stretching or flexion of elbows, shoulders, and neck. Abdomen compression should be avoided to facilitate intermittent positive pressure ventilation and limit barotrauma. Moreover, the reduction of the intrathoracic mean pressure leads to improvement of venous return and helps decrease surgical bleeding. As discussed above, the head and the face should be frequently controlled (Figs. 1.5 and 1.6) to avoid harmful compressions on the eyes and ears [82].

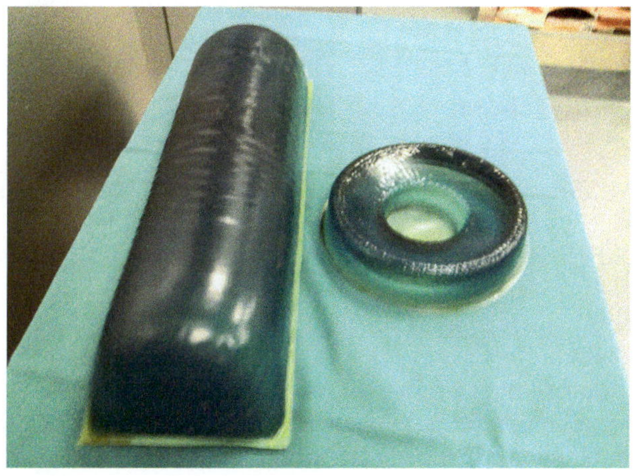

Fig. 1.4 Examples of gel-made devices used for proper intraoperative patient positioning

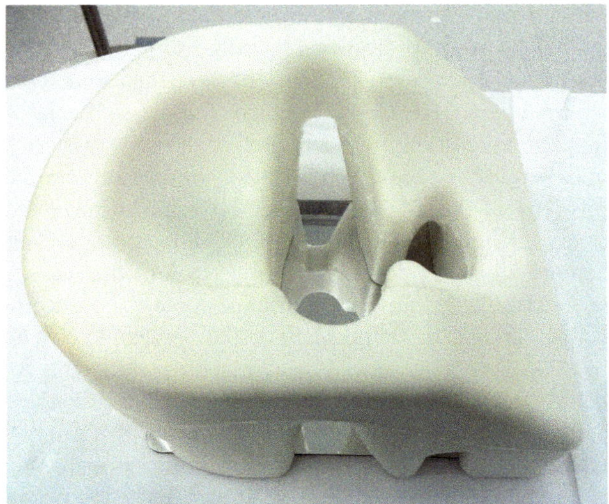

Fig. 1.5 An example of foam-made headrest with mirror

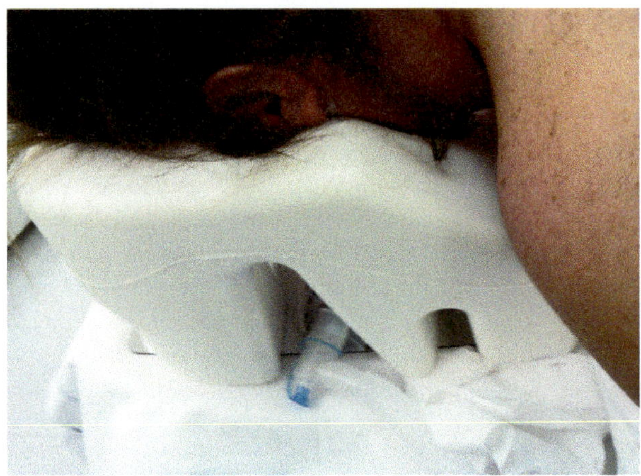

Fig. 1.6 The mirror allows a frequent control of eyes and face placement

Conclusions

MISS has seen great expansion in recent years, thanks to the rapid evolution of bioengineering and to improvements in the knowledge of the physiopathology of the spine. The progress in anesthesiological techniques and drugs, and the availability of modern monitoring devices have allowed to enroll for surgery, and often for fast-track protocols of treatment, even frail older patients or patients with comorbidities.

Performing a minimally invasive surgery, the team should also operate in order to minimize the perioperative side effects and complications and allow a rapid resumption of normal activities of daily living.

Starting with a careful preoperative patient assessment, all the clinical decisions must take into account the prevention of the complications, the optimization of the intraoperative management, multimodal pain control, and customized prevention of PONV.

To achieve optimal results, a skilled anesthesiologist is needed because of the presence, along the way, of several traps and pitfalls, especially during procedures performed under MAC. Above all, the continuous exchange of information among the team members is a key factor to a successful operation.

References

1. Schubert A, Deogaonkar A, Lotto M, Niezgoda J, Luciano M. Anesthesia for minimally invasive cranial and spinal surgery. J Neurosurg Anesthesiol. 2006;18(1):47–56.
2. Bettelli G. Anaesthesia for the elderly outpatient: preoperative assessment and evaluation, anaesthetic technique and postoperative pain management. Curr Opin Anaesthesiol. 2010;23(6):726–31.
3. Takahashi H, Yokoyama Y, Iida Y, Terashima F, Hasegawa K, Saito T, Suguro T, Wada A. Incidence of venous thromboembolism after spine surgery. J Orthop Sci. 2012;17(2):114–7.
4. Epstein NE. Preoperative, intraoperative, and postoperative measures to further reduce spinal infections. Surg Neurol Int. 2011;2:17.
5. Bible JE, Biswas D, Devin CJ. Postoperative infections of the spine. Am J Orthop (Belle Mead NJ). 2011;40(12):E264–71.
6. Baldini G, Carli F. Anesthetic and adjunctive drugs for fast-track surgery. Curr Drug Targets. 2009;10(8):667–86.
7. White PF, Eng M. Fast-track anesthetic techniques for ambulatory surgery. Curr Opin Anaesthesiol. 2007;20(6):545–57.
8. Bettelli G. High risk patients in day surgery. Minerva Anestesiol. 2009;75(5):259–68.
9. Ankichetty S, Chung F. Considerations for patients with obstructive sleep apnea undergoing ambulatory surgery. Curr Opin Anaesthesiol. 2011;24(6):605–11.
10. American Diabetes Association. Executive summary: standards of medical care in diabetes – 2012. Diabetes Care. 2012;35 Suppl 1:S4–10.
11. Joshi GP, Chung F, Vann MA, Ahmad S, Gan TJ, Goulson DT, Merrill DG, Twersky R, Society for Ambulatory Anesthesia. Society for Ambulatory Anesthesia consensus statement on perioperative blood glucose management in diabetic patients undergoing ambulatory surgery. Anesth Analg. 2010;111(6):1378–87.
12. Hammill BG, Curtis LH, Bennett-Guerrero E, O'Connor CM, Jollis JG, Schulman KA, Hernandez AF. Impact of heart failure on patients undergoing major noncardiac surgery. Anesthesiology. 2008;108(4):559–67.
13. Auron M, Harte B, Kumar A, Michota F. Renin-angiotensin system antagonists in the perioperative setting: clinical consequences and recommendations for practice. Postgrad Med J. 2011;87(1029):472–81.
14. Biondi-Zoccai GG, Lotrionte M, Agostoni P, Abbate A, Fusaro M, Burzotta F, Testa L, Sheiban I, Sangiorgi G. A systematic review and meta-analysis on the hazards of discontinuing or not adhering to aspirin among 50,279 patients at risk for coronary artery disease. Eur Heart J. 2006;27(22):2667–74. PubMed PMID.
15. Burger W, Chemnitius JM, Kneissl GD, Rücker G. Low-dose aspirin for secondary cardiovascular prevention – cardiovascular risks after its perioperative withdrawal versus bleeding risks with its continuation – review and meta-analysis. J Intern Med. 2005;257(5):399–414.
16. CAPRIE Steering Committee. A randomised, blinded, trial of clopidogrel versus aspirin in patients at risk of ischaemic events (CAPRIE) CAPRIE Steering Committee. Lancet. 1996;348(9038):1329–39.

17. Chassot PG, Marcucci C, Delabays A, Spahn DR. Perioperative antiplatelet therapy. Am Fam Physician. 2010;82(12):1484–9.
18. Steib A, Hadjiat F, Skibba W, Steib JP, French Spine Surgery Society. Focus on perioperative management of anticoagulants and antiplatelet agents in spine surgery. Orthop Traumatol Surg Res. 2011;97(6 Suppl):S102–6.
19. American College of Cardiology/American Heart Association Task Force on Practice Guidelines (Writing Committee to Revise the 2002 Guidelines on Perioperative Cardiovascular Evaluation for Noncardiac Surgery), and other Societies, Fleisher LA, Beckman JA, et al. ACC/AHA 2007 guidelines on perioperative cardiovascular evaluation and care for noncardiac surgery: executive summary: a report of the American College of Cardiology/American Heart Association Task Force on Practice Guidelines (Writing Committee to Revise the 2002 Guidelines on Perioperative Cardiovascular Evaluation for Noncardiac Surgery). Anesth Analg. 2008;106(3):685–712.
20. Bettelli G. Preoperative evaluation in geriatric surgery: comorbidity, functional status and pharmacological history. Minerva Anestesiol. 2011;77(6):637–46.
21. Chung F, Mezei G, Tong D. Pre-existing medical conditions as predictors of adverse events in day-case surgery. Br J Anaesth. 1999;83(2):262–70.
22. Møller AM, Villebro N, Pedersen T, Tønnesen H. Effect of preoperative smoking intervention on postoperative complications: a randomised clinical trial. Lancet. 2002;359(9301):114–7.
23. Spieth PM, Güldner A, de Abreu MG. Chronic obstructive pulmonary disease. Curr Opin Anaesthesiol. 2012;25(1):24–9.
24. Porhomayon J, El-Solh A, Chhangani S, Nader ND. The management of surgical patients with obstructive sleep apnea. Lung. 2011;189(5):359–67.
25. Abrishami A, Khajehdehi A, Chung F. A systematic review of screening questionnaires for obstructive sleep apnea. Can J Anaesth. 2010;57(5):423–38.
26. Joshi GP, Ankichetty SP, Gan TJ, Chung F. Society for Ambulatory Anesthesia consensus statement on preoperative selection of adult patients with obstructive sleep apnea scheduled for ambulatory surgery. Anesth Analg. 2012. doi:10.1213/ANE.0b013e318269cfd7.
27. Buvanendran A, Thillainathan V. Preoperative and postoperative anesthetic and analgesic techniques for minimally invasive surgery of the spine. Spine (Phila Pa 1976). 2010;35(26 Suppl):S274–80.
28. Sharma S, Balireddy RK, Vorenkamp KE, Durieux ME. Beyond opioid patient-controlled analgesia: a systematic review of analgesia after major spine surgery. Reg Anesth Pain Med. 2012;37(1):79–98.
29. Elvir-Lazo OL, White PF. The role of multimodal analgesia in pain management after ambulatory surgery. Curr Opin Anaesthesiol. 2010;23(6):697–703.
30. LeBlanc KA, Bellanger D, Rhynes VK, Hausmann M. Evaluation of continuous infusion of 05% bupivacaine by elastomeric pump for postoperative pain management after open inguinal hernia repair. J Am Coll Surg. 2005;200(2):198–202.
31. Liu SS, Richman JM, Thirlby RC, Wu CL. Efficacy of continuous wound catheters delivering local anesthetic for postoperative analgesia: a quantitative and qualitative systematic review of randomized controlled trials. J Am Coll Surg. 2006;203(6):914–32.
32. Li Q, Zhang Z, Cai Z. High-dose ketorolac affects adult spinal fusion: a meta-analysis of the effect of perioperative nonsteroidal anti-inflammatory drugs on spinal fusion. Spine (Phila Pa 1976). 2011;36(7):E461–8.
33. Blumenthal S, Min K, Marquardt M, Borgeat A. Postoperative intravenous morphine consumption, pain scores, and side effects with perioperative oral controlled-release oxycodone after lumbar discectomy. Anesth Analg. 2007;105(1):233–7.
34. Loftus RW, Yeager MP, Clark JA, Brown JR, Abdu WA, Sengupta DK, Beach ML. Intraoperative ketamine reduces perioperative opiate consumption in opiate-dependent patients with chronic back pain undergoing back surgery. Anesthesiology. 2010;113(3):639–46.
35. van Middendorp DJ, Pull Ter Gunne DA, Drmed PM, Cohen DD, Hosman DA, van Laarhoven PC. A methodological systematic review on surgical site infections following spinal surgery

part 2: prophylactic treatments. Spine (Phila Pa 1976). 2012. doi:10.1097/BRS.0b013e31825f6652.

36. Lazennec JY, Fourniols E, Lenoir T, Aubry A, Pissonnier ML, Issartel B, Rousseau MA, French Spine Surgery Society. Infections in the operated spine: update on risk management and therapeutic strategies. Orthop Traumatol Surg Res. 2011;97(6 Suppl):S107–16.

37. Meredith DS, Kepler CK, Huang RC, Brause BD, Boachie-Adjei O. Postoperative infections of the lumbar spine: presentation and management. Int Orthop. 2012;36(2):439–44.

38. Takahashi H, Wada A, Iida Y, Yokoyama Y, Katori S, Hasegawa K, Shintaro T, Suguro T. Antimicrobial prophylaxis for spinal surgery. J Orthop Sci. 2009;14(1):40–4.

39. Kahn SR, Lim W, Dunn AS, Cushman M, Dentali F, Akl EA, Cook DJ, Balekian AA, Klein RC, Le H, Schulman S, Murad MH, American College of Chest Physicians. Prevention of VTE in nonsurgical patients: Antithrombotic Therapy and Prevention of Thrombosis, 9th ed: American College of Chest Physicians Evidence-Based Clinical Practice Guidelines. Chest. 2012;141(2 Suppl):e195S–226.

40. Gould MK, Garcia DA, Wren SM, Karanicolas PJ, Arcelus JI, Heit JA, Samama CM, American College of Chest Physicians. Prevention of VTE in nonorthopedic surgical patients: Antithrombotic Therapy and Prevention of Thrombosis, 9th ed: American College of Chest Physicians Evidence-Based Clinical Practice Guidelines. Chest. 2012;141(2 Suppl):e227S–77.

41. Smith JS, Fu KM, Polly Jr DW, Sansur CA, Berven SH, Broadstone PA, Choma TJ, Goytan MJ, Noordeen HH, Knapp Jr DR, Hart RA, Donaldson 3rd WF, Perra JH, Boachie-Adjei O, Shaffrey CI. Complication rates of three common spine procedures and rates of thromboembolism following spine surgery based on 108,419 procedures: a report from the Scoliosis Research Society Morbidity and Mortality Committee. Spine (Phila Pa 1976). 2010;35(24):2140–9.

42. Kim YJ, Lee JW, Park KW, Yeom JS, Jeong HS, Park JM, Kang HS. Pulmonary cement embolism after percutaneous vertebroplasty in osteoporotic vertebral compression fractures: incidence, characteristics, and risk factors. Radiology. 2009;251(1):250–9.

43. Stricker K, Orler R, Yen K, Takala J, Luginbühl M. Severe hypercapnia due to pulmonary embolism of polymethylmethacrylate during vertebroplasty. Anesth Analg. 2004;98(4):1184–6.

44. Monticelli F, Meyer HJ, Tutsch-Bauer E. Fatal pulmonary cement embolism following percutaneous vertebroplasty (PVP). Forensic Sci Int. 2005;149(1):35–8.

45. Lim KJ, Yoon SZ, Jeon YS, Bahk JH, Kim CS, Lee JH, Ha JW. An intraatrial thrombus and pulmonary thromboembolism as a late complication of percutaneous vertebroplasty. Anesth Analg. 2007;104(4):924–6.

46. Krueger A, Bliemel C, Zettl R, Ruchholtz S. Management of pulmonary cement embolism after percutaneous vertebroplasty and kyphoplasty: a systematic review of the literature. Eur Spine J. 2009;18(9):1257–65.

47. Gan TJ, Meyer TA, Apfel CC, Chung F, Davis PJ, Habib AS, Hooper VD, Kovac AL, Kranke P, Myles P, Philip BK, Samsa G, Sessler DI, Temo J, Tramèr MR, Vander Kolk C, Watcha M, Society for Ambulatory Anesthesia. Society for Ambulatory Anesthesia guidelines for the management of postoperative nausea and vomiting. Anesth Analg. 2007;105(6):1615–28, table of contents.

48. Apfel CC, Läärä E, Koivuranta M, Greim CA, Roewer N. A simplified risk score for predicting postoperative nausea and vomiting: conclusions from cross-validations between two centers. Anesthesiology. 1999;91(3):693–700.

49. Apfel CC, Kranke P, Katz MH, Goepfert C, Papenfuss T, Rauch S, Heineck R, Greim CA, Roewer N. Volatile anaesthetics may be the main cause of early but not delayed postoperative vomiting: a randomized controlled trial of factorial design. Br J Anaesth. 2002;88(5):659–68.

50. Kolodzie K, Apfel CC. Nausea and vomiting after office-based anesthesia. Curr Opin Anaesthesiol. 2009;22(4):532–8.

51. Yogendran S, Asokumar B, Cheng DC, Chung F. A prospective randomized double-blinded study of the effect of intravenous fluid therapy on adverse outcomes on outpatient surgery. Anesth Analg. 1995;80(4):682–6.

52. Henzi I, Walder B, Tramèr MR. Dexamethasone for the prevention of postoperative nausea and vomiting: a quantitative systematic review. Anesth Analg. 2000;90(1):186–94.
53. Melton MS, Klein SM, Gan TJ. Management of postdischarge nausea and vomiting after ambulatory surgery. Curr Opin Anaesthesiol. 2011;24(6):612–9.
54. Ormel G, Romundstad L, Lambert-Jensen P, Stubhaug A. Dexamethasone has additive effect when combined with ondansetron and droperidol for treatment of established PONV. Acta Anaesthesiol Scand. 2011;55(10):1196–205.
55. Dogan U, Yavas G, Tekinalp M, Yavas C, Ata OY, Ozdemir K. Evaluation of the acute effect of palonosetron on transmural dispersion of myocardial repolarization. Eur Rev Med Pharmacol Sci. 2012;16(4):462–8.
56. Apfel CC, Zhang K, George E, Shi S, Jalota L, Hornuss C, Fero KE, Heidrich F, Pergolizzi JV, Cakmakkaya OS, Kranke P. Transdermal scopolamine for the prevention of postoperative nausea and vomiting: a systematic review and meta-analysis. Clin Ther. 2010;32(12):1987–2002.
57. Halloran K, Barash PG. Inside the black box: current policies and concerns with the United States Food and Drug Administration's highest drug safety warning system. Curr Opin Anaesthesiol. 2010;23(3):423–7.
58. Gan TJ, Gu J, Singla N, Chung F, Pearman MH, Bergese SD, Habib AS, Candiotti KA, Mo Y, Huyck S, Creed MR, Cantillon M, Rolapitant Investigation Group. Rolapitant for the prevention of postoperative nausea and vomiting: a prospective, double-blinded, placebo-controlled randomized trial. Anesth Analg. 2011;112(4):804–12.
59. Goddard M, Smith PD, Howard AC. Spinal anaesthesia for spinal surgery. Anaesthesia. 2006;61(7):723–4.
60. Bhananker SM, Posner KL, Cheney FW, Caplan RA, Lee LA, Domino KB. Injury and liability associated with monitored anesthesia care: a closed claims analysis. Anesthesiology. 2006;104(2):228–34.
61. Metzner J, Posner KL, Lam MS, Domino KB. Closed claims' analysis. Best Pract Res Clin Anaesthesiol. 2011;25(2):263–76.
62. Ekstein M, Gavish D, Ezri T, Weinbroum AA. Monitored anaesthesia care in the elderly: guidelines and recommendations. Drugs Aging. 2008;25(6):477–500.
63. Ghisi D, Fanelli A, Tosi M, Nuzzi M, Fanelli G. Monitored anesthesia care. Minerva Anestesiol. 2005;71(9):533–8. PubMed PMID.
64. White PF, White LM, Monk T, Jakobsson J, Raeder J, Mulroy MF, Bertini L, Torri G, Solca M, Pittoni G, Bettelli G. Perioperative care for the older outpatient undergoing ambulatory surgery. Anesth Analg. 2012;114(6):1190–215.
65. López AM, Valero R, Brimacombe J. Insertion and use of the LMA Supreme in the prone position. Anaesthesia. 2010;65(2):154–7.
66. Sharma V, Verghese C, McKenna PJ. Prospective audit on the use of the LMA-Supreme for airway management of adult patients undergoing elective orthopaedic surgery in prone position. Br J Anaesth. 2010;105(2):228–32.
67. López AM, Valero R, Hurtado P, Gambús P, Pons M, Anglada T. Comparison of the LMA Supreme™ with the LMA Proseal™ for airway management in patients anaesthetized in prone position. Br J Anaesth. 2011;107(2):265–71.
68. Gupta A, Stierer T, Zuckerman R, Sakima N, Parker SD, Fleisher LA. Comparison of recovery profile after ambulatory anesthesia with propofol, isoflurane, sevoflurane and desflurane: a systematic review. Anesth Analg. 2004;98(3):632–41, table of contents.
69. Collins L, Prentice J, Vaghadia H. Tracheal intubation of outpatients with and without muscle relaxants. Can J Anaesth. 2000;47(5):427–32.
70. Han JU, Cho S, Jeon WJ, Yeom JH, Shin WJ, Shim JH, Kim KH. The optimal effect-site concentration of remifentanil for lightwand tracheal intubation during propofol induction without muscle relaxation. J Clin Anesth. 2011;23(5):379–83.
71. Fotopoulou G, Theocharis S, Vasileiou I, Kouskouni E, Xanthos T. Management of the airway without the use of neuromuscular blocking agents: the use of remifentanil. Fundam Clin Pharmacol. 2012;26(1):72–85.

72. Fink H, Hollmann MW. Myths and facts in neuromuscular pharmacology New developments in reversing neuromuscular blockade. Minerva Anestesiol. 2012;78(4):473–82.
73. Cottrell JE, Hartung J. Developmental disability in the young and postoperative cognitive dysfunction in the elderly after anesthesia and surgery: do data justify changing clinical practice? Mt Sinai J Med. 2012;79(1):75–94.
74. Tang J, White PF, Wender RH, Naruse R, Kariger R, Sloninsky A, Karlan MS, Uyeda RY, Karlan SR, Reichman C, Whetstone B. Fast-track office-based anesthesia: a comparison of propofol versus desflurane with antiemetic prophylaxis in spontaneously breathing patients. Anesth Analg. 2001;92(1):95–9.
75. Song D, Joshi GP, White PF. Fast-track eligibility after ambulatory anesthesia: a comparison of desflurane, sevoflurane, and propofol. Anesth Analg. 1998;86(2):267–73.
76. Sloan TB, Heyer EJ. Anesthesia for intraoperative neurophysiologic monitoring of the spinal cord. J Clin Neurophysiol. 2002;19(5):430–43.
77. Nitzschke R, Hansen-Algenstaedt N, Regelsberger J, Goetz AE, Goepfert MS. Intraoperative electrophysiological monitoring with evoked potentials. Anaesthesist. 2012;61(4):320–35.
78. Asouhidou I, Katsaridis V, Vaidis G, Ioannou P, Givissis P, Christodoulou A, Georgiadis G. Somatosensory evoked potentials suppression due to remifentanil during spinal operations; a prospective clinical study. Scoliosis. 2010;5:8.
79. Roth S. Perioperative visual loss: what do we know, what can we do? Br J Anaesth. 2009;103 Suppl 1:i31–40.
80. American Society of Anesthesiologists Task Force on Perioperative Visual Loss. Practice advisory for perioperative visual loss associated with spine surgery: an updated report by the American Society of Anesthesiologists Task Force on Perioperative Visual Loss. Anesthesiology. 2012;116(2):274–85.
81. Lee LA, Roth S, Posner KL, Cheney FW, Caplan RA, Newman NJ, Domino KB. The American Society of Anesthesiologists Postoperative Visual Loss Registry: analysis of 93 spine surgery cases with postoperative visual loss. Anesthesiology. 2006;105(4):652–9; quiz 867–8.
82. St-Arnaud D, Paquin MJ. Safe positioning for neurosurgical patients. AORN J. 2008;87(6):1156–68; quiz 1169–72.

Chapter 2
Diagnostic Imaging of Degenerative Spine Diseases: The Technical Approach

Cesare Colosimo, Marco Pileggi, Alessandro Pedicelli, Germano Perotti, and Alessandro Maria Costantini

Introduction

The assessment of spinal degenerative diseases with diagnostic imaging – as well as other fields of application – has seen remarkable development with technological progress, in particular regarding computed tomography (CT) and magnetic resonance imaging (MRI). Only 20 years ago, conventional radiography was considered the basis of degenerative spine diagnostic imaging and we proceeded to second-line investigations choosing between CT and MRI based on radiographic findings and clinical evidence. Today, the situation has changed radically thanks to the greater availability of CT and MRI, the relative cost reduction, and the greater scanning speed.

In practice today, faced with clinical situations indicative of degenerative spine disease, the first diagnostic imaging method is increasingly the MRI. This choice has the great advantage of avoiding exposure to ionizing radiation and of reducing the overall time required for diagnosis, thanks to the exploratory capacity of MRI as regards the extension of the field of view, its ability to demonstrate degenerative disease in the vertebrae, discs, joints, and ligaments, and its effects on the "content," that is, the spinal cord, roots, and meningeal sheaths.

In light of the growing availability and accessibility of MRI, we can outline the main clinical and radiological scenarios. First, MRI is sufficient for diagnosis and covers clinical needs alone; no further investigation is needed. Second, MRI is

C. Colosimo, MD (✉) • M. Pileggi, MD • A. Pedicelli, MD • A.M. Costantini, MD
Department of Bioimaging and Radiological Sciences,
Institute of Radiology, Catholic University, Rome, Italy
e-mail: colosimo@rm.unicatt.it

G. Perotti, MD
Department of Bioimaging and Radiological Sciences,
Nuclear Medicine Institute, Catholic University, Rome, Italy

Department of Bio-Imaging, Radiology/Neuroradiology Institute – Nuclear Medicine Institute, Catholic University of Sacred Heart, Polyclinic A Gemelli, School of Medicine, Largo A Gemelli 8, Rome 00168, Italy

P.P.M. Menchetti (ed.), *Minimally Invasive Surgery of the Lumbar Spine*,
DOI 10.1007/978-1-4471-5280-4_2, © Springer-Verlag London 2014

diagnostic, but there is a clinical and radiological need for a complementary targeted CT on a specific area of interest or to define pre-surgical bone status. In selected cases, it will be possible to proceed further with a dynamic radiographic study, as the most simple, effective, and least expensive method of demonstration of any instabilities. Third, the MRI, CT, and X-ray refine the diagnosis, but – albeit exceptionally – there is a need for interventional procedures for diagnostic purposes or as a first step towards the choice of interventional procedures. In this context, there may also be a need to perform intrathecally contrast-enhanced studies (sacculo-radiculography/myelography-CT), discography, or biopsies. Fourth, the MRI is contraindicated (e.g., due to the presence of an incompatible pacemaker) and the CT replaces the MRI in the diagnostic algorithm. If there is a need to study the "content," it becomes necessary to perform a CT-myelography. This is a schematization that moves from the superiority and acceptance to the MRI, sometimes not indicated, but auto-prescribed by the patient and offering the highest sensitivity and specificity.

This chapter, prior to those dedicated to degenerative diseases of the cervicodorsal spine and the lumbosacral spine, respectively, will briefly present the current status of diagnostic imaging techniques used in the assessment of degenerative spinal diseases. For historical reasons, we start with the section on X-rays, followed by those on CT and MRI, and thus the residual use of intrathecal contrast studies and other "invasive" methods. Finally, we present a few words on the – marginal – use of nuclear medicine techniques.

Radiography

The conventional X-ray examination represents the starting point in the study of the spine. Analogical techniques (which made use of direct exposure of film to X-rays) are now only still used by small peripheral radiology centers and were gradually or completely replaced by digital computed radiography (CR) or digital radiography (DR) systems [1]. Although digital systems are more functional and more cost-effective, from the point of view of quality, analogical images remain significantly better than digital ones. Analogical images are better in the study of subtle bone changes, while they have a marginal role, due to their limited contrast resolution, in the study of soft tissue (discs, ligaments).

CR systems are based on phosphor plates sensitive to X-rays, which replace cassettes and analogical films in all respects. After exposure, the cassette is transferred to a digitizer that reads the contained information and creates a digital image that, when saved in DICOM (Digital Imaging and Communication in Medicine) format, can be printed, saved on digital media (DVD, CD), or sent to the PACS (Picture Archiving and Communicating System) for reporting. Unlike CR, DR systems use detectors panels that are placed directly on the radiological table, on dedicated systems, or on portable devices. The high-resolution images are then directly processed by the computer and made available in a few seconds to be subsequently sent to the PACS system for reporting or other digital media, as described for CR systems.

DR systems are much faster than CR systems in making the image available and, overall, both systems (CR and DR) are less sensitive to exposure errors than analogical systems. In addition, overall, digital systems allow reduced doses and number of patient exposures compared to analogical systems.

However, it must be emphasized that the role of conventional radiography in the study of spinal degenerative disease has undergone a critical reevaluation and is currently controversial [2, 3]. Its generalized and routine use was unjustified, dictated more by medico-legal reasons or by the anxiety that patients transmit to the doctor, rather than by legitimate clinical questions.

Given that the examination of basic orthogonal projections alone is often not diagnostic unless accompanied by additional projections (oblique, transbuccal, etc.) – with a significant increase of the dose to the patient – the use of conventional radiography should be reduced in favor of methods such as MRI and CT scans, which until a few years ago were considered "second line" tools. Herein, radiological study techniques are considered separately as regards their use for the cervical, thoracic, and lumbar spine.

Cervical Spine

The routine study in two orthogonal projections has substantially lost value in the diagnosis of degenerative cervical spine diseases. Increasingly often, clinicians directly prescribe MRI and/or CT studies to patients with cervical brachialgia or neck pain, due to their ability to comprehensively display the bony structures and soft tissues (ligaments and discs, bone marrow) with marginal use of radiological examinations. The standard digital radiological examination of the degenerative spine (Fig. 2.1a, b) can still provide useful information on the bone spinal structures, such as on degenerative changes (i.e., spondylosis, osteophytes, irregular morphology of bodies, calcification of ligaments and discs) that are often not directly implicated as the cause of pain. However, X-rays provide more limited and indirect information on the disc (herniations) and possible stenosis of the spinal canal. Although the literature proposes the supine study position, it is useful to study the patient in upright position, at least in the lateral view, which can provide information concerning possible spinal instability (listhesis). The examination is performed in the two orthogonal planes (anteroposterior and latero-lateral), trying as much as possible, especially in the lateral view, to explore the bodies up to C7 (often masked by the shoulder girdle).

If properly performed, oblique views may be of some utility in evaluating the degenerative spine, for the study of the intervertebral foramina, the uncinate processes, and the facet joints, although all of this information can be provided more comprehensively by CT.

Given their complex implementation and their sometimes poor results, "swimmer's" projections and the transbuccal projection for the study of the odontoid process are replaced by CT scan.

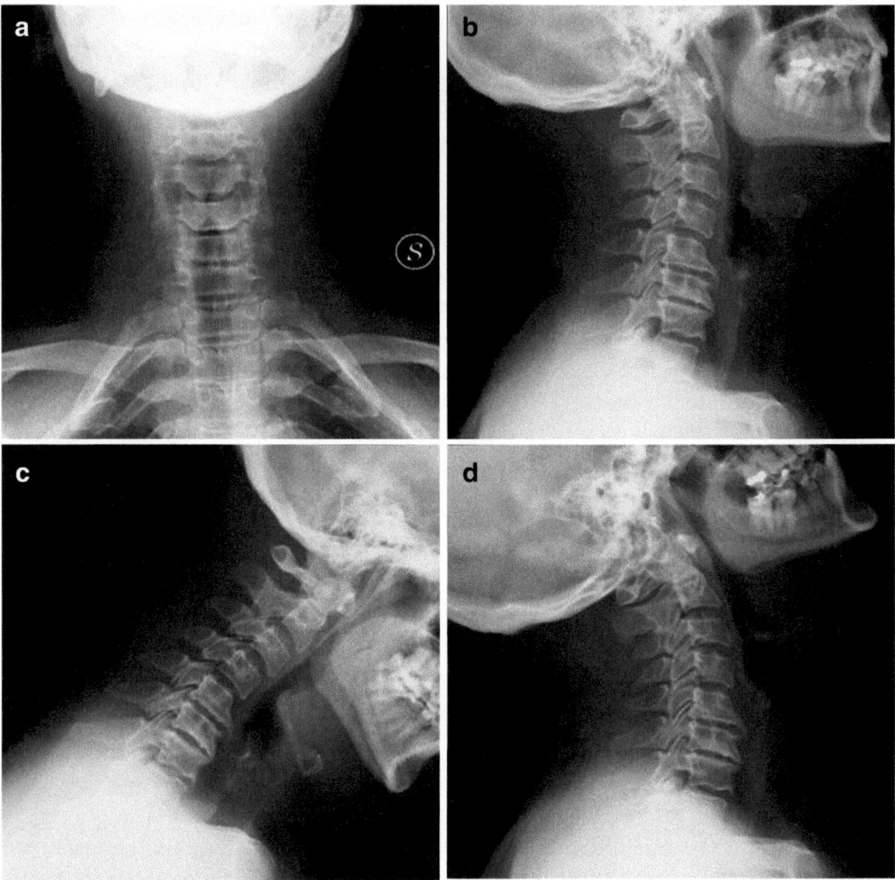

Fig. 2.1 Standard X-ray study of the cervical spine. Antero-posterior (**a**) and lateral (**b**) radiograms, performed in the orthogonal planes, in standing position. Spondyloarthrosis is evident at C5-C7 levels. "Functional" X-ray in flexion (**c**) and extension (**d**)

The "functional" radiological study of the cervical spine (Fig. 2.1c, d), still offers full diagnostic validity in evaluating instability, so as to propose the use of flexion-extension X-rays in upright standing in the routine study for the demonstration of instability [4]. In functional radiograms, the anterior atlantoaxial space (between the posterior margin of the anterior arch of the atlas and the anterior surface of the odontoid process) should never be more than 3 mm in adults and 4 mm in children; an enlarged distance, measured directly on the radiogram, implies the diagnosis of anterior atlantoaxial subluxation.

On the other hand, vertical atlantoaxial subluxations involve a cranial displacement of the odontoid process in relation to certain reference lines, such as, for example, that of Chamberlain, drawn from the posterior edge of the hard palate to the posterior margin of the foramen magnum. If the odontoid process exceeds it by more than 3 mm, we speak of a vertical atlantoaxial subluxation.

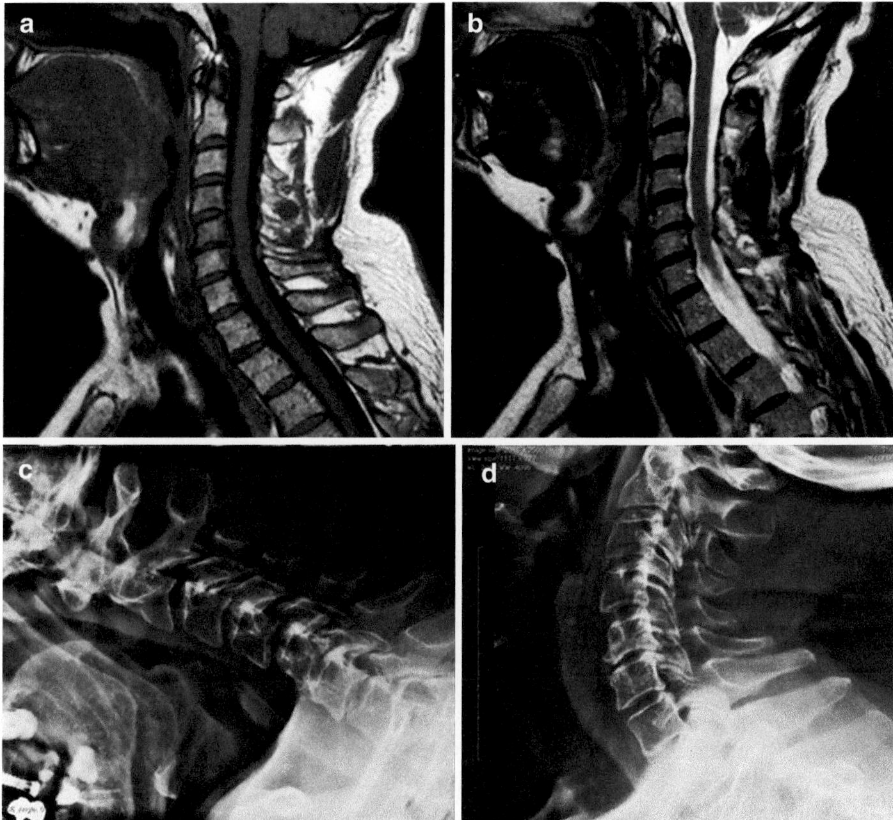

Fig. 2.2 Cervical spondylosis: MRI vs. functional X-ray study. MRI study performed in sagittal plane with T1 TSE (**a**) and T2 TSE (**b**) weighted images. Focal central disc protrusion at C5–C6 level, without cord compression. Plain radiographic functional study in flexion (**c**) and extension (**d**) lateral view, showing minimal hypermobility at C4–C5 level on flexion image

The occurrence of cervical instability in a degenerative spine, demonstrated in the functional radiological study, can alone be the cause – or contributing cause – of pain and must be supplemented, especially by MRI, in suspected ligament laxity/injury (Fig. 2.2).

Thoracic Spine

The study of the thoracic spine is less commonly performed because of the limited involvement of this part of the spine in degenerative changes. It is usually prescribed by the clinician to obtain an overview of the spine and is performed in the supine position in two orthogonal projections (anteroposterior and lateral). As mentioned for the cervical tract, the information obtained has inherent limitations for the cervicodorsal junction (due to the superimposition of the shoulder girdle) and the dorsolumbar junction (because the X-ray beam is positioned at the level of the inter-nipple line, resulting in minimum projective deformations of the last thoracic and first lumbar vertebral bodies). No diagnostic information can be obtained about the width of the spinal canal, discs – if non-calcified – and of course the intraspinal content (spinal cord).

Dynamic radiological examinations are rarely carried out on thoracic spine, but are still applied ("lateral bending") in the comprehensive thoracic/lumbar spine evaluation when bending instability is suspected [5].

Lumbar Spine

As stated above, the X-ray study of the lumbar spine is no longer routinely applied in degenerative diseases and is more commonly used selectively after an evaluation with an MRI and/or CT scan, often with functional issues [6]. It is traditionally performed in the supine position, with frontal and lateral projections, with an incident beam of about 2 cm from the iliac crests [7] (Fig. 2.3a, b). The use of complementary projections, such as oblique, no longer seems justified, as they are replaced by multiplanar CT reconstructions, which certainly provide better information. However, conventional radiology is still useful in evaluating lumbar instability.

"Dynamic studies," which are easy to perform and low cost [8], are performed primarily in an upright position, acquiring radiographs in full flexion and in full extension in the lateral projection [9, 10] (Fig. 2.3c, d).

Some authors [11] report a better evaluation of vertebral translation with the patient in the supine than in the upright position, probably related to the reduced spinal motion determined by the paraspinal and abdominal musculature in the upright position. In addition, the pain that often accompanies such maneuvers in the upright position is less than in the supine position.

Flexion-extension X-rays in the lateral projection allow the measurement of sagittal vertebral translation and of vertebral rotation in the sagittal plane (defined as the variation of the angle formed by the intersection of the lines drawn between the two opposite endplates in full flexion and extension). These measurements, however, may suffer overestimation errors, unless the criteria [12] of a rigorous and standardized measurement technique and high-quality radiographs are met. According to some authors, the estimation error generated could lead to unjustified surgical stabilization procedures. The "cut-off" data for the determination of instability are about 10° for sagittal rotation and 4 mm for sagittal translation [13]. It must nevertheless be taken into account that, in a small percentage of asymptomatic patients, the dynamic examination may find values higher than those of reference above. In these individuals, spinal hypermobility is fully compensated by the muscle and vertebral structures. Side bending or lateral bending can also be radiological indicators of instability [14].

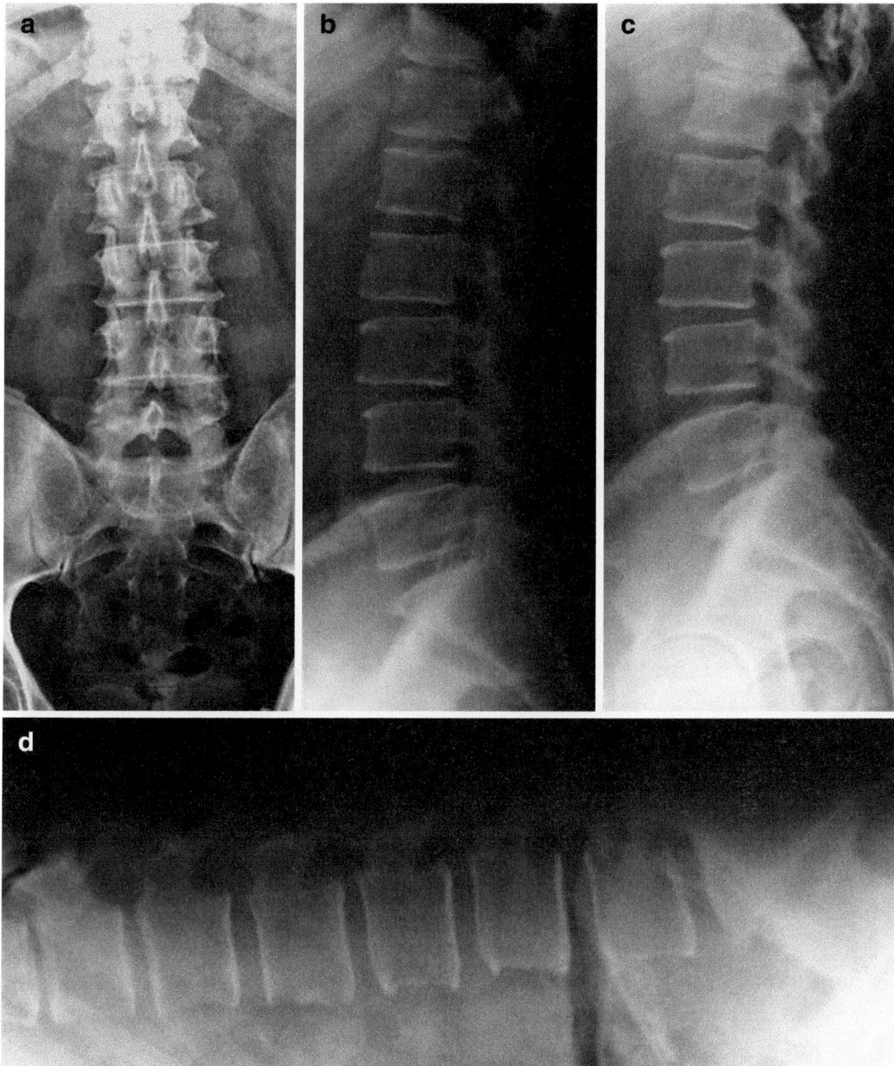

Fig. 2.3 Standard X-ray study of the lumbar spine. Antero-posterior (**a**) and lateral (**b**) radiograms, in standing position. Degenerative radiographic findings can be appreciated at L5–S1 level. "Functional" study performed on the same patient in extension (**c**) and flexion (**d**) lateral views shows no sign of instability

The characteristic findings for determining lateral instability are represented by the misalignment of the spinous processes, laterolisthesis, loss of motility, and excessive widening of the vertebral interbody space during lateral flexion [8]. Some authors argue that lateral bending provides complementary information in flexion-extension studies and that it should be performed whenever there is a suspicion of instability, especially in the case of negative flexion-extension test.

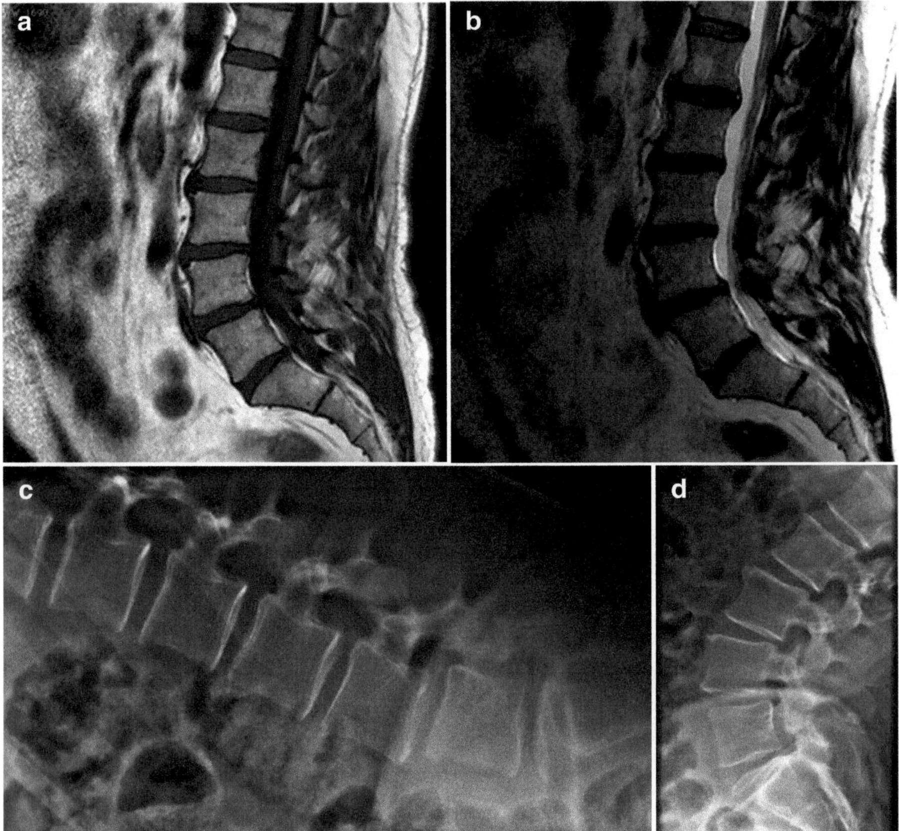

Fig. 2.4 Lumbar instability: MRI vs. functional X-ray study. MRI study performed in sagittal plane with T1 TSE (**a**) and T2 TSE (**b**) weighted images. Multiple disc protrusions, more evident at L4–L5, with minimal deformity of the ventral surface of the thecal sac. No significant listhesis is seen on supine MRI study. Radiographic functional study (lateral view) in flexion (**c**) and extension (**d**) in standing position demonstrates a listhesis at L4–L5 level, increasing on flexion image

We can conclude that the value of functional studies is still debated, but most surgeons require them, for integration of CT or MRI study, and believe in their usefulness as an indicator of instability (Fig. 2.4).

Computed Tomography (CT)

After its introduction, computed tomography became a gold standard in the study of the spine [15]. In the past decade, the introduction of multidetector CT scanners (MDCT) has completely changed the role of the MDCT in spinal studies. The outdated "single-layer" machines with long scan times, thick slices (3 mm), and a reduced exploratory capacity have given way to MDCT, which allows reduced

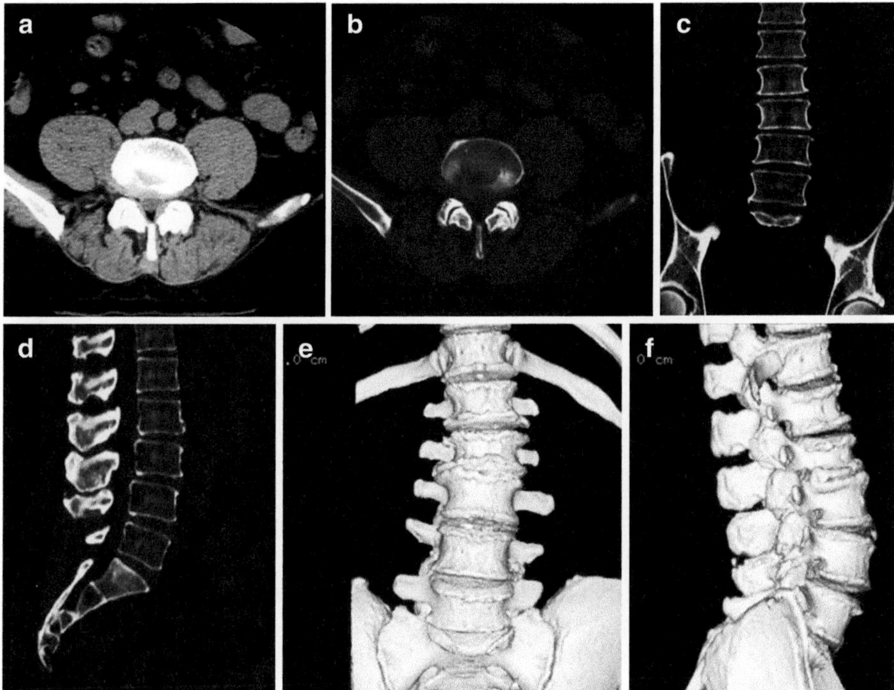

Fig. 2.5 Computed tomography (CT) of lumbar spine. CT axial images, with soft tissue (**a**) and bone (**b**) windows. In (**a**) a wide-based annular disc protrusion, associated to minimal facet changes (**b**). Reformatted coronal (**c**) and sagittal (**d**) images better visualize the bone structures. (**e, f**) 3D shaded surface display

acquisition times (in the order of seconds), submillimeter acquisition/reconstruction thicknesses (0.5–0.6 mm), and the possibility to include the entire spine in a single scan. Modern MDCT equipment can have up to 256 detectors, with an increase in spatial resolution, which reaches values much higher than those of MRI. An MDCT study of the spine provides for the acquisition of axial slices perpendicular to the longitudinal spinal axis, with slice thicknesses chosen according to different equipment and directions; thickness of 0.6–0.7 mm with reconstruction per 1 mm and increases of 0.5–0.6 are satisfactory parameters for most clinical questions. The obtained images, measured using soft tissue (Fig. 2.5a) and bone reconstruction algorithms (Fig. 2.5b), together with the use of convolution filters (high-resolution filters that provide a better spatial resolution but a worse imaging signal/noise ratio, or a standard filter that is a good compromise between spatial resolution and imaging signal/noise ratio), allow an optimal visualization of the bony structures of the vertebral body, such as cortical integrity, and a satisfactory visualization of the intervertebral discs, especially in the lumbar spine, thanks also to the richness of fat tissue in the epidural area, compared to the cervical and thoracic regions. On the other hand, they appear to be totally inadequate in the study of bone marrow and ligaments, which remains the exclusive prerogative of MRI. Axial MDCT acquisitions can be reconstructed and easily viewed in the sagittal and coronal planes, thanks to the new reconstruction algorithms and increased computing power of workstations, with a significant improvement in ease of interpretation (Fig. 2.5c, d).

Three-dimensional (3D) reconstructions appear to be of little diagnostic value, but may give the clinician a better overview, especially in surgery planning [16]. In this regard, the best 3D techniques are those reconstructed with the shaded surface display (SSD) that, while maintaining its inherent limitations (loss of spatial resolution and contrast), provide, however, a marked improvement in the quality of the images [17] (Fig. 2.5e, f). The use of contrast media, especially in the study of the degenerative spine, provides limited additional information and only in selected instances (such as post-surgical evaluations changes and infectious diseases). MDCT is the reference method in the study of the postoperative spine because of its multiplanarity, the scanning speed, and the reduced artifacts derived from orthopedic implants (compared to MRI). It is essential that the study be performed by a "dedicated radiologist," able to distinguish normal surgical sequelae from complications (early or late).

A special use of CT is that of CT fluoroscopy [18], which allows obtaining real-time images during interventional procedures, such as those of nerve block, CT discography, and vertebral and soft tissue biopsies.

The so-called "twist test" is a functional study that is performed on CT to determine the presence of possible lumbar instability.

It consists of placing the patient in a supine position on the CT table, having him/her turn his back first to the right and then to the left, and performing a scan through the interapophyseal joints between two adjacent vertebrae. The test demonstrates an abnormal increase of motility and of the distance of the interapophyseal joints (exhibiting a vacuum phenomenon) during the rotation of the trunk, data that are not appreciable in the functional radiographic tests [19, 20]. Although this test can show the presence of a lumbar vertebral instability, it is not used routinely because of the significant exposure to ionizing radiation it entails.

With regard to CT studies performed using the so-called "axial loader," we refer the reader to the chapter on MRI in which they are discussed.

The superiority of MDCT, however, involves a strong focus on radiation-protection problems, as the radiation dose delivered to the patient is not negligible. It is estimated that, on average, approximately 8.2 mSv are administered for a lumbar MDCT examination and about 3.4 mSv for an examination of the cervical spine. The radiologist must try to reduce the exposure dose (for example, by using automatic programs, reducing the milliamperage, etc.), and to suggest the use of alternative imaging tools (such as MRI) to the clinician.

Magnetic Resonance Imaging (MRI)

Spinal MRIs in general – and those of the degenerative spine in particular – are based on the use of high-field equipments (equal to or greater than 1.5 T), powerful and efficient gradient systems, and phased-array receiving coils. The area to be explored

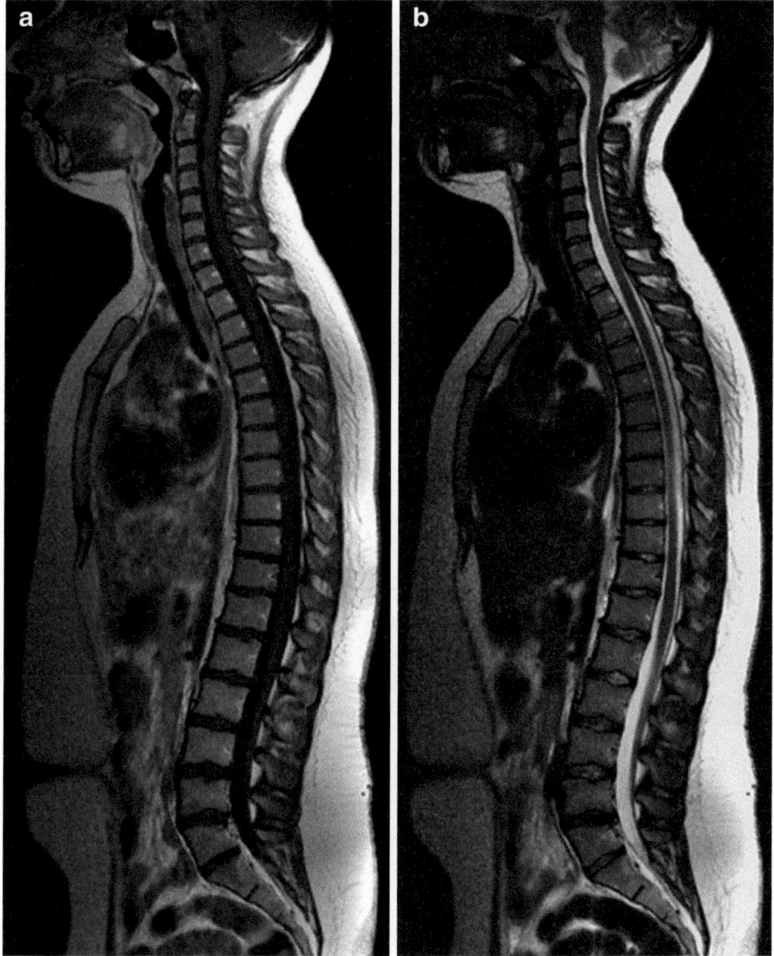

Fig. 2.6 MRI evaluation of the entire spine TSE sagittal T1 (**a**) and TSE sagittal T2 (**b**)

can be the entire spine, but the examination is usually limited to only one region, based on the symptoms and/or previous diagnostic tests and/or other imaging techniques. As already mentioned for X-rays and CTs, with MRIs the study techniques are modified according to the area to be examined. However, both in the cases in which the entire spine study is indicated, and in the more common cases of "segmental" studies, a standard examination method can be indicated, forming the basis of the study.

An MRI of the spine for degenerative diseases (Figs. 2.6, 2.7, and 2.8) should include sagittal and axial T1- and T2-weighted images (T1WI and T2WI) as well as coronal (T1WI or T2WI) [21]. Depending on the imaging sequence, the repetition times (TR) and echo times (TE) to obtain T1 and T2 images may vary. In general, however, for T1, in Spin-Echo (SE) and Turbo Spin-Echo (TSE) sequences, they range between TR of 400–700 ms and TE of 15–30 ms, while the variability grows

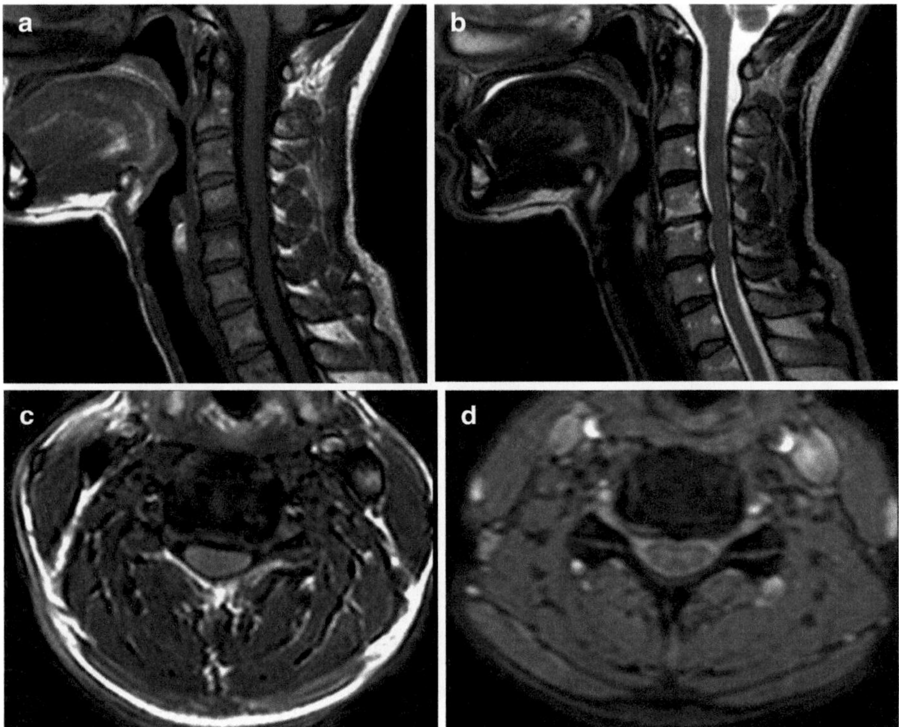

Fig. 2.7 MRI evaluation of the cervical spine in degenerative disease. TSE sagittal T1 (**a**), TSE sagittal T2 (**b**) weighted images; GRE axial T1 (**c**), GRE axial T2 3D with water selection (**d**). Degenerative disc disease with spondylosis are shown at C4–C5 and C5–C6 level. Note the evidence of central gray matter intensity on axial T2 3D image

in the case of T2WI, almost constantly for TSE, with TR ranging between 1,500 and 3,000 ms and effective TE of 120–150 msec. The sagittal images must have an anatomical coverage sufficient to fully include the foramina on both sides, using a number of slices that depends on the slice thickness. In most cases, the sagittal sequences are obtained using a Spin-Echo (SE) technique or, more often, Turbo Spin Echo (TSE), with 2D acquisition and slice thicknesses between 3 and 4 mm.

For axial images, the choice of sequences is more complicated, because it is more related to the anatomical area (and, therefore, determined by the need to avoid pulse/movement artifacts), and because it is largely based on the clinically suspected pathology or visualized through sagittal images. In the case of axial images, especially of T2WI, 3D sequences are frequently used, both with TSE and with Gradient Echo (GRE) techniques. 3D sequences are preferred in particular when the area of interest is small, for example, in the case of two or at most three intersomatic levels (Fig. 2.9). Meanwhile, TSE and SE sequences are performed according to the rules previously defined for sagittal images. In the case of axial GRE sequences, T1 and T2 weighting depends mainly on the selection of the "flip angle," with T2WI

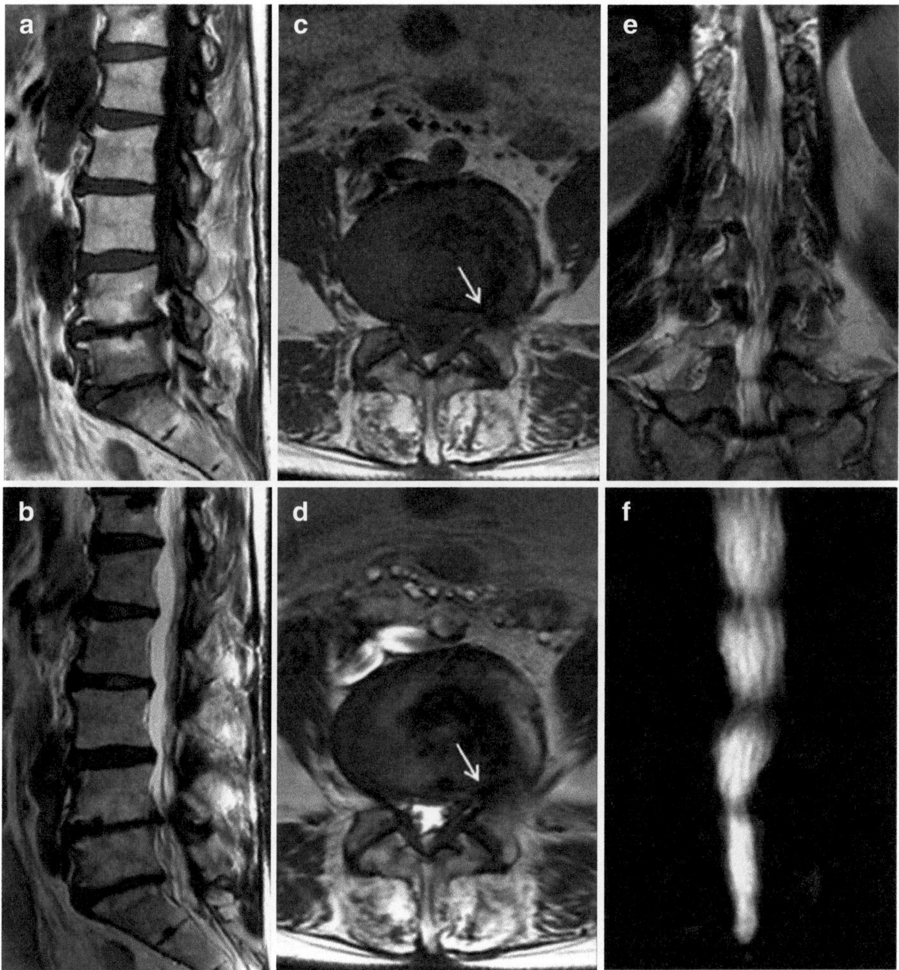

Fig. 2.8 MRI evaluation of the lumbar spine in degenerative disease. TSE sagittal T1 (**a**), TSE sagittal T2 (**b**), TSE axial T1 (**c**), BFE axial T2 (**d**), TSE coronal T2 (**e**), TSE (2D) coronal myelogram (**f**). There are diffuse degenerative disc and facet changes, especially at L4–L5 and L5–S1 levels. At L4–L5 spondylosis, disc protrusion and facet disease result in left L5 lateral recess stenosis with deformity of the thecal sac (*white arrows*)

(T2*) based on the choice of short flip angles (<30 ms) and T1WI with large flip angles. Coronal images are (or should be) part of all MRI studies of the spine, as multiplanarity represents an inherent essential advantage of MRI, and because it enhances the exploratory potential of MRI, allowing, for example, the visualization of paravertebral changes/diseases that are otherwise missed. In the case of coronal images, both T1 or T2 images can be obtained.

The sagittal, axial, and coronal images should be considered the basis of all spinal MRIs, but can – and in some cases must – be supplemented by more specific

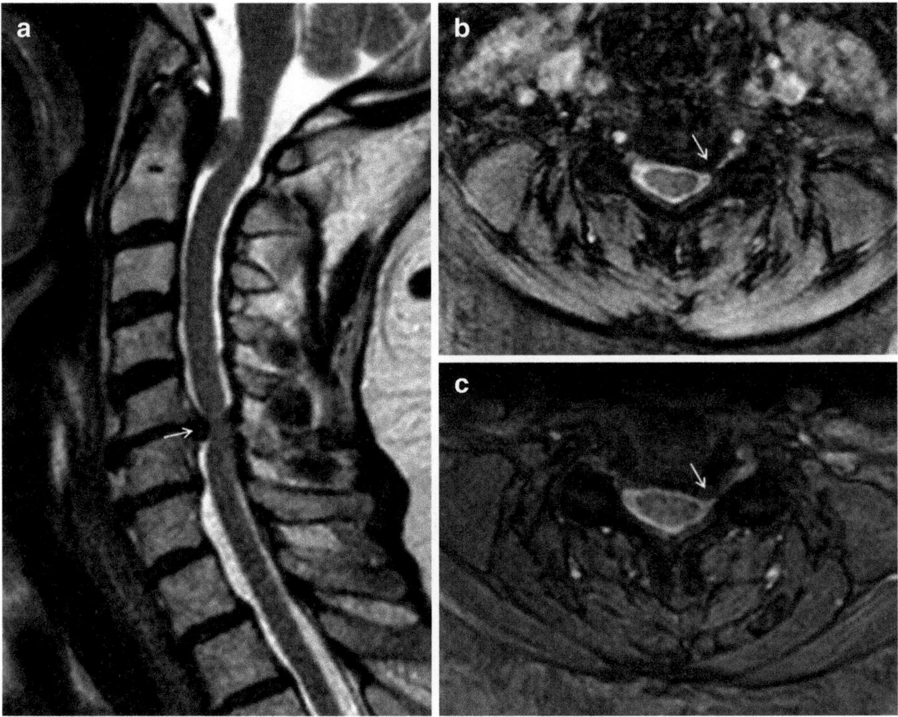

Fig. 2.9 C5–C6 disc herniation; different axial T2 image sequences. TSE sagittal T2 (**a**), GRE axial T2 3D with water selection (**b**), GRE axial T2 2D with water selection. Disc herniation is shown on sagittal T2 image; the soft tissue left postero-lateral herniated disc (*white arrows*) is better demonstrated on axial T2 2D (**c**) than on axial T2 3D (**b**), in which there is no significant contrast between spondylosis and herniated disc

scanning planes and sequences, selected to complete the study and optimize the diagnosis. For example, oblique scanning (or reconstruction if there are 3D acquisitions) planes can be added according to the axis of emergence of the cervical or lumbar roots and/or according to other structures of clinical interest (Fig. 2.10). In other cases, the angle of the axial images may have to be changed. These are typically obtained along the axis of the discs, but sometimes instead along the orientation of the lamina (for example, if we need to prove/exclude spondylolysis).

Fat-suppression images are frequently used in degenerative spinal diseases. Fat signal suppression can be achieved with the short tau inversion recovery (STIR) technique or with a TSE sequence, using spectral suppression (SPIR, SPAIR). The main advantage of these sequences is in the optimal demonstration of bone edema and fluid components on T2WI in which the signal of the fat is cancelled. In this way, for example, we can recognize and characterize algodystrophic or Modic [22, 23] type "discogenic" changes, edema resulting in instability and/or typical of vertebral fractures. The choice of suppression on T2WI (STIR or SPIR/SPAIR) is largely dependent on the equipment used and the efficiency of suppression in

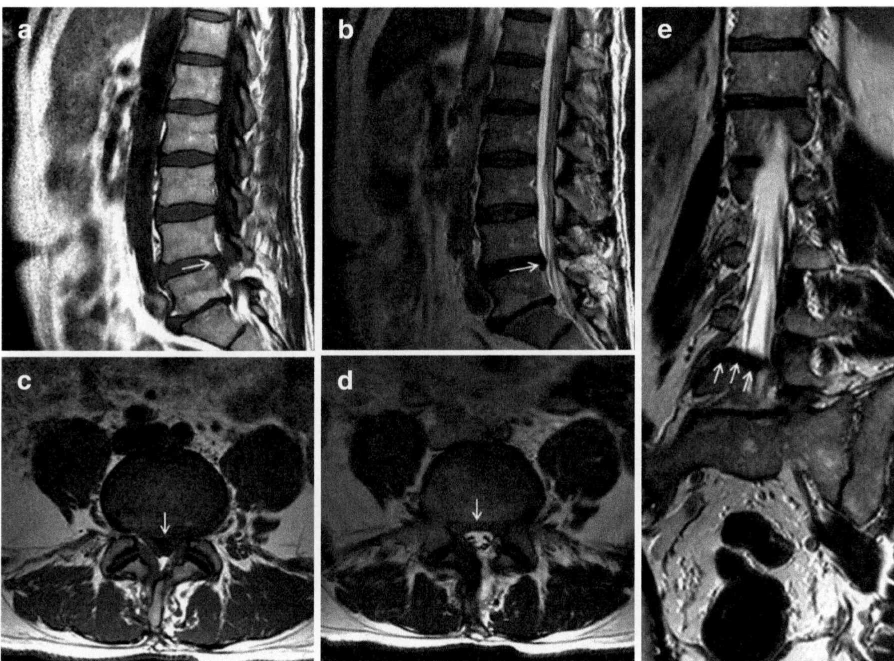

Fig. 2.10 Recurrent L4–L5 left postero-lateral disc herniation; usefulness of coronal oblique acquisition. TSE sagittal T1 (**a**), TSE sagittal T2 (**b**), TSE axial T1 (**c**), BFE axial T2 (**d**), TSE oblique coronal T2 (**e**). The recurrent herniated disc (*white arrows*) is shown on all imaging planes; note the evidence of the lesion on oblique coronal T2 image (**e**)

different locations/areas, but in general the rule is that STIR is preferred for large fields of view and SPIR/SPAIR for small fields of view. This usually leads to favoring the STIR in sagittal and coronal images and the SPIR/SPAIR in axial images (Fig. 2.11). It must also be considered that the quality of suppression is usually better in the lumbar and cervical spine compared to the thoracic spine, because the presence of respiratory artifacts and abundant air (in the lungs) degrades the result in the thoracic spine. When faced with ligament changes/injuries, obtaining high-resolution proton density (PD) images with fat suppression has also proved useful. These sequences not only optimally display the longitudinal ligaments (anterior and posterior) but also the ligamenta flava, the interspinous ligaments, and the most complex ligaments in the craniocervical junction.

Fat-suppressed T1WI is instead almost always obtained using the spectral technique (SPIR) and its use is mostly combined with the intravenous administration of contrast agent (based on gadolinium). The use of intravenous contrast agent in extradural spinal diseases should necessarily lead to the use of SPIR sequences, because, without suppression, the evidence of contrast enhancement (CE) in fat-rich cancellous bone is very limited.

In addition to the need to suppress the fat, the study of the degenerative spine can greatly benefit from the use of sequences that optimize the contrast between the

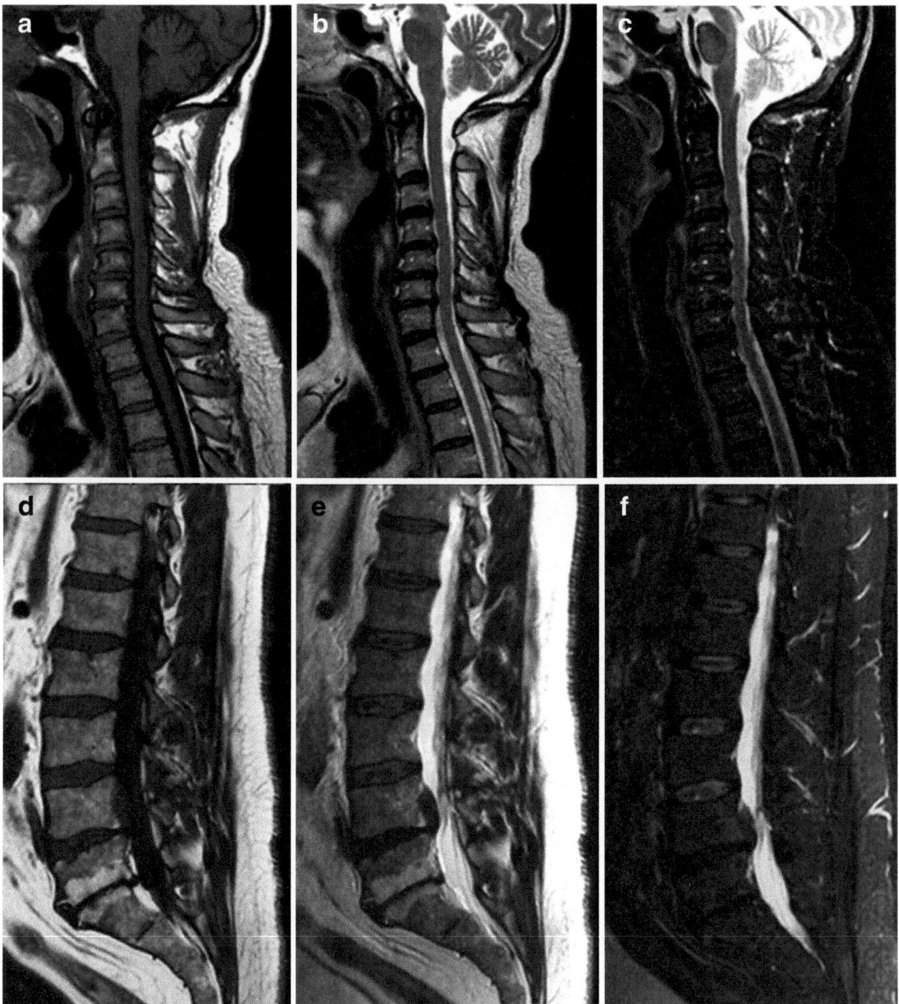

Fig. 2.11 STIR sagittal images in spinal degenerative disease. Patient 1: TSE sagittal T1 (**a**), TSE sagittal T2 (**b**), STIR sagittal T2 (**c**). Degenerative C4–C5, C–5–C6, C6–C7 disc disease without vertebral signal changes. Patient 2: TSE sagittal T1 (**d**), TSE sagittal T2 (**e**), STIR sagittal T2 (**f**). Large L4–L5 extruded, cranially migrated, herniated disc. Modic 3 signal changes are seen at L5–S1, completely suppressed by STIR sequence (confirming fat-like signal). Note, in both patients, the optimal homogeneity of fat-suppressed images using STIR acquisitions

bony and the discal/ligamentous structures. These sequences are very useful in defining, for example, how much of a protrusion in cervical spondylosis is caused by osteophytes ("hard," calcified) and how much by true disc herniation ("soft"). These are mainly GRE T2* sequences, which facilitate distinction by increasing the contrast between the hypointensity of the bone and the (hyper-) intensity of the disc (Fig. 2.12). According to the findings, the axial or the sagittal plane may be favored.

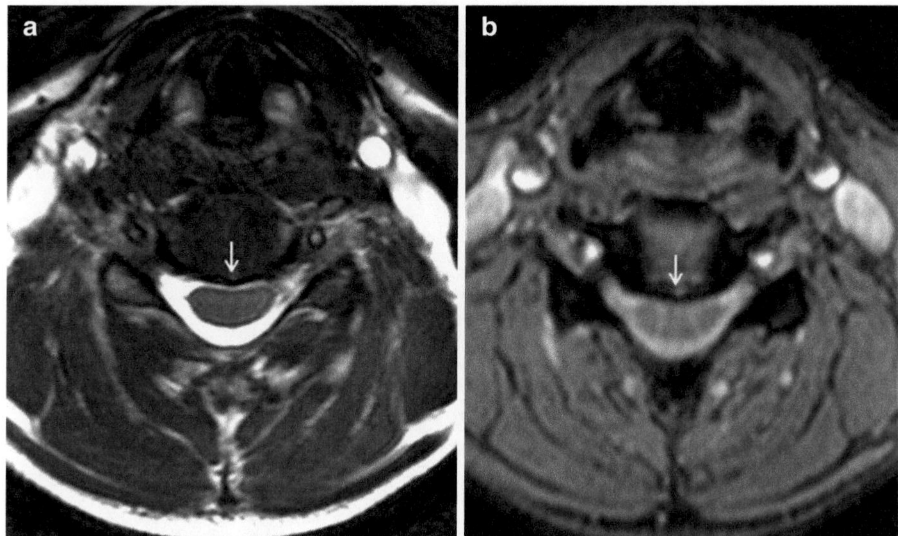

Fig. 2.12 Tiny C4–C5 central disc herniation; BFE 2D vs. GRE 3D axial T2 image sequences. Note how the minimal central focal disc protrusion (*white arrows*) is better differentiated on GRE T2 3D (**b**) than on BFE T2 2D (**a**)

The use of T2* sequences with fat suppression in 3D high-resolution acquisition optimally marks out the body from the disc, enhances the demonstration ligaments, and, above all, allows an optimal quality of the study on the orientation/integrity of the fibers of the annulus fibrosus. With this technique, for example, we can directly see the interruption of the fibers of the ring that allows the expulsion of a herniated disc (Fig. 2.13).

MRI myelography represents a useful enrichment of the previously described morphological sequences. Its definition comes from a representation similar to that of myelography/saccoradiculography and is obtained using different sequences – 2D and 3D – mostly based on the TSE acquisition, which increase and enhance the CSF signal and decrease the signal of solid tissue (bone, disc, ligaments, spinal cord, spinal nerves). In this way, similar to other "fluid-enhanced" MRIs (MR-cisternography, MR-urography, MR-cholangiopancreatography), we obtain an enhancement of the CSF signal and see – in negative, as a filling defect – the intrathecal spinal nerves and the spinal cord with excellent demonstration of the radicular cervical, thoracic, and, mainly, lumbar root sleeves. MRI-myelography can be achieved with 3D volume study (Fig. 2.14a–c), or, especially in the lumbar and cervical spine, with multiple individual acquisitions according to different angles of view (Fig. 2.14d–f).

In the case of multiple 2D acquisitions, the so-called "single shot TSE" is often used, in which a single TR is used to completely fill the K-space (so that the entire set of images is obtained in just a few seconds). It is important to note that the MRI myelographic images, and more generally those strongly T2WI (with very high TR

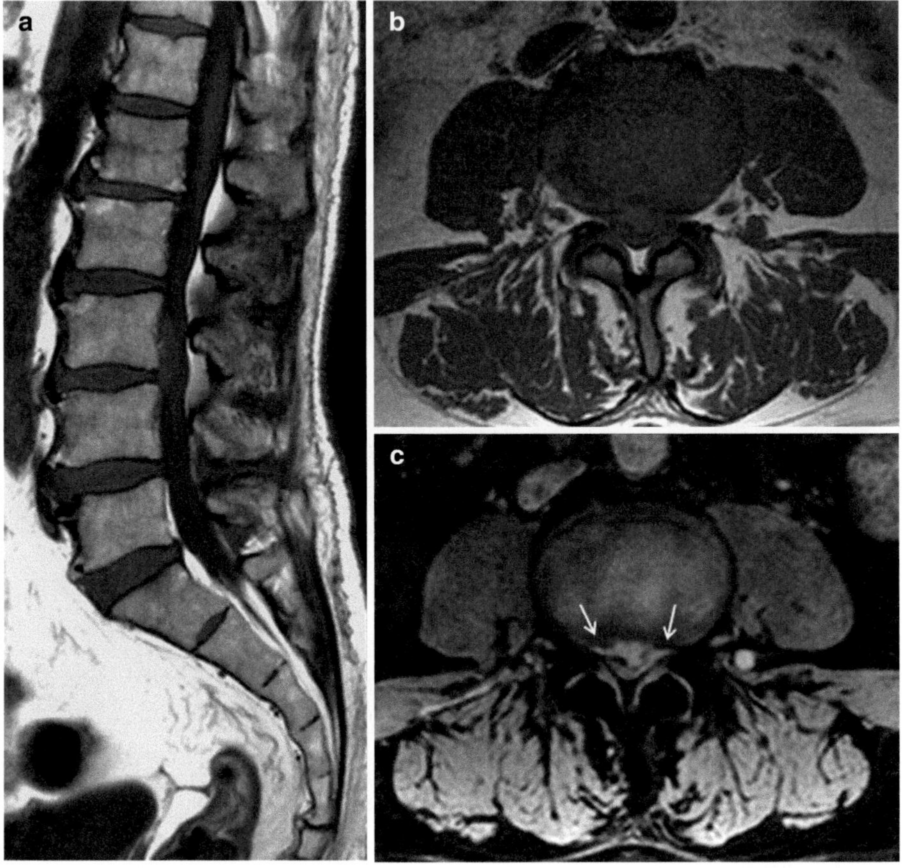

Fig. 2.13 Large L3–L4 cranially migrated/extruded disc herniation. TSE sagittal T1 (**a**), TSE axial T1 (**b**), GRE axial intermediate 3D with water selection (**c**). The large herniated disc is optimally demonstrated on all imaging sequences; note how on (**c**) water selection provides excellent evidence of the tear in the annulus fibrosus, allowing the extrusion of the disc material (*white arrows*)

and TE), increase the fluids/solids contrast, but offer little or no intraparenchymal contrast, and thus are not suitable, for example, for detecting intramedullary lesions.

The use of magnetic resonance angiography (MRA) in degenerative diseases is limited and marginal. It is mostly used when we want to demonstrate the effect of spondylosis and unco-arthrosis on the course of the vertebral arteries in the transverse processes. For these requirements, we can use the so-called phase-contrast MRA (3D, velocity-encoding between 20 and 40 ms) or the so-called "contrast enhanced" technique, based on a bolus of paramagnetic contrast agent.

In degenerative diseases of the spine, the administration of a contrast agent during MRI is used only rarely, mostly in cases where there is a different suspicion

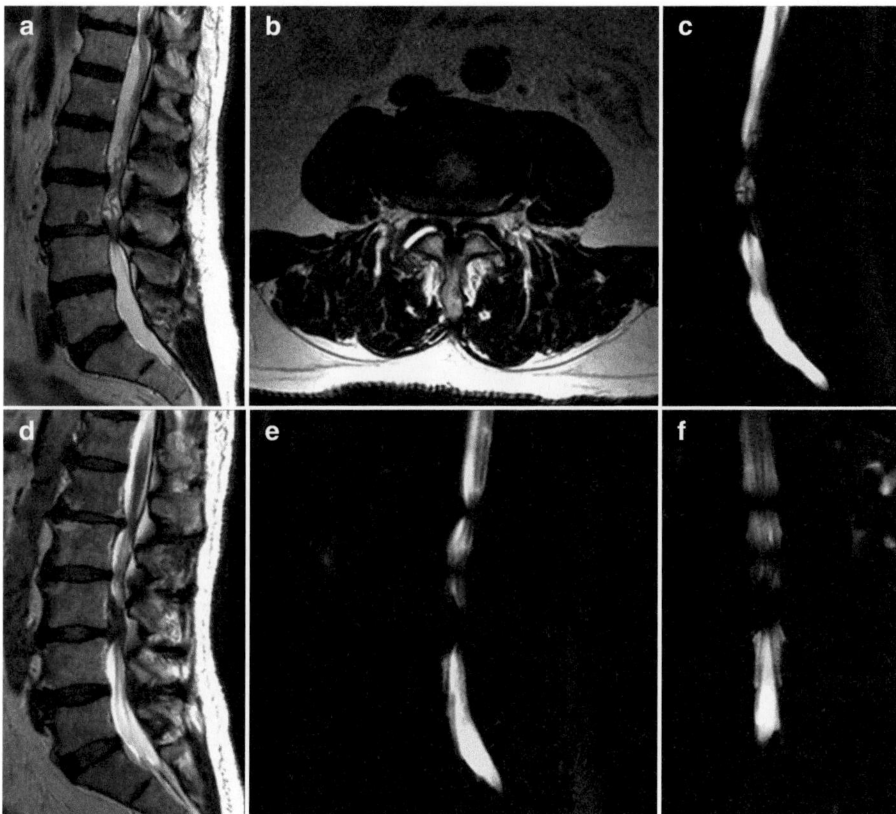

Fig. 2.14 MR-myelography using 3D or 2D acquisition; two different patients. Patient 1: TSE sagittal T2 (**a**), TSE axial T2 (**b**), oblique sagittal myelogram extracted by 3D MR myelogram (**c**). Severe L3–L4 stenosis with facet subluxation and instability with complete effacement of the thecal sac; note the complete lack of CSF on axial image as well as the varicoid appearance of roots cranially to the stenosis. Patient 2: TSE sagittal T2 (**d**), oblique sagittal (**e**) and coronal (**f**) MR myelographic images obtained by multiple 2D acquisitions. The large L3–L4 herniated disc results in complete obliteration of CSF space in the compressed thecal sac

(i.e., for exclusion of neoplastic and infectious diseases) or in postoperative studies. In fact, it is certainly true that the contrast agent modifies the diagnosis of degenerative diseases in a few selected cases. It is equally true that the use of contrast agent (combined with fat suppression) increases the evidence of degenerative vertebral, discal, and ligament changes. The contrast enhancement (CE) can better define herniated discs (and differentiate them from the adjacent venous congestion), confirms the diagnosis of infectious or "chemical" discitis, and strengthens the diagnosis of interapophyseal arthrosis/arthritis [24] (Fig. 2.15)

To complete the brief presentation on the MRI study technique, it is worth recalling that "axial load" studies, performed with MRI and/or CT scans, have been introduced in clinical practice [25, 26]. These studies mainly use the so-called "axial

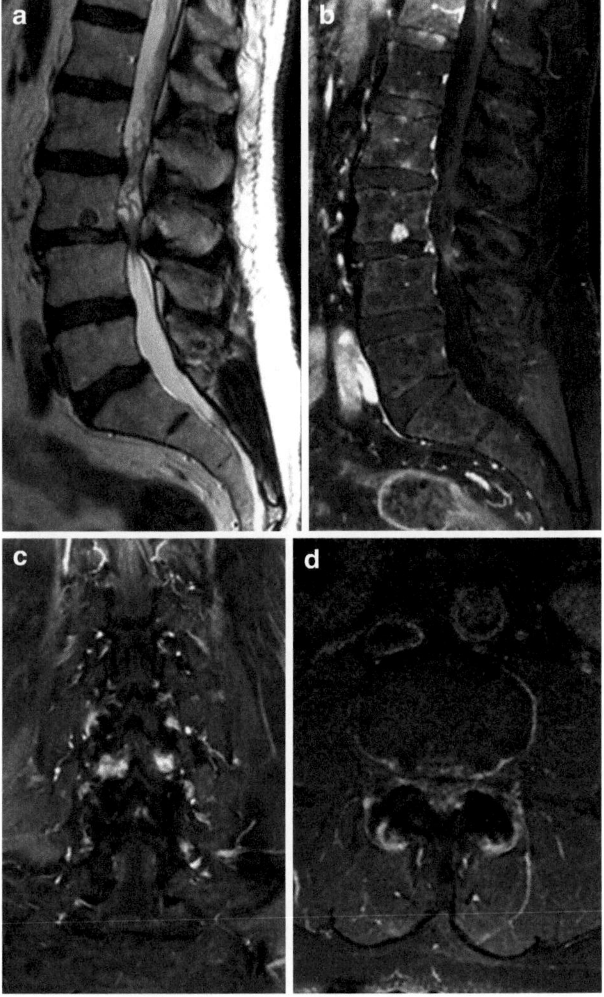

Fig. 2.15 L3–L4 spinal stenosis and instability; the contribution of contrast-enhanced fat-suppressed (fs) T1 images. TSE sagittal T2 (**a**), T1 fs sagittal (**b**), T1 fs coronal (**c**) and T1 fs axial (**d**) images with contrast agent. Note how the contrast enhancement marks both the subchondral disc changes as well as the bilateral facet joint degenerative disease

loader," that is, a mechanical system that aims to simulate the functional load on the spine (especially the lumbar) through the use of an apparatus that, with the patient supine, exerts scalable pressure on the shoulders, usually selected based on the body weight of the patient. The use of the axial loader has been supported by many authors and is supposed to serve the dual purpose of highlighting signs of instability under load and of increasing the sensitivity of MRI, revealing root/ganglion compressions that are not evident with the patient supine and that become manifest under load. The authors had the opportunity to use the axial loader in both CT and MRI scans, and consider the system unreliable. In fact, the loading conditions created by the axial loader do not bring into play the muscular dynamics and do not reproduce the situation of the upright position. This risks creating many false positives and highlighting discal protrusions/herniations that are not responsible for clinical symptoms or deserving of treatment (surgery). Think, for example, how many disc herniations are without corresponding clinical symptoms. The authors believe rather that, in the case of a symptomatic patient (without evidence of radicular compression and instability in the classic MRI), we can proceed to an MRI using the new reclining systems (intermediate field) that allow MRI studies in the upright position and have achieved a good level of image quality (although still lower than that of conventional high-field MRI). In the case of clinical or MRI suspicion of instability and unavailability of reclining MRI (the technology is not still currently accessible), the authors still prefer "dynamic" (flexion/extension) X-ray in the upright position, also because of the lower costs of such a choice.

Invasive Diagnostic Tools

Until the introduction of CT, myelography enjoyed a widespread use, especially in the diagnosis of lumbar radiculopathy and spondylotic myelopathy. With the advent and improvement of CT, the indication for intrathecal contrast-enhanced studies became limited and changed greatly, aiming mainly to demonstrate the effects of degenerative disease on the "content" and shifting the focus of imaging to CT-myelography. However, the impact of MRI has virtually eliminated the use of CT-myelography, which is limited primarily to patients with pacemakers or other absolute contraindications to MRI, for whom it is necessary to find the causes of spinal cord or radicular impairment. In fact, some authors continue to perform myelography and CT-myelography studies even in patients who can undergo an MRI, supporting the effectiveness and reliability of the technique and claiming the importance of the dynamic study (e.g., standing up, with dynamic flexion and extension tests).

Gas myelography has been completely abandoned and in cases in which we perform myelography/CT myelography, the introduction of contrast agents is almost exclusively via lumbar puncture, by administration of iodinated nonionic contrast agents of low osmolarity. When it is important to obtain dynamic myelographic studies, 10 cc of contrast agent are usually administered at a concentration of 300–350 mg I/ml and we proceed to radiography in two orthogonal and in oblique projections. After achieving the collection of the contrast agent in the areas of clinical interest, with an appropriate position and inclination of the patient table, and after the X-ray documentation, we proceed to the acquisition of CT myelography. In most common cases in which the indication is derived from the impossibility of use of MRI, an evaluation by CT myelography is instead sufficient. In these cases, the use of a smaller amount of contrast agent is preferred, and especially with lower iodine concentration. A lower contrast agent concentration is useful both to reduce side effects and to have a less increased density, as the opposite would disturb the detection of thinner intraspinal structures in the CT myelography. Indeed, it is essential to obtain a good contrast agent dilution in the CSF, to obtain a more homogeneous opacification, and this is achieved with multiple changes of position and rotations of the patient [27, 28].

Discography may provide valuable information in patients with unexplained chronic back pain regarding a possible discogenic origin of the pain. Discography is the only imaging procedure for the assessment of back pain that directly tries to correlate the patient's pain response to internal disc morphology. It is more sensitive than MR in the detection of internal disc disruption. The technique consists of percutaneously placing a needle into a disc, injecting a low volume of iodinated contrast agent (1.5–3.0 ml) into the nucleus polposus, and then assessing the patient immediate pain response. The main value is in the clinical assessment of patient's response to pain; the second value is in disc morphology assessment (discogram) by radiography and CT scans, based on the Modified Dallas Discogram Scale (Grade 0–5) [29].

There are other spinal contrast agent injections. A very low volume of nonionic iodinated contrast agent (0.5–1 ml) is injected during fluoroscopy-guided percutaneous spinal procedures. These include selective nerve root block, in order to document the correct needle position into the nerve root sleeve before injection of the therapeutic agents, and facet or sacro-iliac joint injection, in order to document the correct intra-synovial position of the needle before injection of the therapeutic agents. A larger volume of diluted contrast agent (2–3 ml) is injected during epidural block procedures, in order to visualize (by a lateral-view fluoroscopic image) the correct position of the needle tip evidenced by spread of the agent within the epidural space, before injection of the therapeutic agents.

Nuclear Medicine

The role of nuclear medicine in the characterization of bone degenerative lesions, in particular in the spine, is definitely limited. In the great majority of cases, the detection of changes is an incidental finding in the course of bone scans with diphosphonates, performed for the identification of skeletal metastases in cancer patients or for the diagnosis of benign bone tumors. In such cases, we typically see a symmetrical uptake of the radiopharmaceutical in the interapophyseal facet joints of the lumbar vertebrae, especially L5 (Fig. 2.16), in patients with lumbar osteoarthritis associated with "lower back pain," or "mid-cervical-lateral-focus" at the level of a cervical vertebral body in patients with neck pain [30].

However, bone scintigraphy retains an important role in the differential diagnosis between benign and malignant changes, especially in the case of single skeletal metastasis and/or in the few patients in whom the CT and MRI give equivocal results or do not allow a reliable disease characterization. The sensitivity of bone scintigraphy (greater than 70 % in different series) can be increased up to 90 % with the use of hybrid SPECT (single-photon emission tomography)/CT imaging. The hybrid method allows the integration of the functional information of bone scintigraphy with the morphological information of a MDCT. SPET/CT allows a better localization of the radiopharmaceutical uptake compared to the planar images of bone scintigraphy alone, especially in the spine. Indeed, uptakes localized in the

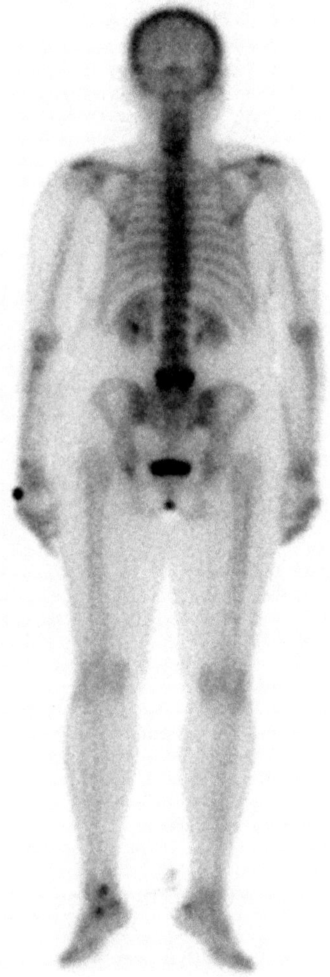

Fig. 2.16 Whole body ^{99m}Tc-MDP bone scintigraphy, posterior view: increased uptake of the radiopharmaceutical at the level of the articular facets of L5, expression of degenerative process

vertebral pedicle have a higher likelihood of malignancy compared to the same finding in the facet joints or in the vertebral body (88 % vs. 21–57 %) [31].

Nuclear medicine functional imaging continues to be essential in differentiating degenerative changes from inflammatory changes, in particular as regards spondylodiscitis. The most frequently used methods are SPET/CT with ^{67}Ga-citrate and, more recently, ^{18}F-FDG (fluoro-deoxy-glucose) PET (positron emission tomography)/CT [32]. A recent review has shown that SPET/CT with ^{67}Ga-citrate has a sensitivity equal to MRI (92 %) but higher specificity (92 vs. 77 %), especially in cases where the MRI proves not definitive (Fig. 2.17). ^{18}F-FDG (fluoro-deoxy-glucose) PET (positron emission tomography)/CT has sensitivity, specificity, and accuracy of 100, 87, and 96 %, respectively, in spinal infections, and is used especially in mild spondylitis and discitis, particularly if associated with concurrent infection of the adjacent soft tissues [33].

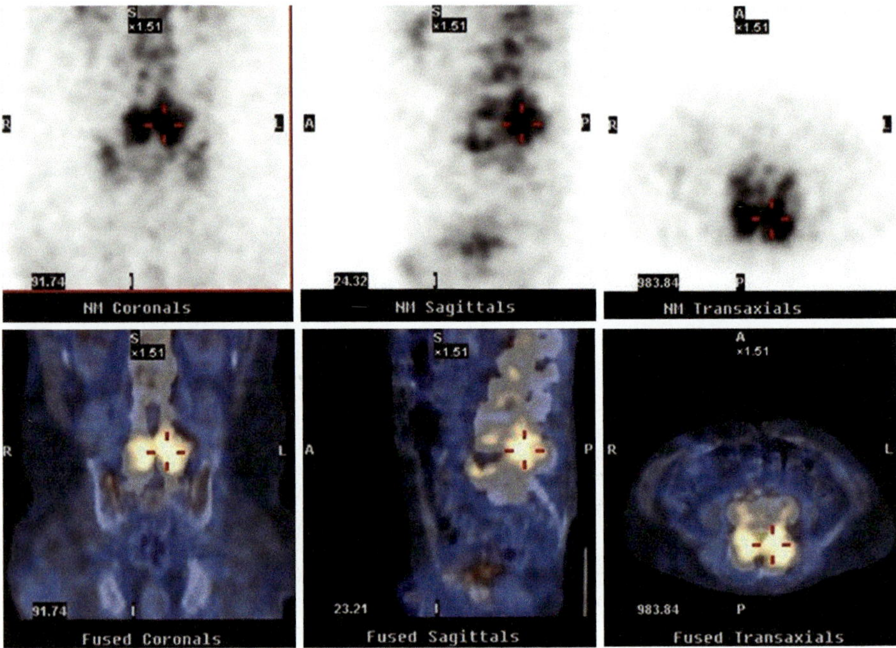

Fig. 2.17 67Ga-citrate SPET and SPET/CT fused images (axial, coronal, and sagittal view): intense accumulation of the radiopharmaceutical at the level of L5, due to an active infectious process (spondylitis)

Conclusion

Imaging has become the basis for the diagnosis and choice of treatment in degenerative spinal disease. The imaging assessment has rapidly changed over the past 20 years, with a drastic reduction in the role and appropriateness of radiographs and the predominant use of MRI. In practice, in most clinical situations of degenerative spinal diseases, the first imaging tool is now the MRI and it is only on the basis of the MRI findings that the indication for a targeted complement by CT or by radiographic study is proposed, which increasingly must include a functional/dynamic study (Fig. 2.18). It is essential that MRI allows us to obtain a certain diagnosis in order to reduce the time and cost of diagnosis, as well as to limit the use of imaging tools that require radiation exposure. It therefore becomes essential that, during the MRI study, the radiologist, starting from the standard images/sequences in multiple planes, integrates in the MRI procedure the specific sequences that will allow solving the clinical problems of the patient and, if appropriate, contribute to suggesting the subsequent diagnostic procedure.

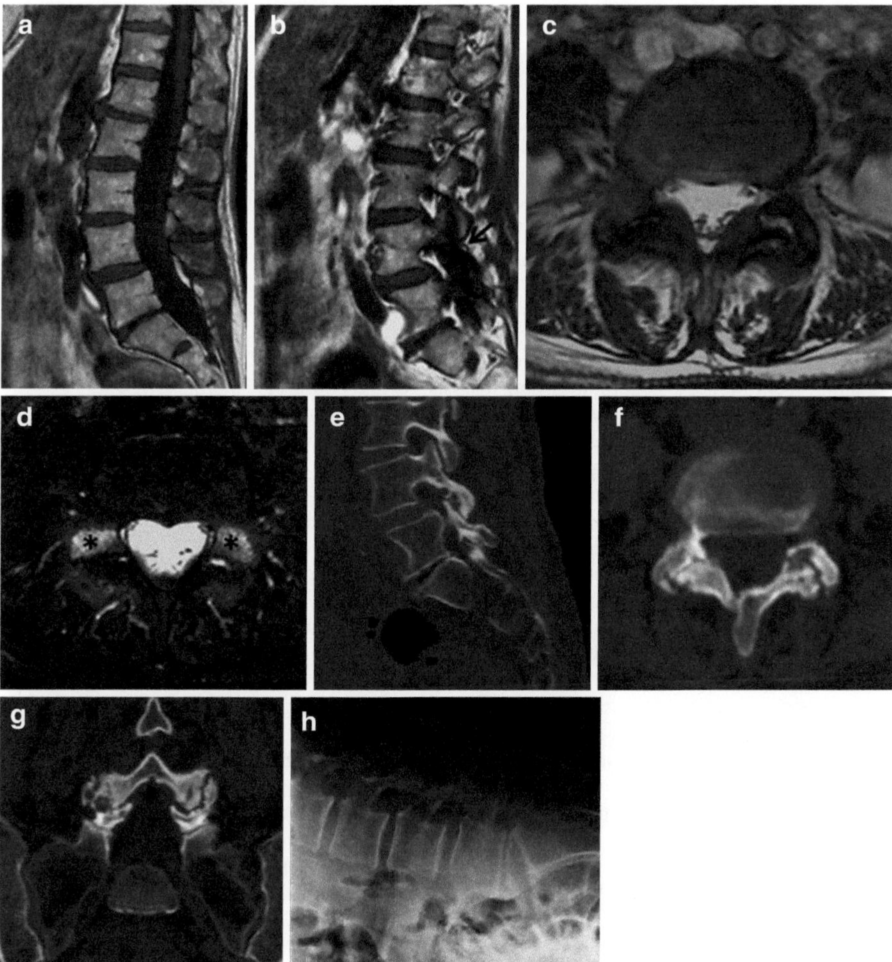

Fig. 2.18 Exhaustive imaging assessment of lumbar spine instability. TSE mid-line sagittal T1 (**a**), parasagittal (**b**), BFE axial T2 (**c**), TSE axial fat-suppressed (SPAIR, **d**), sagittal (**e**), axial (**f**) and coronal (**g**) CT reconstructions, X-ray lateral projection, flexion study (**h**). Sagittal T1 images show longstanding disc L5–S1 degenerative disease, minimal L4–L5 listhesis, and obvious signal modification of articular pillars (*arrow*); on axial BFE image there are obvious irregularities of interpophyseal joint surfaces with some subluxation on the left side. The acquisition of T2 axial fat-suppressed SPAIR images increases the evidence of bone edema (*). On the basis of MRI findings, the patient's evaluation has been completed by MDCT and functional/dynamic upright X-ray study. CT study optimally depicts the facet joint modifications with ankylosis and subchondral erosions. The upright flexion lateral X-ray demonstrates evident instability with L4–L5 degenerative spondylolisthesis

References

1. Boos N, Aebi M. Spinal disorders. Fundamentals of diagnosis and treatment. New York: Springer; 2008.
2. Fullenlove T, Williams AJ. Comparative roentgen findings in symptomatics and asymptomatics backs. Radiology. 1957;68:572–4.
3. Gehweiler JA, Daffner RH. Low back pain: the controversy of radiologic evaluation. AJR Am J Roentgenol. 1983;140:109–12.
4. Wood KB, Popp CA, Transfeldt EE, Geissele AE. Radiographic evaluation of instability in spondylolisthesis. Spine. 1994;19:1697–703.
5. Pitkanen M, Manninen HI. Sidebending versus flexion-extension radiographs in lumbar spinal instability. Clin Radiol. 1994;49:109–14.
6. Leone A, Costantini AM, Guglielmi G, Tancioni V, Moschini M. Degenerative disease of the lumbosacral spine: disk herniation and stenosis. Rays. 2000;25(1):35–48. Review.
7. Scavone JG, Latshaw RF, Weidner WA. Anteroposterior and lateral radiographs: an adequate lumbar spine examination. AJR Am J Roentgenol. 1981;136:715–7.
8. Dupuis PR, Yong-Hing K, Cassidy JD, Kirkaldy-Willis WH. Radiological diagnosis of degenerative lumbar spinal instability. Spine. 1985;10:262–6.
9. Dvorak J, Panjabi MM, Chang D, Theiler R, Grob D. Functional radiographic diagnosis of the lumbar spine: flexion-extension and lateral bending. Spine. 1991;16:562–71.
10. Hayes MA, Howard TC, Grue CR, Kopta JA. Roentgenographic evaluation of lumbar spine flexion-extension in asymptomatic individuals. Spine. 1989;14:327–31.
11. Lowe RW, Hayes TD, Kaye J, Bagg RJ, Luekens CA. Standing roentgenograms in spondylolisthesis. Clin Orthop Relat Res. 1976;117:80–4.
12. Shaffer WO, Spratt KF, Weinstein J, Lehmann TR, Goel V. The consistency and accuracy of roentgenograms for measuring sagittal translation in the lumbar vertebral motion segment. Spine. 1990;15:741–50.
13. Boden SD, Wiesel SW. Lumbosacral segmental motion in normal individuals: have we been measuring instability properly? Spine. 1990;15:571–6.
14. Kirkaldy-Willis WH, Farfan HF. Instability of the lumbar spine. Clin Orthop Relat Res. 1982;165:110–23.
15. Cacayorin ED, Kieffer SA. Applications and limitations of computed tomography of the spine. Radiol Clin North Am. 1982;20(1):185–206.
16. Rothman SLG, Glenn WV. Multiplanar CT of the spine. Baltimore: University Park Press; 1985. Chapters 1–4, p. 1–112, chapters 16–17, p. 477–504.
17. Perrone L, Politi M, Foschi R, Masini V, Reale F, Costantini AM, Marano P. Post-processing of digital imaging. Rays. 2003;28(1):95–101. Review.
18. Fast A, Goldsher D. Navigating the adult spine: Bridging clinical practice and neuroradiology. New York: Demos; 2007.
19. Larde D, Mathieu D, Frija J, Gaston A, Vasile N. Spinal vacuum phenomenon: CT diagnosis and significance. J Comput Assist Tomogr. 1982;6:671–6.
20. Czervionke LF, Daniels DL. Degenerative disease of the spine. In: Atlas SW, editor. Magnetic resonance imaging of the brain and spine. New York: Raven; 1991.
21. Colosimo C, Gaudino S, Alexandre AM. Imaging in degenerative spine pathology. Acta Neurochir Suppl. 2011;108:9–15.
22. Modic MT, Masaryk TJ, Ross JS, Carter JR. Imaging of degenerative disk disease. Radiology. 1988;168:177–86.
23. Modic MT, Ross JS. Lumbar degenerative disk disease. Radiology. 2007;245:43–61.
24. Colosimo C, Cianfoni A, Di Lella GM, Gaudino S. Contrast-enhanced MR imaging of the spine: when, why and how? How to optimize contrast protocols in MR imaging of the spine. Neuroradiology. 2006;48:18–33.
25. Saifuddin A, Blease S, MacSweeney E. Axial loaded MRI of the lumbar spine. Clin Radiol. 2003;58(9):661–71.

26. Kinder A, et al. Magnetic resonance imaging of the lumbar spine with axial loading: a review of 120 cases. Eur J Radiol. 2012;81(4):e561–4.
27. Fenton DS, Czervionke LF. Image-guided spine intervention. Philadelphia: Saunders (Elsevier); 2003.
28. Williams AL, Murtagh FR. Handbook of diagnostic and therapeutic spine procedures. St. Louis: Mosby (Elsevier); 2002.
29. Sachs BL, Vanharanta H, Spivey MA, et al. Dallas discogram description: a new classification of CT/discography in low back disorders. Spine. 1987;12:287.
30. Scharf S. SPECT/CT imaging in general orthopedic practice. Semin Nucl Med. 2009;39(5):293–307.
31. Reinartz P, Schaffeldt J, Sabri O, Zimny M, Nowak B, Ostwald E, Cremerius U, Buell U. Benign versus malignant osseous lesions in the lumbar vertebrae: differentiation by means of bone SPET. Eur J Nucl Med. 2000;27:721–6.
32. Treglia G, Focacci C, Caldarella C, Mattoli MV, Salsano M, Taralli S, Giordano A. The role of nuclear medicine in the diagnosis of spondylodiscitis. Eur Rev Med Pharmacol Sci. 2012;16 Suppl 2:20–5.
33. Rosen RS, Fayad L, Wahl RL. Increased 18F-FDG uptake in degenerative disease of the spine: characterization with 18F-FDG PET/CT. J Nucl Med. 2006;47:1274–80.

Chapter 3
Radiofrequency Lumbar Facet Joint Denervation

Charles A. Gauci

Lumbar Facet Joint Pain

Pain originating from the facet or zygapophyseal joints is responsible for about 15 % of all low back pain complaints [1].

The facet joints are true synovial joints and pain can be precipitated by various causes such as facet joint degeneration, intervertebral disc degeneration, postural abnormalities such as lumbar scoliosis, and problems arising from the bony structures such as collapse (due to osteoporosis or pathological fractures) or defects (e.g., spondylolisthesis). It can also come about as the result of repeated minor trauma.

These conditions result in arthritic changes in the facet joints, which in turn leads to inflammation and swelling. This stretches the joint capsule and creates pain.

Clinically, the patient presents with axial low back pain which is ill-defined and poorly localized with frequent vague (i.e., nonsegmental) radiation into the groin or thigh.

It tends to be posture-related and is usually worse at rest (sitting/standing) but helped by mobility. The pain can be quite bad at night and is frequently accompanied by early morning pain and/or stiffness.

On examination, the patient exhibits pain on extension, rotation, and lateral flexion of the lumbar spine; there is frequently tenderness over the affected facet joint(s) although this may be difficult to elicit in a well-built muscular patient. Sometimes there is hypersensitivity to light touch over the painful area.

In the absence of any concomitant pathology such as a prolapsed intervertebral disc, there are usually no abnormal neurological findings or specific changes on the MRI scan.

Degenerative changes of the joints themselves may or may not be seen on imaging, but there is no correlation between the degree of any degeneration and the pain.

C.A. Gauci, MD, KHS, FRCA, FIPP, FFPMRCA
Department of Pain Management, Whipps Cross University Hospital, London E11, UK
e-mail: charles.gauci@btinternet.com

P.P.M. Menchetti (ed.), *Minimally Invasive Surgery of the Lumbar Spine*,
DOI 10.1007/978-1-4471-5280-4_3, © Springer-Verlag London 2014

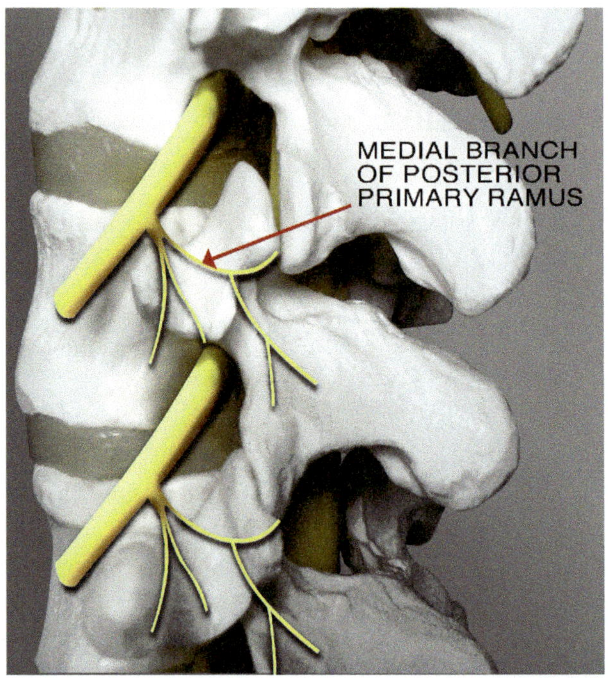

Fig. 3.1 Medial branch, lumbar posterior primary ramus

The diagnosis is made on the basis of the history, examination, and a diagnostic block, done under X-ray control.

The diagnostic block can be either an intra-articular block or, preferably, a medial branch block, using a short-acting local anesthetic such as 2 % lidocaine.

A positive diagnostic block is essential for reaching a diagnosis [2].

Radiofrequency (RF) facet denervation is currently considered the standard treatment of facet-mediated persistent pain [3].

Lumbar Facet Joint Denervation

There are various techniques used to carry out lumbar facet joint denervation.

The following description is reproduced with permission from *Manual of RF Techniques, 3rd Edition*, by Dr. Charles A. Gauci and published by CoMedical, the Netherlands, 2011.

Anatomy

Be very familiar with the medial branch of the posterior primary ramus—this is your target! (Fig. 3.1)

Table 3.1 For facet denervation, target the medial branches at the levels you want to treat together with the medial branch to the level above

Facet joint	Target medial branches of posterior primary rami of
L1/L2	T12, L1, L2
L2/L3	L1, L2, L3
L3/L4	L2, L3, L4
L4/L5	L3, L4, L5
L5/S1	L4, L5, S1

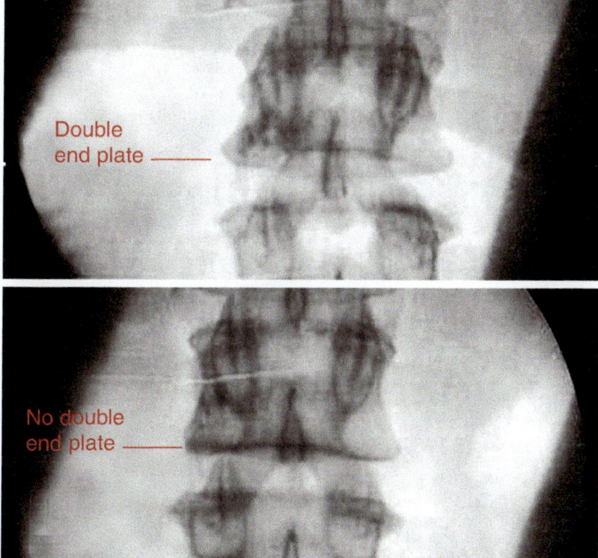

Fig. 3.2 Posteroanterior X-ray view of lumbar spine showing double end plate and its plate removal

For facet denervation, target the medial branches at the levels you want to treat together with the medial branch to the level above (Table 3.1).

Position of Patient

The patient should be lying prone on a radiolucent table; stand on the left side of the patient if you are right-handed and vice versa if you are left-handed.

With the C-arm image intensifier in the posteroanterior axis, obtain a clear view of the lumbar vertebrae; if necessary, adjust the position of the image intensifier so as to obliterate any double end plates. It is done by angling the image intensifier, which is in the posteroanterior axis, very slightly caudally. This maneuver results in the lower border becoming a single line on X-ray screening (Fig. 3.2). Occasionally, the double end plate is removed by moving the axis of the C-arm image intensifier very slightly cranially.

The best place to start trying to locate the medial branch of the posterior primary ramus is the point where it enters the groove on the back of the vertebral lamina.

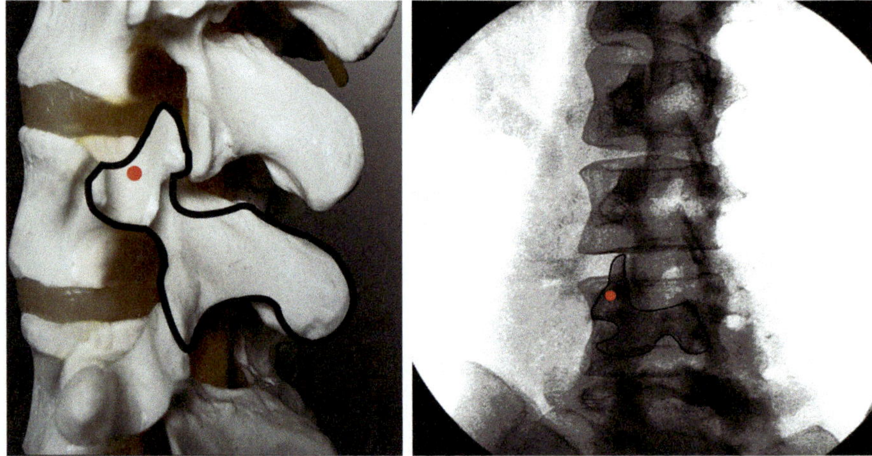

Fig. 3.3 "Eye of the Scottie dog"

Fig. 3.4 Target!

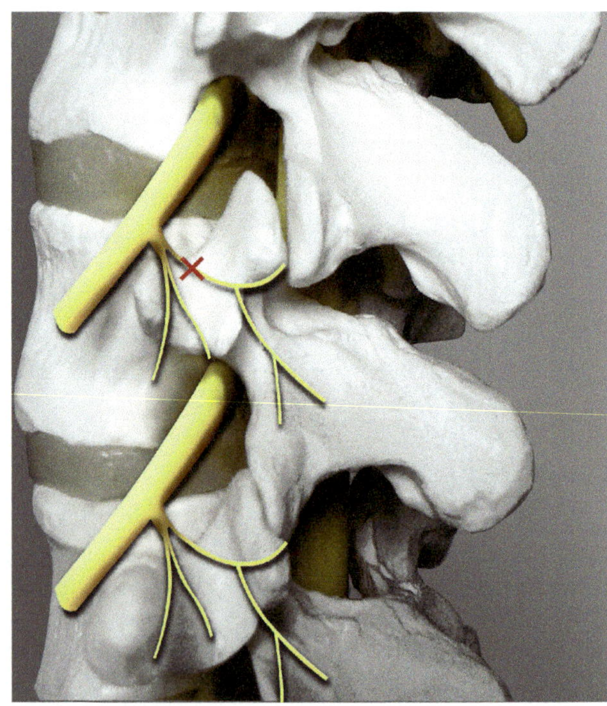

For this you need to move the image intensifier from its initial posteroanterior axis (corrected for "double end plates") obliquely away from the patient so as to obtain a good view of the so-called Scottie dog. Your preliminary target is the "eye of the dog" (Fig. 3.3); this point overlies the medial branch (Fig. 3.4).

Fig. 3.5 Tunnel vision

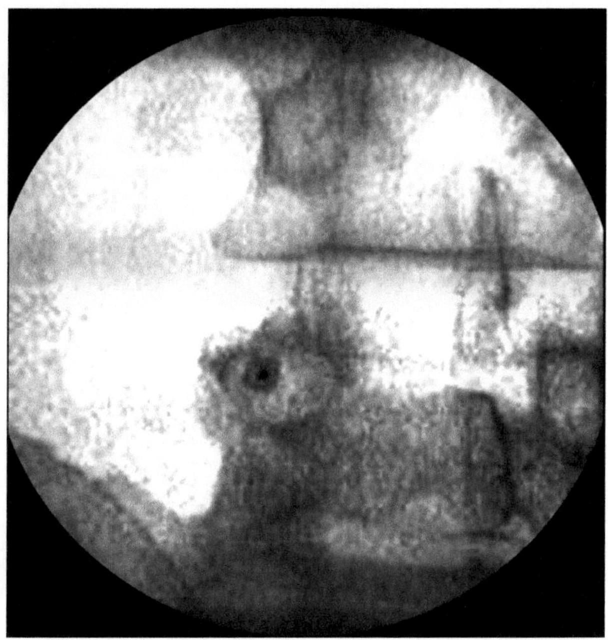

Technique

Use a 25# needle to infiltrate the superficial tissues only; do not go down as far as bone, as you will anesthetize the medial branch and be unable to locate it by stimulation.

Insert a 22#, 100.5 mm (5 mm exposed tip) RF needle along the angle of the X-ray beam so as to hit the "eye of the Scottie dog" in tunnel vision (Fig. 3.5).

Replace the RF needle stilette with the thermocouple electrode and try to locate the medial branch by sensory stimulation, using the following parameters on your machine:

Frequency: 50 Hz
Pulse width: 1 ms
Voltage: up to 0.5 V

NB if you only manage to locate the nerve at a voltage greater than 0.5 V, keep looking! You are unlikely to produce an effective lesion here.

If you cannot locate the nerve on bone, then slip forward off bone and into the groove close to the intervertebral foramen (Fig. 3.6) and try again. If you still cannot locate the nerve, advance deeper *and very slowly* checking the position of your needle in the lateral axis (Fig. 3.7). The tip of your needle must *never* lie anterior to an imaginary line passing through the posterior margin of the intervertebral foramen (Fig. 3.8). *If you lesion anterior to this point, you run the double risk of causing neuritis and of damaging the motor root.*

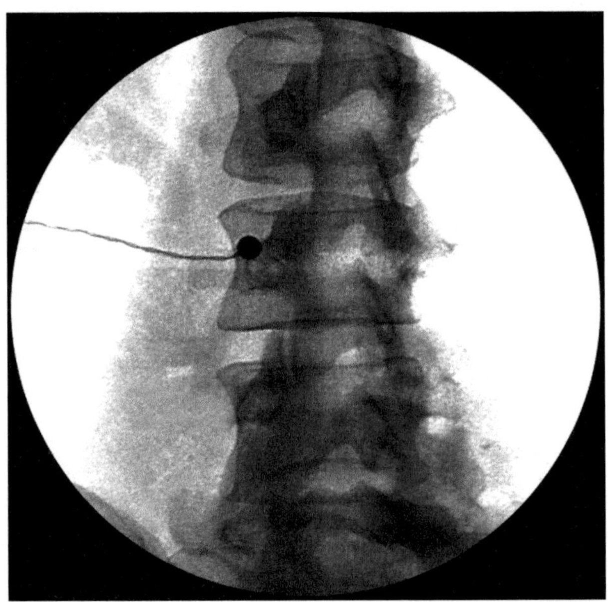

Fig. 3.6 Needle in groove

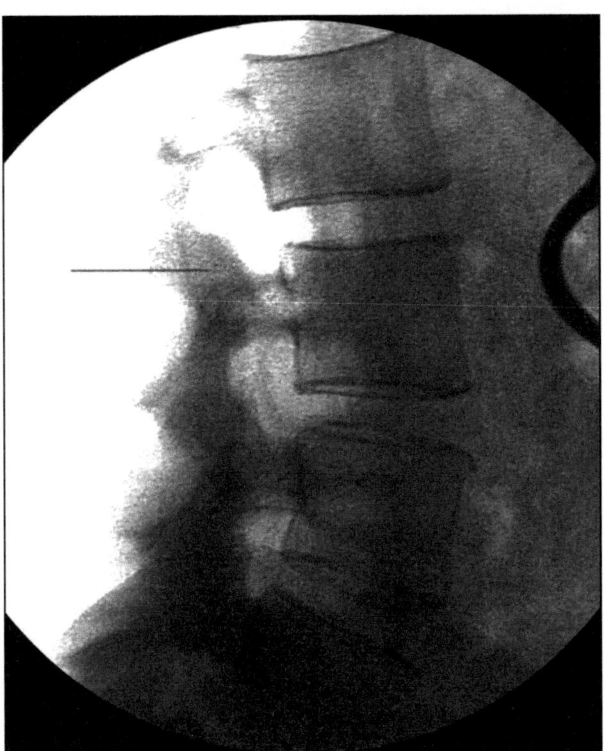

Fig. 3.7 View of needle in lateral axis-1

Fig. 3.8 Danger zones!

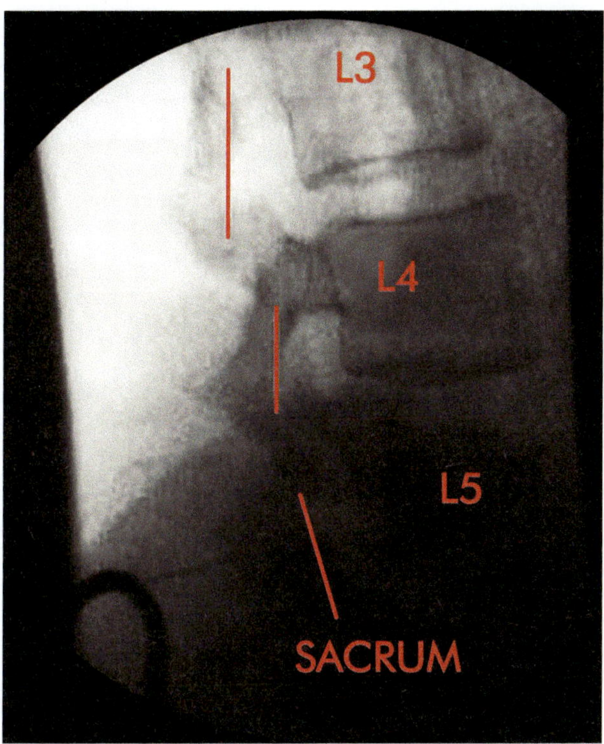

As you gain experience in the technique, you may decide to slip forward into the groove from the "eye of the Scottie dog" as a matter of routine. After identification of the nerve in the groove means that you are using the shaft of the needle as opposed to its tip, and many workers consider it to be a better way of obtaining a permanent lesion (*see* section on "The Physics of Radiofrequency and Pulsed Radiofrequency").

Once you have achieved localization by sensory stimulation, test for motor stimulation using the following parameters on your machine:

Frequency: 2 Hz
Pulse width: 1 ms
Voltage: double the sensory threshold but at least 1 V

NB it is very common to see localized contractions around the needle area (due to stimulation of the multifidus muscle by the motor component of the medial branch); these can safely be ignored. You are on the lookout for rhythmical contractions in the lower limb. Should these appear, reposition the needle.

You are now ready to carry out a lesion.
Preset the timer to 60 s.
Preset the temperature maximum to 85 °C.
Remove the thermocouple electrode and inject 1 ml of 2 % lidocaine through the needle.
Replace the electrode.

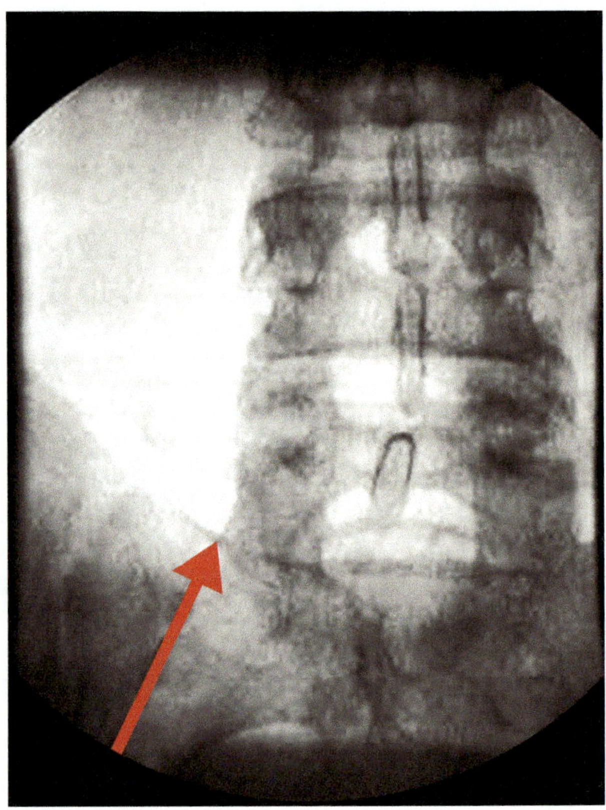

Fig. 3.9 Radiographic landmark on A-P view for L5 medial branch. *Red arrow* indicates the target point for detect L5 medial branch

Switch your machine to *lesion* mode and gradually increase the power, which will in turn cause a temperature rise.

When the temperature reaches 80 °C, switch the timer on, in order to create the lesion. When the lesion has been performed, remove the electrode and inject 1 ml of a mixture of 0.5 % bupivacaine plus a depot steroid preparation in order to reduce postprocedure discomfort.

The Medial Branch of the L5 Posterior Primary Ramus

Your target here is slightly different. With the image intensifier in the posteroanterior axis, visualize the sacrum; your target is the junction between the superior articular process and the upper surface of the lateral part of the sacrum (Fig. 3.9); very often you can locate the medial branch here without needing to move the image intensifier off the posteroanterior axis; instead, you may find it useful to angle your needle, departing from strict "tunnel vision."

Hunt for the nerve as already outlined above.

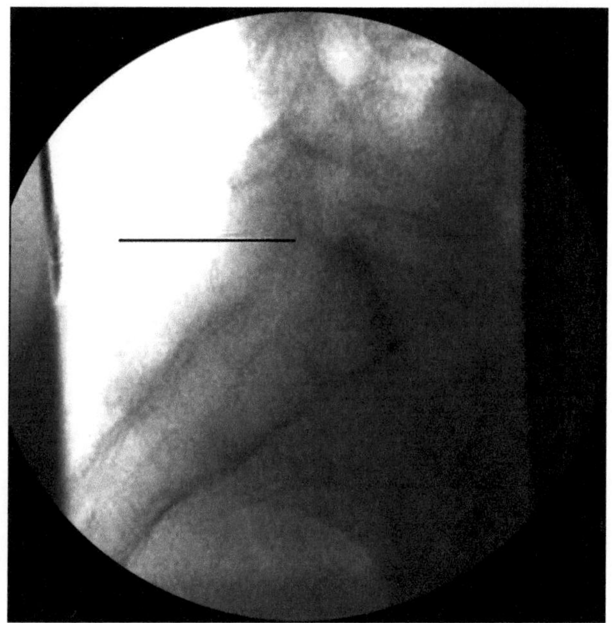

Fig. 3.10 View of needle in lateral axis-2

If you cannot locate the nerve on bone, then slip forward off bone and into the groove close to the intervertebral foramen and try again. If you still cannot locate the nerve, advance deeper *and very slowly* checking the position of your needle in the lateral axis. The tip of your needle must *never* lie anterior to an imaginary line passing through the posterior margin of the L5 intervertebral foramen (Fig. 3.10). If you lesion anterior to this point, you run the double risk of causing neuritis and of damaging the motor root.

As you gain experience in the technique, you may decide to slip forward into the groove from bone as a matter of routine. After identification of the nerve in the groove means that you are using the shaft of the needle as opposed to its tip, and many workers consider it to be a better way of obtaining a permanent lesion (*see* section on "The Physics of Radiofrequency and Pulsed Radiofrequency").

Branch from S1

This lies just lateral to the S1 foramen (Fig. 3.11); you do not need a motor test at this point.

Aftercare

Warn the patient about temporary numbness and limb weakness due to the local anesthetic; do not discharge the patient until you are certain that he/she can walk unaided.

Warn the patient about residual soreness, which may last for a couple of weeks; this usually readily responds to NSAID therapy.

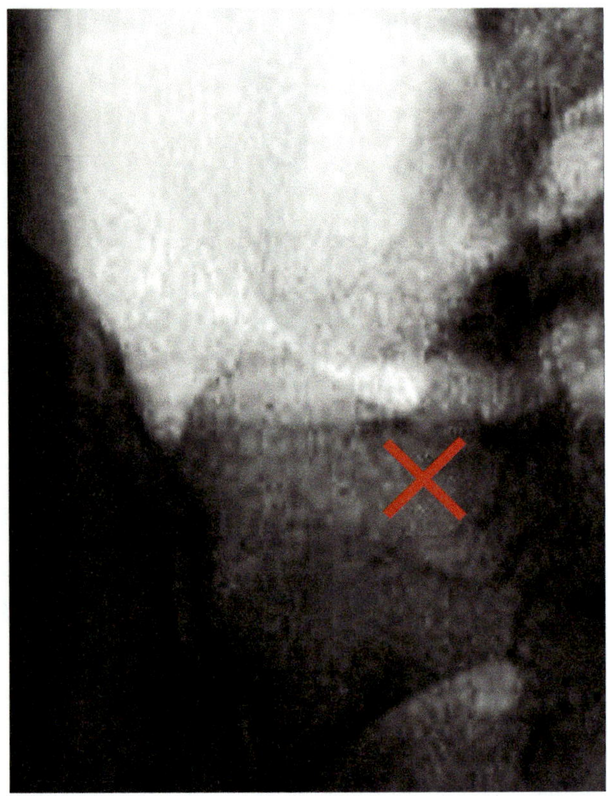

Fig. 3.11 Radiographic landmark for detect the Contribution of S1 to L5/S1 facet joint (*cross mark*)

Evidence

The most recent reviews of the evidence for radiofrequency facet joint denervation are contained in papers written by van Zundert et al. [3] and by Cohen et al. [4].

The technique was given a score of *1B+* (positive recommendation) in a recently published practice guideline for interventional pain management.

The Physics of Radiofrequency and Pulsed Radiofrequency

The following account is reproduced with permission from *Manual of RF Techniques, 3rd. Edition*, by Dr. Charles A. Gauci and published by CoMedical, the Netherlands, 2011.

Section 1

Dr. Eric R. Cosman, Jr., MEng, PhD; Dr. Charles A. Gauci, MD, FRCA, FIPP, FFPMRCA; and Prof. Eric R. Cosman, Sr., PhD

Radiofrequency (RF) lesioning refers to the delivery of high-frequency electrical current in the RF range ($\approx$500 kHz) to patient tissue via an RF electrode to induce a biological effect, such as the thermal destruction of nerves that carry painful impulses. RF methods used in pain management today can be subdivided by the following broad characteristics, each of which involves different physical and clinical considerations.

- *Waveform/Set Temperature*

  - *Thermal RF (TRF)*: The sustained tissue temperature exceeds 42 °C grossly. A continuous RF (CRF) waveform and tissue temperatures in the range of 70–90 °C are typical. The clinical objective is gross thermal nerve ablation. This category includes "cooled RF" methods, where the electrode is internally cooled, but induced tissue temperatures are neurolytic.
  - *Pulsed RF (PRF)*: The tissue temperature is held at or below 42 °C on average. RF is delivered in short high-intensity bursts so that the RF electric field strength is increased without gross heating. The clinical objective is neural modification by electric and thermal fields (Cosman and Cosman 2005), but the pain-relief mechanism remains under scientific investigation, as described later on in this book by Cahana et al.

- *Electrode Polarity*

  - *Monopolar RF*: Current passes between a needle electrode and a large-area reference ground pad. RF current intensities are highest near the needle electrode's uninsulated tip. In monopolar thermal RF, an ellipsoidal heat lesion is generated (Fig. 3.12). With proper full adhesion of the ground pad to the skin, current densities are low over the pad's large area, and thus nearby tissue is not typically elevated to lesion levels.
  - *Bipolar RF*: Current passes between two needle-electrode tips, and the current density is high at both locations. Thus, in bipolar thermal RF, a heat lesion is generated near both tips. When parallel tips are brought close together, the electric field is focused between the tips and a large "strip" lesion is formed (Fig. 3.18).

Monopolar thermal RF is the most common and basic form of RF treatment and has been used widely in pain management and neurosurgery since the earliest RF generators were built by B. J. Cosman, S. Aranow, and O. A. Wyss in the early 1950s (Sweet and Mark 1953; Cosman and Cosman 1974, 1984). In the 1990s, monopolar pulsed RF was introduced by Sluijter, Cosman, Rittman, and van Kleef (1998) and is used where conventional thermal RF is contraindicated (e.g., neuropathic pain) or could be potentially hazardous (e.g., DRG lesioning). Bipolar thermal RF between parallel electrodes has been used in pain management for the last decade (Ferrante et al. 2001; Burnham et al. 2007), but only recently has the large size of bipolar RF lesions been fully appreciated (Cosman and Gonzalez 2011). A pioneering application of bipolar pulsed RF has been reported, and this was in the treatment of carpel tunnel syndrome pain (Ruiz-Lopez 2008).

In one author's clinical experience (CAG), there are some basic rules which should be followed in RF lesioning. Thermal RF should be used only for treatment of

Fig. 3.12 Monopolar thermal RF: electric field (*above*), steady-state tissue temperatures (*below*), and the heat lesion boundary (*black*)

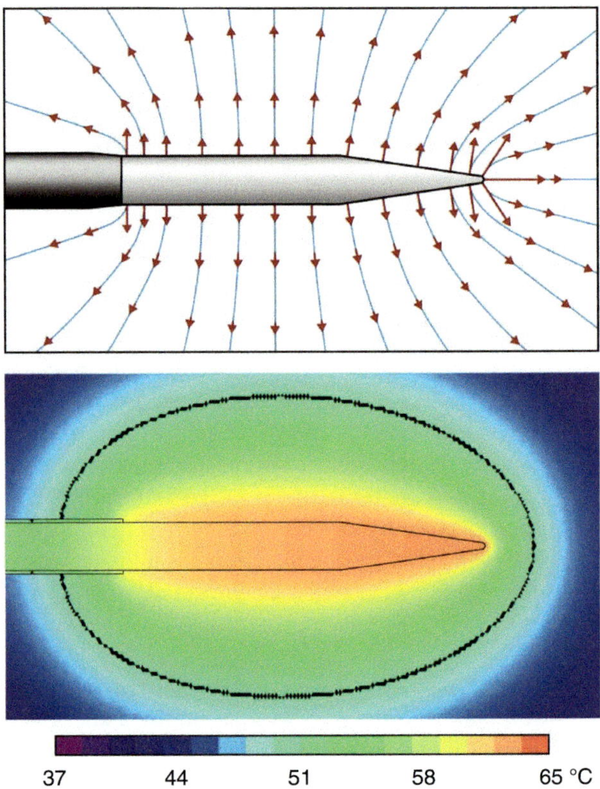

nociceptive pain. RF should not be used in patients with marked psychological overlay and/or drug dependency. RF should not be used in patients with total body pain. You should ensure that the patient has realistic expectations since the total abolition of pain may not be possible. You should exhaust all other nondestructive forms of treatment first and achieve unequivocal benefit from preliminary prognostic blocks.

Monopolar Thermal RF

Using standard equipment, the steps for monopolar RF lesioning in the spine typically include the following steps:

1. Place the ground pad on the skin near the treatment site.
2. Place the RF cannula percutaneously near the target nerve.
3. Stimulate: The RF electrode delivers sensory and motor nerve stimulation to ensure that the cannula's tip is near the target nerve and distant from nontarget nerves.
4. Inject anesthetic through the cannula to prevent pain during lesioning.
5. Lesion: The electrode delivers RF current to the cannula's tip and the nearby nerve(s) are lesioned with temperature control.

The RF cannula is typically a hollow 22G, 21G, 20G, 18G, or 16G needle that is fully insulated except at the tip. The cannula's hollow interior accepts either (a) a stilette to make the cannula solid for insertion, (b) injected fluid anesthetics and steroids, or (c) a 28G thermocouple (TC) electrode for tip temperature measurement and delivery of stimulation and RF currents. In some applications, such as cordotomy, DREZ, brain, and even spinal lesioning, the electrode and cannulae are integrated into a single device. X-ray guidance is typically used to position the cannula nearby the target nerve by reference to bony landmarks. Once positioned, the cannula's stilette is removed and is replaced by the electrode. The operator then seeks the nerve by sensory stimulation, which are low-voltage electrical pulses delivered at 50 Hz (pulses per second). A stronger sensory response at a lower voltage indicates the cannula's tip is closer to the nerve. In the clinical experience of one author (CAG), the cannula needs to be within 3 mm of the nerve in order to create an adequate heat lesion, and a stimulation level of at most 0.6 V is indicative of this.

The operator should always ensure that the cannula/electrode is not dangerously close to any motor nerve in the vicinity of the sensory nerve he/she is trying to lesion. To accomplish this, low-frequency motor stimulation pulses are delivered at 2 Hz. In the clinical experience of one author (CAG), if no muscle twitch in the territory of the nerve is noted at twice the voltage strength necessary to achieve sensory stimulation, it can be safely assumed that there are no motor paths within 3 mm of the needle and that, consequently, there is no risk of damage to any motor nerve. When working on spinal nerves, e.g., medial branches of posterior primary rami, one should not worry about localized contractions close to the area of needle insertion; one is concerned with motor twitches at more distant sites, e.g., the arm or the leg.

When the operator is satisfied that the needle is safely in position, RF current is delivered to the electrode and cannula. Frictional heating occurs near the cannula's uninsulated tip due to tissue electrolytes being pulled to and fro by the RF current alternating at approximately 500 kHz (500,000 cycles per second). While heating occurs only in the tissue and not within the electrode, within a few seconds of sustained RF heating, the temperature measured in the electrode/cannula's tip registers the maximum tissue temperature (Cosman and Cosman 2003; Cosman 2010) (Fig. 3.12). This occurs due to coherent heat diffusion into the electrode tip from all sides. This maximum temperature can be directly controlled by the operator. It must be cautioned that for cooled RF, where the electrode is cooled by internally circulating water, the electrode does not measure the maximum tissue temperature; rather, the maximum tissue temperature occurs at a variable location remote of the electrode and can far exceed the temperature measured within or nearby the electrode (Wright 2007). As the current is applied at the destructive levels typical of thermal RF, a well-circumscribed heat lesion appears. It will grow until a steady state is reached; at this point, the passage of current only maintains the temperature. Little further spread takes place at the edge of the lesion, since (a) the electric field and rate of heating decrease with distance from the electrode and (b) the rate of RF heating within the lesion volume is roughly balanced by the rate of heat diffusion into the surrounding tissue, heat diffusion into the electrode shaft, and blood-flow cooling.

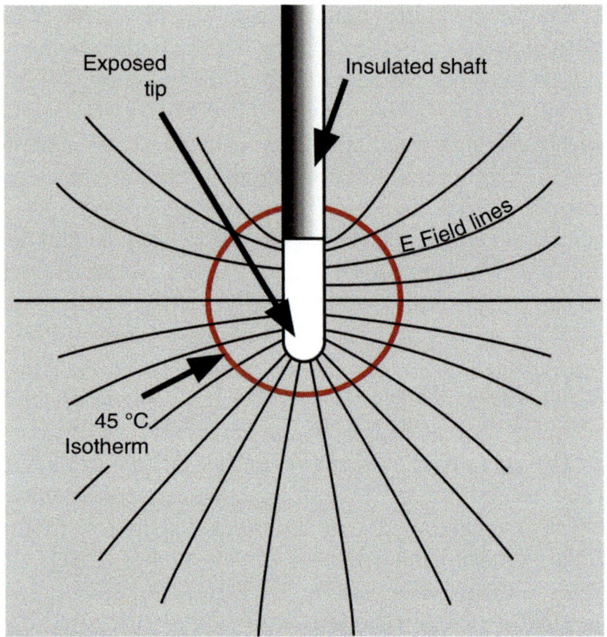

Fig. 3.13 Monopolar thermal RF lesion zone and the 45 °C isotherm (Adapted from Cosman and Cosman (1984))

The heat lesion is shaped like a match head (Fig. 3.12) and is commonly defined as the tissue regions for which the temperature exceeds 45–50 °C for at least 20 s (Brodkey 1964; Dieckmann 1965; Smith 1981; Cosman and Cosman 1974, 1984). Though permanent neurological damage occurs when tissue is exposed to temperatures exceeding 42 °C over longer durations (Cosman et al. 2009), for practical purposes, when we talk about lesion size, we mean the volume of tissue within the 45 °C isotherm (Fig. 3.13). According to Abou-Sherif et al. (2003), thermal RF produces the following effects in the rat sciatic nerve at 6–8 weeks: Wallerian degeneration in all nerve fibers, physical disruption of the basal laminae, focal disruption of the perineurium, degranulation of mast cells, recruitment of exogenous macrophages, local muscle necrosis, delayed axonal regeneration, and prolonged changes in the microvascular bed (vascular stasis) with extravasation of erythrocytes, this latter resembling the ischemic changes of reperfusion injury.

The heat lesion extends maximally around the shaft of the cannula, with a diameter that ranges from 2 to 10 mm depending on the cannula's diameter/gauge, the tip temperature, and lesion time (Fig. 3.14). The lesion extends 1–2 mm both ahead of the tip and up the shaft, yielding a total length 2–3 mm longer than the tip length (Cosman and Cosman 1984). Because of this geometry, many physicians prefer "parallel"/"side-on" cannula placement for monopolar thermal RF lesioning so that the nerve is positioned at the side of the cannula tip where the lesion extends maximally. In the alternative "perpendicular"/"point-on" approach, the nerve is placed directly ahead of the cannula tip, thus exposing a smaller volume of the nerve to neurolytic temperatures.

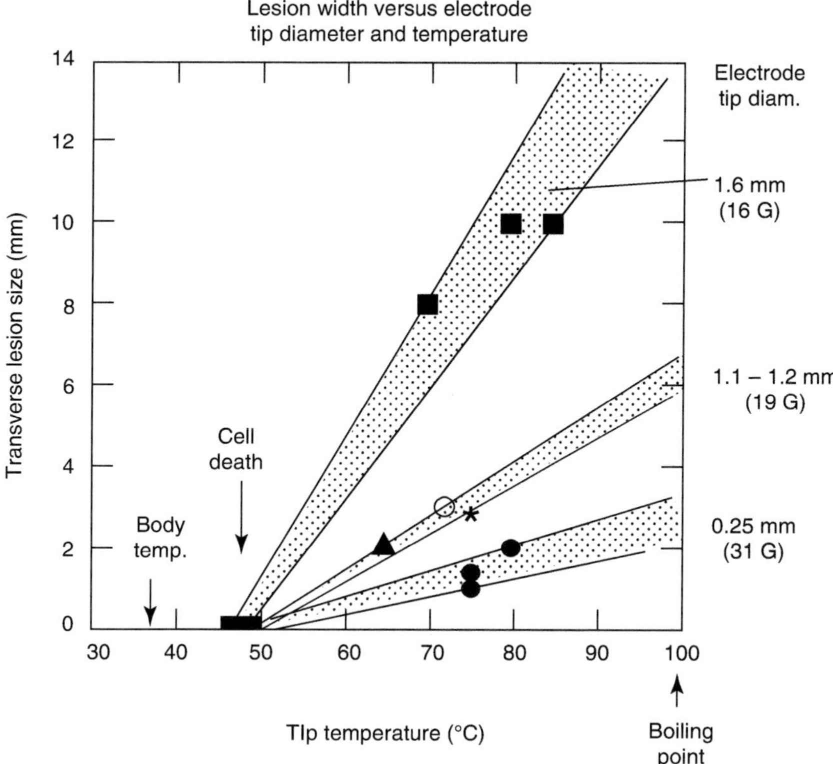

Fig. 3.14 Postmortem monopolar thermal RF lesion width around the electrode shaft for different electrode diameters/gauges and tip temperatures (Adapted from Cosman et al. (1988))

For a given electrode/cannula tip temperature, if lesion size is plotted against exposure time, it will be observed that the size increase is relatively linear over the early part of the curve, but then begins to slow as the steady state is approached (Fig. 3.15). For electrode/cannula of the sizes used in pain management, the steady-state lesion size is not reached until 30–90 s after the tip temperature reaches its set value. Thus, the tip should be held at the desired temperature for this duration of time to ensure that the lesion has reached its full spread for that temperature. The steady-state lesion size (Fig. 3.16) is strongly influenced by the tip temperature and electrode/cannula diameter (Fig. 3.14). All other things being equal, a larger heat lesion will be produced by a larger electrode tip and a higher tip temperature (assuming that boiling does not shut down RF current flow). Additionally, several factors can affect lesion size and dynamics, including variations in tissue densities, proximity to bone, and proximity to CSF (especially in trigeminal lesions), blood vessels, etc.

It is advisable to keep the tissue temperature below boiling (100 °C). Boiling can lead to uncontrolled gas discharges, burning steam that travels up the electrode's shaft to the skin, irregular lesion geometry, and charring at the electrode tip. In one

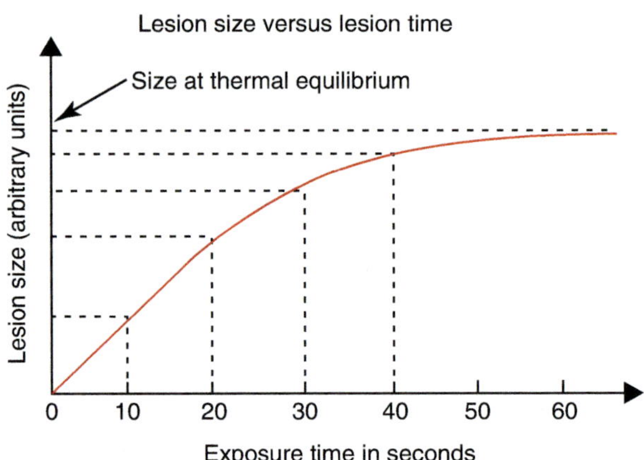

Fig. 3.15 Schematic plot of thermal RF lesion size vs. exposure time to RF current (Adapted from Cosman and Cosman (1974))

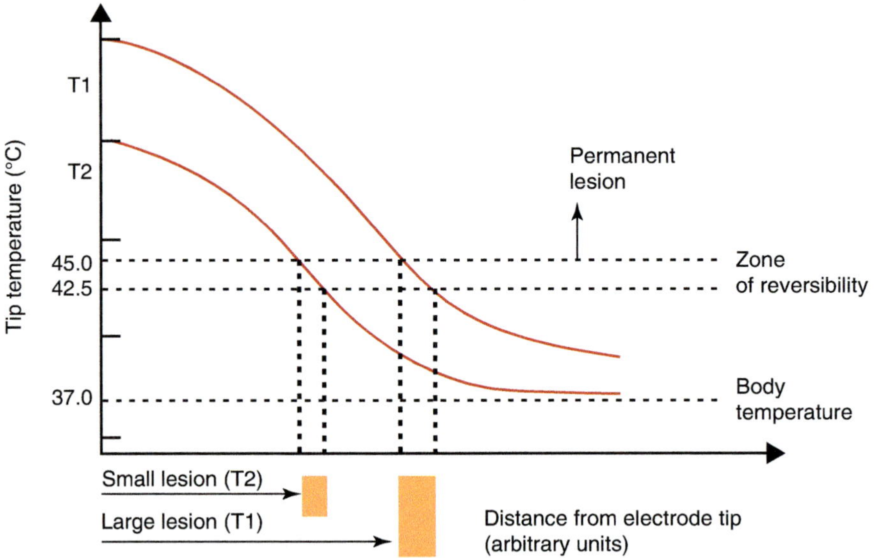

Fig. 3.16 Effect of tip temperature on RF lesion size (Adapted from Cosman and Cosman (1974))

author's clinical practice (CAG), the lesion temperature is held below 85 °C to give a broad temperature margin relative to 100 °C.

The resistance to the flow of electrical current from the tip of the cannula, the impedance, can be measured and should be observed by the operator. A very high impedance, or open circuit, can indicate that the electrode or ground pad is not in proper contact with the patient or that the cables are disconnected. A rising, high impedance can also indicate that the tissue is boiling at the cannula's tip, since electrical current cannot easily traverse boiling gas bubble; this is an important safety check in case the temperature sensor is broken or misplaced outside the cannula's tip (Cosman 2010). A very low impedance, or short circuit, can indicate a failure of the RF equipment or direct contact between the electrode and the ground pad or

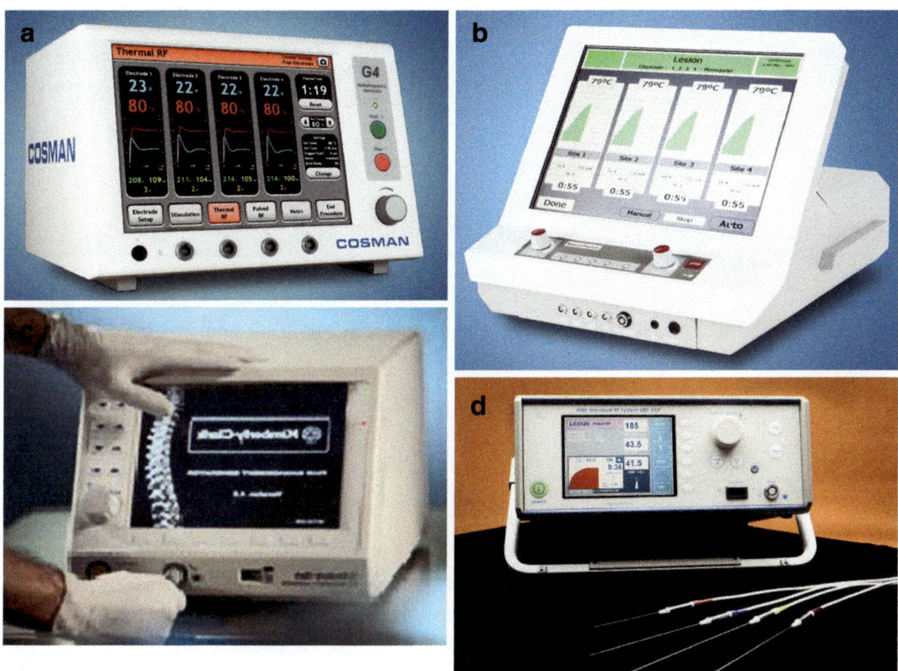

Fig. 3.17 RF Generators (a) The Cosman G4 four-electrode RF generator (b) NeuroTherm NT2000 RF lesion generator (c) Kimberly-Clark Pain Management System (d) Diros OWL URF-3AP Multi-Lesion

contact with a large metallic implant. Impedance can also be of use in certain procedures since it can indicate the tissue type in which the cannula's tip is positioned. For example, during a percutaneous cordotomy, the impedance will be 400 Ω when the tip is in the extradural tissues, fall to 200 Ω as the needle tip enters the CSF, and then rise to over 800 Ω as the needle tip enters the spinal cord. When working in the intervertebral disc, the impedance is usually very high in the outer annulus, falling to less than 200 Ω in the nucleus pulposus.

For facet denervations, some physicians use "pole needles." These are non-temperature-monitoring, tissue-piercing electrodes with integrated, flexible, fluid injection lines. They are used when it is felt that the electrode position must not be perturbed through stimulation, injection, and lesioning. Typically, 20 V is applied with the expectation of producing an 80 °C heat lesion. However, in vivo clinical experiment shows that the tip temperature is not consistently 80 °C but rather can range from values less than 80 °C to those exceeding boiling (Buijs et al. 2004; Gultuna et al. 2011). As such, when pole needles are used, one should halt RF delivery if an impedance rise is observed that indicates tissue boiling; and when precise lesion control is required, one should use temperature-monitoring injection electrodes.

Four standard radiofrequency lesion generators in common use around the world are shown in Fig. 3.17.

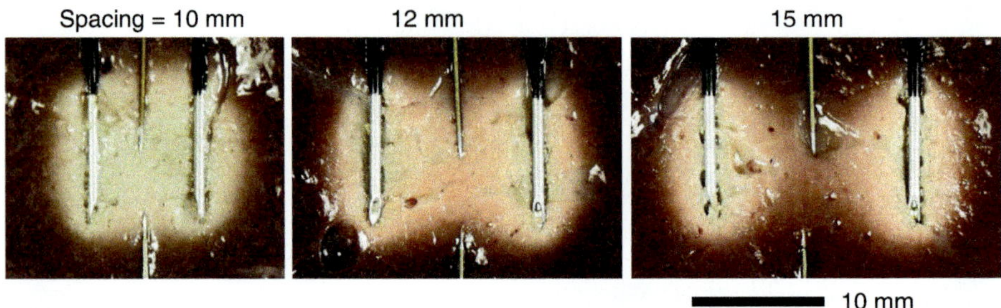

Fig. 3.18 Bipolar lesion size for 20 gauge, 10 mm tip length, 90 °C, 3 min, and increasing spacing: strip $12 \times 15 \times 8$ mm^3 (*left*), strip $10 \times 17 \times 5$ mm^3 (*middle*), and two Ellipsoids $12 \times 7 \times 7$ mm^3 (*right*)

Bipolar Thermal RF

Whereas a monopolar configuration drives RF current between an electrode's exposed tip and a distant ground pad, a bipolar configuration drives RF current between two nearby electrode tips. As bipolar electrode tips are brought closer together, the resulting thermal lesion shape transitions from that of two volumes surrounding each tip separately to that of a single volume connecting the tips (Fig. 3.18). The connected geometry and larger total lesion volume are strongly influenced by a focusing of the electric and current density fields between closely spaced electrode tips. Bipolar electrodes can be arranged collinearly or in parallel, but parallel arrangements produce the largest lesion size increases (Cosman et al. 1984). Important features of parallel bipolar heat lesions include:

- *Large*: Bipolar RF lesions are larger than cooled RF lesions as used in pain management (Figs. 3.19 and 3.20, *left*). The size of one bipolar RF lesion is roughly that of three conventional monopolar RF lesions placed side by side (Fig. 3.20, *right*).
- *Conformal*: Bipolar RF applied to closely spaced electrode tips produces heat lesions shaped like a rounded brick, also known as a "strip lesion." To conform to anatomical constraints, the width and length of the strip can be adjusted nearly independently of each other and the lesion depth (Fig. 3.18). As such, a large lesion can be produced without unnecessary damage to healthy tissue and with reduced risk to sensitive structures. This is not possible for monopolar lesions around a cylindrical electrode since the lesion width and depth are the same.
- *Connected strip lesions*: By leapfrogging electrodes (Ferrante et al. 2001), brick-like strip lesions can be placed side by side without gaps to produce an elongated lesion zone that has consistent height and thickness (Figs. 3.20, *middle*; 3.21). This is not possible for cooled and conventional monopolar RF without positioning electrodes very close together.
- *Robust*: Strip lesions can be generated reliably for parallel tip spacings of 10 mm, tip temperature 90 °C, and lesion time 3 min. Perturbations of these geometric and RF parameters do not substantially affect lesion size (Cosman and Gonzalez

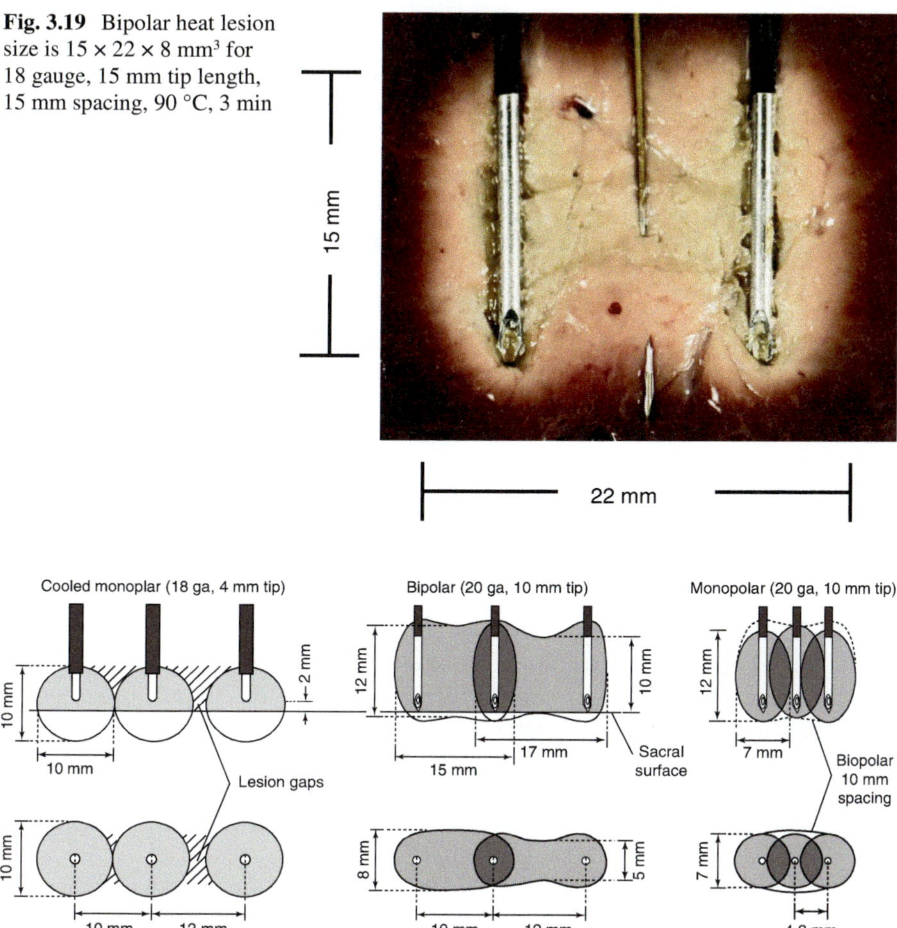

Fig. 3.19 Bipolar heat lesion size is $15 \times 22 \times 8$ mm^3 for 18 gauge, 15 mm tip length, 15 mm spacing, 90 °C, 3 min

Fig. 3.20 Comparison of bipolar RF lesion size with that of cooled and conventional monopolar RF

2011; Fig. 3.18). The tip temperature and lesion time used for bipolar RF are greater than those used for monopolar RF since it is desired that larger heat lesions are formed.

As an example, all these features are illustrated by the RF palisade approach to sacroiliac joint (SIJ) denervation (Fig. 3.21). In this approach, four to five large bipolar RF lesions are placed side by side like bricks in wall to traverse the region between the dorsal sacral foramina and SIJ line in which sacral lateral branch nerves form the SIJ's dorsal innervation. While each lesion is large in the inferior-superior direction, its depth is constrained in the left-right direction, thus reducing the risk of damage to the sacral nerve roots. Because lesion size is robust to variations in tip spacing and because adjacent lesions overlap, the total lesion zone has a consistent thickness and height from the sacral surface.

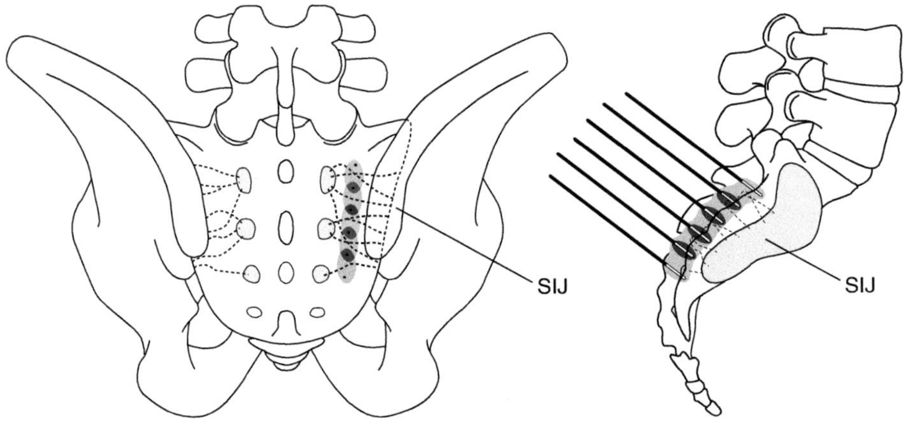

Fig. 3.21 Palisade sacroiliac joint denervation

Bipolar RF lesions of the sizes shown in Fig. 3.18 have been used success-fully in pain management (Ferrante et al. 2001; Burnham et al. 2007; Cosman and Gonzalez 2011). Ex vivo experiments by Cosman and Gonzalez (2011) document further flexibility in the size and shape of bipolar lesions. Indeed, bipolar lesions with dimensions exceeding 2 cm can be readily created with standard RF equipment. As for all RF lesioning, before the clinical use of novel bipolar configurations, a physician must consult lesion-size studies to determine whether that configuration is appropriate for the target anatomy. The proximity of target nerves to nontarget nerves, blood vessels, skin surface, and other sensi-tive structures imposes an upper bound on the safe size of any heat lesion, espe-cially in the spine.

Monopolar Pulsed RF

While making a radiofrequency lesion in the standard thermal RF mode, the tissue which surrounds the tip of the electrode is exposed to a concentrated electric field that induces tissue heating (Fig. 3.12). The electric field (E-field) intensity decreases precipitously with distance from the tip, falling to a low level at distances beyond the extent of a typical heat lesion (Cosman and Cosman 2005). Since the high tem-peratures within the heat lesion volume reliably induce cellular death, it is assumed that the E-field per se has little or no clinical effect in thermal RF.

The introduction of pulsed RF (Sluijter et al. 1998) was motivated by the desire to expose nerves to high electric fields without gross neurodestructive heating, so as to reduce the risk of RF treatment in sensitive anatomy such as the DRG. In the mid-1990s, Cosman and Sluijter modified a standard lesion generator to deliver radiofre-quency voltage bursts at a repetition rate of 2 Hz. Since each burst is only 20 ms long, the intervening inactive period 480 ms allows heat to dissipate into the sur-rounding tissue after exposure to the electric field (Figs. 3.22 and 3.23). As such, the

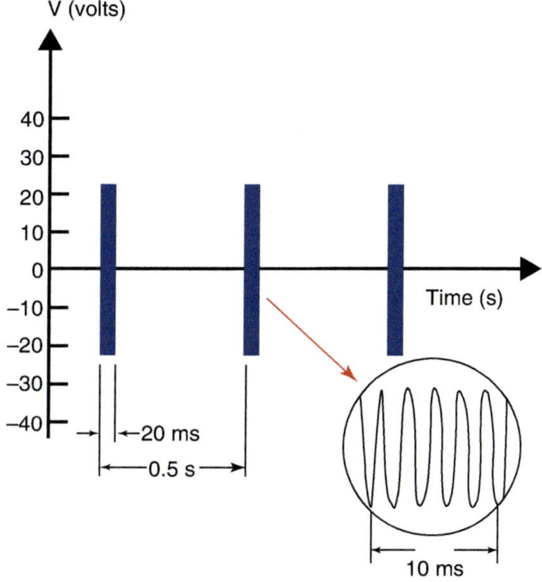

Fig. 3.22 Pulsed RF. *Red arrow* indicates the target point for detect L5 medial branch.

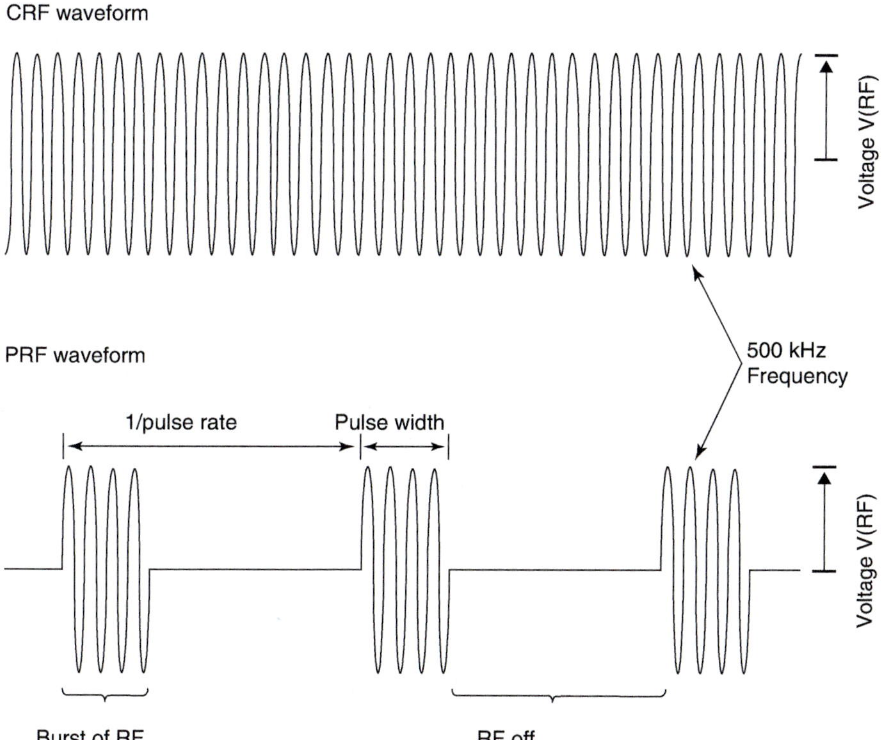

Fig. 3.23 Schematic RF waveforms for CRF and PRF (parameters and times not to scale)

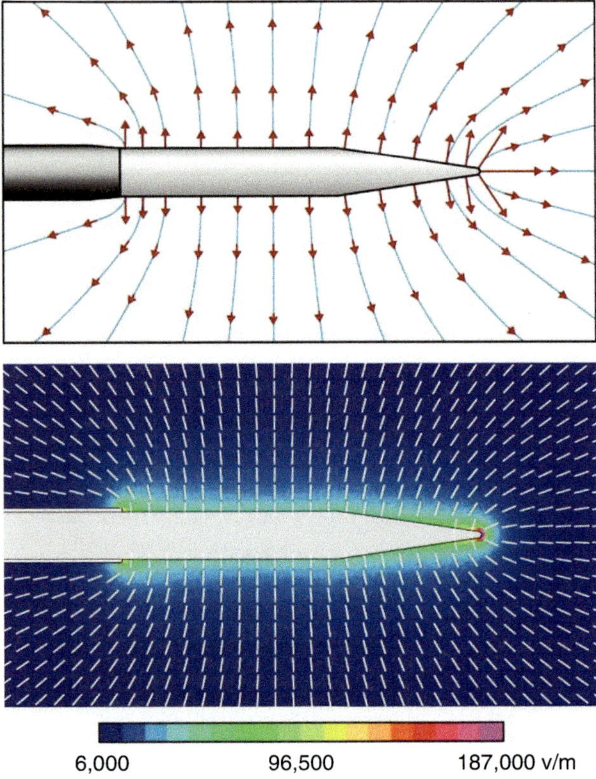

Fig. 3.24 (*Top*) schematic E-field patterns. (*Bottom*) E calculated in tissue for a 22~ electrode at V(RF)=45 V

RF voltage, and thus the E-field strength, can be increased while holding the electrode tip temperature at or below 42 °C, a level assumed not to produce gross neurodestructive effects (Fig. 3.24). Cosman and Cosman (2005) have shown that tissue around the electrode shaft is broadly exposed to high-intensity E-fields without substantial heating. They also showed that the very intense electric fields at electrode's pointed tip cause "hot flashes" during each RF burst. The full details of this physical geometry is given later on in this book, but some salient points are:

- Ahead of the tip: Within ≈0.2 mm of the electrode point, temperature spikes into the neurolytic range and above the measured tip temperature during each burst of RF (Fig. 3.25). At larger distances and between RF bursts, the temperature does not substantially exceed that of the electrode tip. While the electric field is maximal within ≈0.2 mm of the electrode point, it falls off very quickly with distance ahead of the tip so that beyond ≈0.2 mm, its magnitude is smaller ahead of the tip than it is lateral to the shaft (Fig. 3.26).
- Around the shaft: Temperature does not substantially exceed the measured tip temperature. The electric field falls off slowly with distance and exposes tissue to electrical forces that are high in biological terms and that appear to produce a

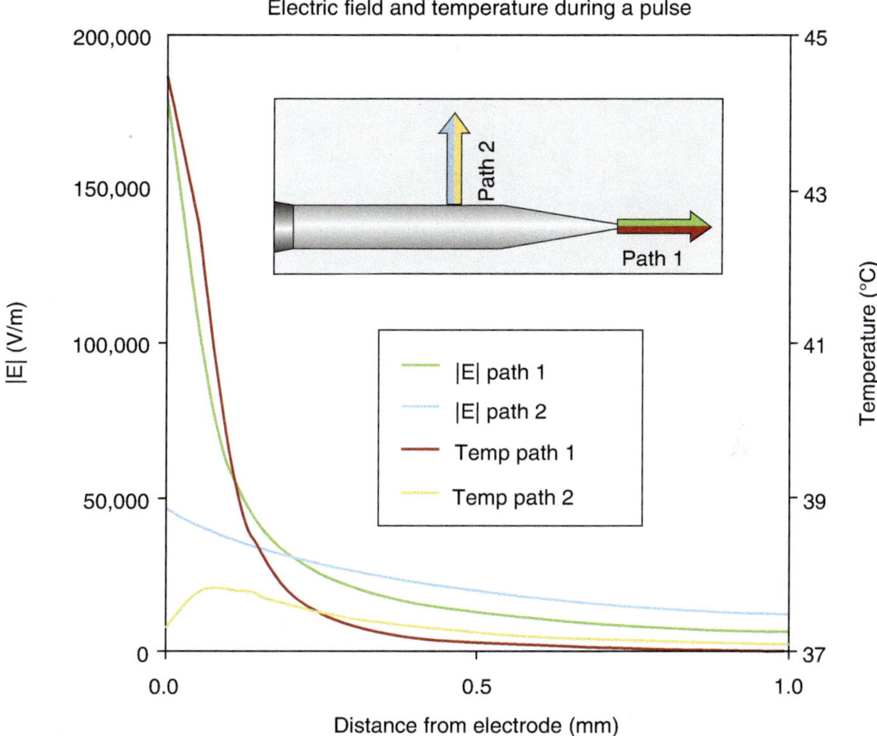

Fig. 3.25 E-smd T-fields during the first PRF pulse for V(RF)=45 V and pulse width=20 ms

disruptive effect (Erdine et al. 2009); as such, its range of influence is broader around the shaft than ahead of the tip (Figs. 3.26 and 3.27).

In typical pulsed RF practice, the generator is set to target pulse voltage=45 V, pulse width=20 ms, and pulse rate=2 Hz. The generator then automatically adjusts the either the pulse voltage, the pulse width, or less commonly the pulse rate to maintain the temperature at or below 42 °C for 120 s. Sluijter (personal communication, 1998) further recommends that the tissue impedance be reduced by the injection of about 1 ml of local anesthetic or normal saline. This is an approach supported by finite-element calculations of the electric field that assume directional saline spread toward the nerve (Cosman and Cosman 2005a). Dr. Bill Cohen (personal communication, 1998) also advocates saline injection and has observed the spread of fluid injection toward the nerve using X-ray contrast.

The clinical effects and pain-relief mechanism of pulsed RF is the subject of ongoing scientific investigation. Though there is growing evidence that pulsed RF has a physical effect on nerves (see Cahana et al. later on in this book), in the absence of an established model of PRF's pain-relief mechanism, what is known about pulsed RF's pain-relief efficacy depends on clinical trials using specific

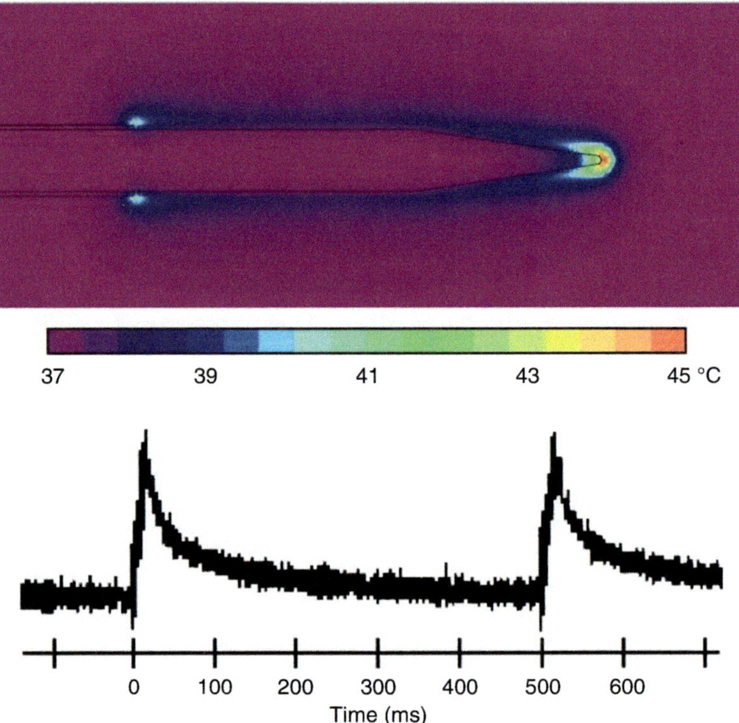

Fig. 3.26 Hot flashes during a PRF pulse

parameters and control algorithms. Since the first publication about the clinical use of pulsed RF in pain management, numerous peer-reviewed clinical studies of pulsed RF technique and pain-relief outcomes have been published, including an RCT related to PRF treatment of cervical radicular pain (Van Zundert et al. 2007). While treatment parameters vary somewhat, these published clinical trials generally use set values voltage=45 V, pulse width=20 ms, pulse rate=2 Hz, and treatment time=120 s, and they all use delivery algorithms that vary either the pulse voltage or the pulse width to maintain the temperature at or below 42 °C. Beyond this, a number of questions about pulsed RF methodology remain unanswered:

Is it better to approach a nerve "side-on" or "point-on" with a PRF electrode?

Many clinicians prefer to use the point-on/perpendicular approach as they feel this allow for more precise targeting, with greater electric field effect. While this may be valid, since the E-field is very large only within a very small distance ahead of the electrode point (≈0.2 mm), and otherwise falls to intensities less than those around the electrode shaft, it is unlikely that the very large E-field at the electrode point accounts for the full clinical effect. Further, since the E-field at the point has destructive intensity and is coincident with high-temperature hot flashes, the point-on approach cannot be having a purely nondestructive effect. On the other hand, since the E-field intensity

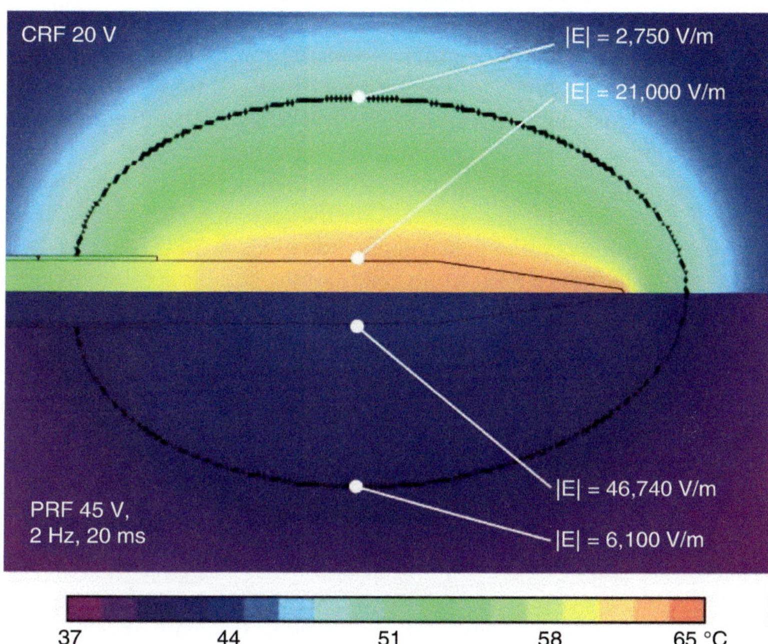

Fig. 3.27 E-fields dominate over T-fields in PRF. The opposite is true for CRF

declines less precipitously lateral to the electrode shaft, the side-on/parallel approach exposes a larger nerve volume to elevated electric fields, with less heating. Recent animal studies by Erdine et al. (2009) show that the side-on approach can disrupt axonal microtubules, microfilaments, and mitochondria. Clinical trials are required to determine the relative efficacy of the side-on and point-on methods.

Can clinical outcomes be improved by changing the typical set values?

Voltage = 45 V, pulse width = 20 ms, pulse rate = 2 Hz, and treatment time = 120 s? These parameters were selected for practical purposes by PRF's inventors, and there is no clinical evidence that they are "ideal" in any sense. Many workers use longer treatment times in excess of 4 min, or pulse width = 10 ms and pulse rate = 4 Hz, as they feel it augments the electric field exposure, also known as E-dose (Cosman and Cosman 2005). While these variations may prove useful, there is currently no clinical proof that any such variations improve outcomes.

Do clinical outcome vary depending on the temperature control algorithm?

Modern RF generators (Fig. 3.17) implicitly incorporate at least one method of PRF temperature control that varies either pulse voltage, pulse width, or pulse rate, while fixing the other parameters. For example, the NeuroTherm NT 1100 generator's promotional literature refers to its particular pulse-rate algorithm by the trade name pulse dose. The Cosman G4 generator incorporates an E-dose setting that allows the operator to select between control algorithms to adjust a nerve's exposure to the E-field. While all clinical studies showing positive PRF outcomes to date employ generators that vary either the voltage or the pulse width to control temperature, they do not compare these control methods. The authors are not aware of any clinical study of PRF outcomes in which temperature is controlled by varying the pulse rate or using pulse dose. There is theoretical reason to believe that pulse-rate/pulse-dose algorithms may be less effective if PRF's mechanism depends on long-term depression (LTD). The LTD hypothesis of PRF pain relief was proposed by Cosman and Cosman (2005) and is based on the idea that PRF stimulates action potentials and thus subthreshold postsynaptic potentials at 2 Hz, which falls within a rate range known to induce LTD using conditioning stimulation (Sandkuler 1997; Bear 2003). Since a pulse-rate/pulse-dose algorithm may reduce the pulse rate substantially below the known LTD range, it may also reduce the LTD effect. Voltage and pulse-width control algorithms do not suffer from this concern. Nevertheless, in the absence of strong model of PRF's mode of action or clinical trials, PRF temperature control algorithms cannot be clinically distinguished.

Section 2

Dr. Eric R. Cosman, Jr., MEng, PhD and Prof. Eric R. Cosman, Sr., PhD

There are two output modes of RF generators that are used today to produce pain relief. The first is the standard, thermal RF mode which uses a continuous sinusoidal waveform RF output, commonly referred to as continuous RF or CRF. The second uses a series of pulsed bursts of RF signal, referred to as pulsed RF or PRF. The amplitude, V(RF), of both these waveforms is measured in units of voltage (V). For voltages commonly used in clinical practice, a continuous RF waveform produces a heat lesion. This means that the neural tissue near the uninsulated, metal electrode tip is heated continuously to destructive temperatures (greater than 45–50 °C) by ionic friction of the RF currents in the tissue. Thus, the CRF lesion volume includes all tissue within the 45–50 °C isotherm boundary, which tends to have an ellipsoidal shape that encompasses the electrode tip. Within this lesion volume, all cell structures are macroscopically destroyed by heat. The action of pulsed RF on neural tissue is different. Because the RF output is delivered in bursts of short duration relative to the intervening quiescent periods, the average temperature of the tissue near the electrode is not raised continuously or as high as for continuous RF at the same RF voltage. Since the PRF voltage is typically regulated to keep the average tip temperature in a nondestructive range, other mechanisms produce the clinically observed pain-relieving effects.

The electric field, E, is the fundamental physical quantity that governs all the actions of RF output on neural tissue, both for pulsed RF and for continuous RF modes. The electric field is created in space around an RF electrode that is connected to the output voltage V(RF) from an RF generator (Fig. 3.13). E is represented by an arrow (vector) at every point in space around the electrode tip, indicative of the magnitude and the direction the force it will produce on charged structures and ions in the tissue. The E-lines indicate the pattern of E in a homogeneous medium. The E-field produces various effects on tissue including oscillations of charges, ionic currents, charge polarizations, membrane voltages, and structure-modifying forces. For continuous RF mode, the dominant consequence of these effects is the production of heat in the tissue caused by frictional energy loss due to the ionic currents that are driven by the E-field. However, for pulsed RF, the effects of E-field are more complex and varied and range from heat flashes, to modification of neuron ultrastructure, to neural excitation phenomena. All of these effects can play a role in neuronal modification, though exactly how they produce antinociception in PRF treatments is an area of active scientific investigation.

To understand any of the E-field effects of pulsed RF, the magnitude of the E-field around an actual electrode in tissue must be determined. This has been calculated for a typical electrode during a PRF pulse (Figs. 3.13, 3.23, and 3.25) using finite-element computational methods (Cosman and Cosman). The quantitative values of E and temperature T at distances from the electrode tip are plotted in (Fig. 7c) for a 22 Ga electrode at V(RF) = 45 V. Near the sharp point of the electrode, the E-field has strength of up to 187,000 V/m. This drops off rapidly with distance from the point. At the side of the electrode, E is 46,740 V/m and drops off more slowly with lateral distance. These are very high E-fields in biological terms and are capable of a variety of modifications of neurons that account for the effects of pulsed RF.

Two consequences of these predictions are supported by experimental and clinical observations. The first is that, as a consequence of the very high E-fields at the electrode tip, there are hot flashes at the electrode tip that can be thermally destructive to neurons. The second is that there are significant nonthermal effects of the E-field on neurons at positions away from the point of the tip that are certainly related to the pain-relieving effects of PRF.

During the brief RF pulse, a hot spot occurs at the tip which can be 15–20 °C above the average tissue temperature of the tissue that remains near body temperature of 37–42 °C. This has been confirmed by ex vivo measurements and finite-element calculations. The intense E-field and hot flashes could be expected to have destructive effects on neural tissue very near the tip point. Evidence for such destruction has been observed in vitro (Cahana et al.). This may play a role in PRF's clinical effect when electrode point is in the nerve or pressing against the nerve. However, it is unlikely that such focal effects can account for all of PRF pain relief, since the region of extremely high E-fields and T hot flashes are likely confined to less than about 0.2 mm radius from the electrode point.

There is evidence that direct, nonthermal effects are important in PRF. It is known that pain relief can be achieved when the side of the electrode tip, not the tip point, is next to an axon or DRG. While the hot flash fluctuations are less than 1 °C at 0.5 mm from the tip in any direction for typical PRF voltages, at lateral distances of greater than 1 mm, the magnitude of the electric field is still large in biological terms. For example, finite-element computation of the E-field for V(RF) = 45 V predict that the E is 20,000 V/m at 0.5 mm and 12,000 V/m at 1.0 mm laterally. Thus, neuronal modifications in this E-field range should be significant.

Comparison of E and T strengths between typical CRF and PRF waveforms shows striking differences between these RF modes (Fig. 7e). Calculations predict that after 60 s of CRF at V(RF) = 20 V, $E = 21{,}000$ V/m and $T = 60\text{--}65$ °C at the lateral tip surface and $E = 2{,}750$ V/m and $T = 50$ °C at 1.8 mm away. In contrast, after 60 s of PRF with V(RF) = 45 V, $E = 46{,}740$ V/m and $T = 42$ °C at the lateral tip surface and $E = 6{,}100$ V/m and $T = 38$ °C at 1.8 mm away. In other words, in PRF, the direct electric field effects are more prominent, whereas in CRF, the thermal fields are more prominent and largely mask the E-field effects.

Combined with the understanding that PRF has a clinical effect even when the electrode is not placed on the nerve directly, these physical observations suggest that the E-field is directly involved in the analgesic effect of PRF. It is known that PRF E-fields produce significant transmembrane potentials on the neuron membrane and organelles (Cosman and Cosman 2005). The E-field can also penetrate the membranes of axon and the DRG soma to disrupt essential cellular substructures and functions. For example, PRF applied to the DRG of rabbits causes pronounced neuron ultrastructural modifications that are seen only under electron microscopy (Erdine et al. 2005) and that are likely to modify or disable the cell's function. Additionally, PRF applied to afferent axons in the rat sciatic nerve with a "parallel"/"side-on" approach causes disruption of microtubules, microfilaments, and mitochondria; the disruption appears to be more pronounced in C fibers than in A-delta and A-beta fibers (Erdine et al. 2009). This would suggest that PRF can produce subcellular, microscopic lesions on neurons in a volume around the electrode, possibly resulting in reduction of afferent pain signals. Blockage of axonal transmission of action potentials has been observed in the sural and sciatic nerves of rats using electrophysiological microelectrode recording on individual teased nerve fibers (Cosman et al. 2009); the blockage occurs at lower voltages for a "perpendicular"/"point-on" approach than it does for a "parallel"/"side-on" approach, likely due to the very high E-field and hot flashes present at the electrode's pointed tip. PRF membrane potentials are also capable of neural excitations (action potentials) by a process called membrane rectification. This excitation has been observed in the sural and sciatic nerves of rats using the aforementioned teased-fiber recording technique (Cosman et al. 2009). Because the PRF pulse rate is similar to that of classical conditioning stimulation (1–2 Hz), it has been proposed that PRF may have a similar action (Cosman and Cosman 2005). Conditioning stimulation is capable of suppressing synaptic efficiency of A-delta and C-fiber afferent nociception signals (Sandkuhler), a phenomenon known as long-term depression (LTD). Therefore, the PRF might be reducing transmission of pain information by LTD of synaptic connections in the dorsal horn. The appropriate exposure of PRF for a given pain syndrome and anatomical target, for either microscopic or LTD mechanisms, should be governed by the PRF "E-dose" (Cosman and Cosman 2005). E-dose provides a parametric measure of E-field strength and integral pulse/time exposure.

Section 3

Prof. A. Cahana, MD, DAAPM, FIPP; Prof. Philippe Richebé, MD, PhD; and Dr Cyril Rivat, PhD

Cosman and Cosman (2005) have shown that pulsed RF (PRF) exposes tissue to higher electric field (E-field) intensities than does continuous/thermal RF (CRF), as illustrated in Fig. 7e. For a CRF heat lesion with tip temperature 65 °C, the E-field strength is 21,000 V/m around the needle, as compared to 46,740 V/m for a PRF lesion with tip temperature 42 °C. At a lateral distance from the shaft roughly coincident with the outer limit of the CRF heat lesion, the CRF E-field strength is 2,700 V/m, whereas the PRF E-field strength is 6,100 V/m. Furthermore, since PRF produces lower temperatures around the shaft, the tissue that would be exposed to neurolytic temperatures in the CRF case is principally exposed to high E-fields in the PRF case. As described earlier, the E-field strength is highest within ≈ 0.2 mm of the pointed needle tip; transient, focal, high-temperature spikes are also present during each RF pulse at this location. On the other hand, since the E-field intensity decreases less precipitously around the shaft than ahead of the tip, it has a higher intensity over a larger range around the shaft than it does directly ahead of the tip.

In the light of all the recent work on pulsed radiofrequency, many workers prefer to use the needle tip ("perpendicular approach") as they feel that this approach allows for more precise targeting. They feel that use of the needle tip combines a reduced heat effect with a greater electric force effect and therefore carries with it a theoretically reduced risk of neuritis than would use of the needle shaft. There is, however, no scientific evidence for this hypothesis!

Sluijter describes four phases in a pulsed radiofrequency procedure, viz.:

- A stunning phase, which provides immediate relief.
- A phase of postprocedure discomfort, which may last for up to 3 weeks.
- A phase of beneficial clinical effect, which is of variable duration.
- A phase of recurrence of pain; we are still in the early days but many cases record 4–24 months of relief.

There is no clinical evidence of any nerve damage with pulsed radiofrequency. Higuchi et al. (2002) have presented experimental evidence that pulsed radiofrequency applied to the rat cervical dorsal root ganglion causes upregulation of the immediate early gene c-fos [4].

With the technological improvements made during the last decade, cellular and ultrastructural effects of PRF and RF have been better evaluated.

Pulsed radiofrequency does seem to have a clinical effect on peripheral nerves. Hamann (2003) pointing out the lack of laboratory evidence for this phenomenon felt that this may be due to changes induced in the function of the Schwann cells [5]. Cahana et al. (2003) have shown that pulsed radiofrequency affects cell cultures only within a range of 1 mm, raising questions as to how close to the target tissue one needs to be with the electrode [6].

Podhajsky et al. (2005) compared histologic effects of CRF, PRF, and continuous heat at 42 °C on DRG and sciatic nerves 2, 7, and 21 days after procedure. PRF did not induce any paralysis or sensory deficits in animals. Only mild edema and some fibroblast activation (collagen deposition in epineural space and subperineural region) around nerve fibers were seen in the PRF group at 2 and 7 days after procedure in sciatic nerve and DRG. At 21 days after PRF, these mild changes were back to normal. RF group showed extensive edema, swollen axons and degeneration of neurons [7]. Erdine et al. (2005) reported an animal study showing PRF induced in DRG neurons only, an enlargement of endoplasmic reticulum, and a mild increase of vacuoles. RF showed at the same level mitochondria degeneration, loss of integrity of nuclear membrane, and highly increased number of vacuoles in the DRG cells [8]. These two studies led to the conclusion PRF does not appear to rely on thermal injury to achieve its clinical effect.

One year later, Hamann et al. (2006) applied pulsed radiofrequency to the sciatic nerve or the L5 dorsal root ganglion in the rat. They studied, at up to 14 days after application, the expression of activating transmission factor 3 (ATF3), an early intermediate gene expressed in response to cell stress. They found that ATF3 was upregulated selectively in the small cells of the dorsal root ganglion after direct application to the ganglion but not after application to the sciatic cells. They concluded that pulsed radiofrequency selectively stresses the population containing the nociceptor cell bodies. It would also appear that the primary effect of pulsed radiofrequency is predominantly on the cell body rather than on its processes. The observation that PRF targets preferentially neurons whose axons are composed of small diameters (A-delta and C fibers) was also reported by in this study [9].

It is only in 2009 that publication started reporting more precise neuronal modulation at the ultrastructural level after PRF. Tun et al. (2009) confirmed by ultrastructural approach that CRF (70 °C), as opposed to PRF (42 °C, 120 s), was responsible for much more neurodestruction in the sciatic nerve [10]. Erdine et al. (2009) published interesting results on electronic microscopy of sensory nociceptive axons showing physical evidence of ultrastructural damage following PRF. The mitochondria, microtubules, and microfilaments showed various degrees of damage and disruption. These damages were more important in C fibers than A-delta than A-beta fibers. This observation was consistent with the clinical effect of PRF which seems to have greater effects on the smaller pain-carrying C- and A-delta fibers [11]. Protasoni et al. (2009) also reported some mild effects of PRF on DRGs at the acute phase of exposure. At light microscopy (LM) few differences appeared after PRF, but at transmission electron microscopy (TEM), myelinated axons appeared delaminated and the organization in bundles was lost. Also, T gangliar cells contained abnormal smooth reticulum with enlarged cisternae and numerous vacuoles. As a conclusion authors said PRF slightly damages myelin envelops of nerve fibers at acute stage. No information came out of this study on long-term effect to know whether or not these effects were persistent or just transient [12].

Pulsed radiofrequency may be useful where conventional RF is contraindicated, e.g., neuropathic pain, and it is safe in locations where conventional RF may be potentially hazardous, e.g., DRG lesioning.

PRF is mostly a neuro-remodelling technique based on neuromodulation as opposed to RF which is mainly based on neurodegeneration to reach its clinical effects.

PRF is virtually painless as no heat is generated.

References

Lumbar Facet Denervation

1. Schwarzer AC, Wang SC, Bogduk N, et al. Prevalence and clinical features of lumbar zygapophysial joint pain: a study in an Australian population with chronic low back pain. Ann Rheum Dis. 1995;54:100–6. doi:10.1.136/ard.54.2.100.
2. Wilde VE, Ford JJ, McMeeken JM. Indicators of lumbar zygapophyseal joint pain: survey of an expert panel with the Delphi technique. Phys Ther. 2007;87:1348–61. doi:10.2522/ptj.20060329.
3. Van Zundert J, Vanelderen P, Kessels A, van Kleef M. Radiofrequency treatment of facet-related pain: evidence and controversies. Curr Pain Headache Rep. 2012;16(1):19–25. doi:10.1007/si 1916-011-0237-8. Published online 18 Nov 2011. PMCID: PMC3258411.
4. Cohen SP, Huang JHY, Brummett C. Facet joint pain-advances in patient selection and treatment. Nat Rev Rheumatol. 2013;9(2):101–16. doi:10.1038/nrrheum.2012.198. Advance on lime publication; 20/11/12.
5. van Kleef M, Vanelderen P, Cohen SP, et al. 12. Pain originating from the lumbar facet joints. Pain Pract. 2010;10(5):459–69. The evidence rating used is a system that considers the potential burden and benefit of the treatment.

Physics: Section 1

6. Cosman Jr ER, Cosman Sr ER. Electric and thermal field effects in tissue around radiofrequency electrodes. Pain Med. 2005;6(6):405–24.
7. Sweet WM, Mark VH. Unipolar anodal electrolyte lesions in the brain of man and cat: report of five human cases with electrically produced bulbar or mesencephalic tractotomies. Arch Neurol Psychiatry. 1953;70:224–34.
8. Cosman BJ, Cosman Sr ER. Guide to radio frequency lesion generation in neurosurgery. Burlington: Radionics; 1974.
9. Cosman Sr ER, Cosman BJ. Methods of making nervous system lesions. In: Wilkins RH, Rengachary SS, editors. Neurosurgery. New York: McGraw-Hill; 1984. p. 2490–9.
10. Cosman ER, Rittman WJ, Nashold BS, Makachinas TT. Radiofrequency lesion generation and its effect on tissue impedance. Appl Neurophysiol. 1988;51:230–42.
11. Sluijter ME, Cosman ER, Rittman WJ, Van Kleef M. The effects of pulsed radiofrequency fields applied to the dorsal root ganglion – a preliminary report. Pain Clin. 1998;11(2):109–18.
12. Ferrante FM, King LF, Roche EA, et al. Radiofrequency sacroiliac joint denervation for sacroiliac syndrome. Reg Anesth Pain Med. 2001;26:137–42.
13. Burnham RS, Yasui Y. An alternate method of radiofrequency neurotomy of the sacroiliac joint: a pilot study of the effect on pain, function, and satisfaction. Reg Anesth Pain Med. 2007;32:12–9.
14. Cosman Jr ER, Gonzalez CD. Bipolar radiofrequency lesion geometry: implications for palisade treatment of sacroiliac joint pain. Pain Pract. 2011;11(1):3–22.

15. Ruiz-Lopez R. Treatment of carpal tunnel syndrome with pulsed radiofrequency. In: Lecture at the invasive procedures in motion conference. Swiss Paraplegic Center, Nottwil; 18–19 Jan 2008.
16. Cosman ER Sr, Cosman ER Jr. RF Electric fields and the distribution of heat in tissue. In: Lecture at the international radiofrequency symposium honoring the 70th birthday of Prof. Menno Sluijter: radiofrequency today. Nottwil; 18–19 Oct 2003.
17. Cosman ER Jr. Physics of radiofrequency. In: Presented at the 15th annual advanced interventional pain conference and practical workshop, and the 17th World Institute of Pain FIPP Examination. Budapest; 31 Aug 2010.
18. Wright RF, Wolfson LF, DiMuro JM, Peragine JM, Bainbridge SA. In vivo temperature measurement during neurotomy for SIJ pain using the Baylis SInergy probe. In: Proceedings of the international spine intervention society 15th annual scientific meeting; Budapest, Hungary. 2007. p. 82–4.
19. Brodkey JS, Miyazaki Y, Ervin FR, Mark VH. Reversible heat lesions with radiofrequency current: a method of stereotactic localization. J Neurosurg. 1964;21:49–53.
20. Dieckmann G, Gabriel E, Hassler R. Size, form, and structural peculiarities of experimental brain lesions obtained by thermocontrolled radiofrequency. Confin Neurol. 1965;26:134–42.
21. Smith HP, McWhorter JM, Challa VR. Radiofrequency neurolysis in a clinical model. Neuropathological correlation. J Neurosurg. 1981;55:246–53.
22. Cosman ER Sr, Cosman ER Jr, Bove G. Blockage of axonal transmission by pulsed radiofrequency fields. In: Proceedings of the society of neuroscience conference. Chicago; 17–21 Oct 2009.
23. Abou-Sherif S, Hamann W, Hall S. Pulsed radiofrequency applied to dorsal root ganglia causes selective increase in ATF-3 in small neurons. In: Proceedings of the peripheral nerve society meeting. Banff; 26–30 July 2003.
24. Buijs EJ, van Wijk RM, Geurts JW, Weeseman RR, Stolker RJ, Groen GG. Radiofrequency lumbar facet denervation: a comparative study of the reproducibility of lesion size after 2 current radiofrequency techniques. Reg Anesth Pain Med. 2004;29(5):400–7.
25. Gultuna I, Aukes H, van Gorp EJ, Cosman ER Jr. Limitations of voltage-controlled radiofrequency and non-temperature-measuring injection electrodes. Submitted for publication; 2011.
26. Cosman Sr ER, Nashold BS, Ovelman-Levitt J. Theoretical aspects of radiofrequency lesions in the dorsal root entry zone. Neurosurgery. 1984;15:945–50.
27. Erdine S, Bilir A, Cosman ER, Cosman ER. Ultrastructural changes in axons following exposure to pulsed radiofrequency fields. Pain Pract. 2009;9(6):407–17.
28. Cosman ER Sr, Cosman ER Jr. RF Electric fields and the distribution of heat in tissue. In: Lecture at the 2nd international symposium on interventional treatment of pain. Swiss Paraplegic Center, Nottwil; 14–15 Jan 2005.
29. Van Zundert J, Patijn J, Kessels A, Lamé I, van Suijlekom H, van Kleef M. Pulsed radiofrequency adjacent to the cervical dorsal root ganglion in chronic cervical radicular pain: a double blind sham controlled randomized clinical trial. Pain. 2007;127(1–2):173–82.
30. Sandkühler J, Chen JG, Cheng G, Randic M. Low frequency stimulation of afferent Aδ-fibers induces long-term depression at primary afferent synapses with substantia gelatinosa neurons in the rat. J Neurosci. 1997;17:6483–91.
31. Bear MF. Bidirectional synaptic plasticity: from theory to reality. Philos Trans R Soc Lond B Biol Sci. 2003;358:649–55.

Physics: Section 2

32. Cosman Jr ER, Cosman Sr ER. Electric and thermal field effects in tissue around radiofrequency electrodes. Pain Med. 2005;6(6):405–24.
33. Cahana A, Vutskits L, Muller D. Acute differential modification of synaptic transmission and cell survival during exposure target position pulsed and continuous radiofrequency energy. J Pain. 2003;4(4):197–202.
34. Erdine S, Yucel A, Cunan A, et al. Effects of pulsed versus conventional radiofrequency current in rabbit dorsal root ganglion morphology. Eur J Pain. 2005;9(3):251–6.

35. Sandkuhler J, Chen JG, Cheng G, Randic M. Low frequency stimulation of the afferent A-delta fibers induces long-term depression at the primary afferent synapses with substantia gelatinosa neurons in the rat. J Neurosci. 1997;17:6483–91.
36. Erdine S, Bilir A, Cosman Sr ER, Cosman Jr ER. Ultrastructural changes in axons following exposure to pulsed radiofrequency fields. Pain Pract. 2009;9(6):407–17.
37. Cosman ER Sr, Cosman ER Jr, Bove G. Blockage of axonal transmission by pulsed radiofrequency fields. In: Proceedings of the society of neuroscience conference. Chicago; 17–21 Oct 2009.

Physics: Section 3

38. Abou-Sherif S, Hamann W, Hall S. Traumatic injury in the PNS induces increased numbers of endoneural mast cells. In: Abstracts 10th world convention on pain. IASP Press. pp 290–1. see also Hamann W, Hall S. RF-lesions in anaesthetized rats. Br J Anaesth. 1992;68:443.
39. Sluijter M, et al. The effects of pulsed radiofrequency fields applied to the dorsal root ganglion – a preliminary report. Pain Clin. 1998;II(2):109–17.
40. Cosman Jr ER, Cosman Sr ER. Electric and thermal field effects in tissue around radiofrequency electrodes. Pain Med. 2005;6(6):405–24.
41. Higuchi Y, Nashold BS, Sluijter M, Cosman E, Pearlstein R. Exposure of the dorsal root ganglion in rats to pulsed radiofrequency currents activates dorsal horn lamina I and II neurons. Neurosurgery. 2002;50(4):850–6.
42. Hamann W. Mechanisms, indications and protocol for pulsed radiofrequency treatment. In: Meeting at St. Thomas' Hospital. London; 2003.
43. Cahana A, Vutskits L, Muller D. Acute differential modulation of synaptic transmission and cell survival during exposure to pulsed and continuous radiofrequency energy. J Pain. 2003; 4(4):197–202.
44. Erdine S, Yucel A, Cimen A, Aydin Podhajsky RJ, Sekiguchi Y, Kikuchi S, Myers RR. The histologic effects of pulsed and continuous radiofrequency lesions at 42°C to rat dorsal root ganglion and sciatic nerve. Spine. 2005;30(9):1008–13.
45. Erdine S, Yucel A, Cimen A, Aydin S, Sav A, Bilir A. Effects of pulsed versus conventional radiofrequency current on rabbit dorsal root ganglion morphology. Eur J Pain. 2005;9:251–6.
46. Hamann W, Abou-Sherif S, Thompson S, Hall S. Pulsed radiofrequency applied to dorsal root ganglia causes a selective increase in ATF3 in small neurons. Eur J Pain. 2006;10:171–6.
47. Tun K, Cemil B, Gurhan A, Kaptanoglu E, Sargon MF, Tekdemir I, Comert A, Kanpolat Y. Ultrastructural evaluation of pulsed radiofrequency and conventional radiofrequency lesions in rat sciatic nerve. Surg Neurol. 2009;72:496–501.
48. Erdine S, Bilir A, Cosman ER, Cosman Jr ER. Ultrastructural changes in axons following exposure to pulsed radiofrequency fields. Pain Pract. 2009;9(6):407–17.
49. Protasoni M, Reguzzoni M, Sangiorgi S, Reverberi C, Borsani E, Rodella LF, Dario A, Tomei G, Dell'Orbo C. Pulsed radiofrequency effects on the lumbar ganglion of the rat dorsal root: a morphological light and transmission electron microscopy study at acute stage. Eur Spine J. 2009; 18:473–8.

Chapter 4
Percutaneous Treatment in Lumbar Disc Herniation

Pier Paolo Maria Menchetti and Walter Bini

Introduction

The conventional surgical approach to disc herniation treatment may cause several complications (relapse, infection, CSF leakage, iatrogenic instability, peridural scar). In order to reduce the incidence rate of the above complications, in the last 30 years, many percutaneous procedures in lumbar disc herniation treatment have been used. All the percutaneous procedures are minimally invasive, and the main purpose is to respect as much as possible the anatomy of spine, reducing postoperative complications with a faster return to daily activities. The development of the percutaneous procedures was driven by the need to improve the efficacy of disc surgery and to reduce morbidity of the open surgical techniques. The goals included sufficient removal of disc material, minimal retraction of the nerve root, meticulous hemostasis, the possibility to approach concomitant pathologies, and the preservation of spinal stability. In addition, minimizing muscle dissection, decreasing postoperative pain, and avoiding general anesthesia in older patients were other objectives. Today, virtual reality, robotic assistance, and CT-scan are already available to surgeons performing minimally invasive spinal surgery, in order to reduce both complications and recovery time respect to surgical open approaches.

The success of the minimally invasive treatments depends exclusively on the appropriate surgical indications, and it is important to know exactly their action, complications, and limits. However, every minimally invasive treatment, in case of persistence of symptoms, permits conventional surgical procedures without any problem. Over the last 30 years, percutaneous lumbar disc herniation treatments

P.P.M. Menchetti, MD, FRCS (US) (✉)
Florence University, Florence, Italy

Department of Orthopaedics, Rome American Hospital, Rome, Italy
e-mail: ppm.menchetti@libero.it

W. Bini, MD, FRCS
Department of Neurosurgery, The City Hospital, Dubai, UAE

P.P.M. Menchetti (ed.), *Minimally Invasive Surgery of the Lumbar Spine*,
DOI 10.1007/978-1-4471-5280-4_4, © Springer-Verlag London 2014

have included several procedures such as chemonucleolysis, percutaneous automated nucleotomy, percutaneous manual and endoscopic nucleotomy, IDET (intra discal electro thermal) therapy, nucleoplasty (coblation), PLDD (percutaneous laser disc decompression), and hydrodiscectomy.

Background

Minimally invasive surgery of spine could have originated in 1963, when Smith [1] begin to use intradiscal injection of chymopapain in patients affected by sciatica. This procedure had a widespread clinical use in the 1970s but lost popularity because of severe complications, such as transverse myelitis and anaphylactic shock. In 1978, Williams [2] modified the operating microscope from brain surgery to discectomy, publishing the first series. The advantages of minimally invasive spinal surgery were shown compared to the traditional surgical approach. The advantages included one-inch incision, improved visualization and illumination, reduced operating time, and shortening of the hospitalization with a faster return to daily activities. The need to improve the efficacy of disc surgery and to reduce morbidity, mortality, and the cost of the procedures provided the impetus for the development of chemonucleolysis and microdiscectomy. Surgical goals included sufficient disc removal, minimal nerve root retraction, excellent hemostasis, ability to detect and evaluate concomitant pathology, and preservation of spinal instability.

In order to find further surgical alternatives to laminectomy and open discectomy, Hijikata [3] in 1975 performed a percutaneous nucleotomy under local anesthesia coupled with a partial resection of the disc material by a posterolateral surgical approach. Intradiscal pressure was strongly reduced with removal of nucleus polposus inside the central portion of the disc, releasing thereby irritation of the nerve root and the pain receptors around the disc herniation. However because of the posterolateral surgical approach and the instrumentations to be improved, a small amount of disc material could be removed. Anatomic structures into the spinal canal could not be directly visualized, but 2–3 g of disc were extracted by initial penetration of the capsule with a fenestrated punch and serial insertion of punch forceps through cannulas of increasing size. After performing discography by introducing Evans blue dye into the disc, only blue-stained material was removed. The percutaneous approach was further developed with modified instrumentation. The outer diameter of the working sheath was enlarged to 6.9 mm and the inner 1–5 mm, allowing the introduction of upbiting and deflecting forceps. Finally, with the introduction of small-caliber glass fiber optics, visualization of the foraminal and extraforaminal regions was possible.

By 1985, Onik and his coworkers [4] developed a blunt-tipped suction cutting probe for automated percutaneous lumbar discectomy in contained disc herniation treatment. The simultaneous cutting and aspirating of the nucleus polposus was monitored under C-arm fluoroscopy. Subsequently, a curved cannula through which a flexible nucleotome could be placed also into the L5–S1 disc space was designed. In 1983, Friedman [5] used a chest tube and speculum introduced into the disc through a 1-in. incision over the iliac crest. Sheppered [6] designed retroacting rongeurs to retrieve material from the posterior region of the disc, but none of the above-mentioned techniques were effective for sequestered fragments or important degenerative changes. Intradiscal pressure studies before and after laser treatment of cadaveric disc were performed by Asher [7] beginning in 1985. Percutaneous intradiscal laser nucleotomy with a special tip pressure transducer was also reported by Yonezawa [8] in 1990, demonstrating that after laser vaporization, the nucleus polposus was replaced with cartilaginous fibrous tissue, obtaining similar changes after open laminectomy an discectomy.

Considering the increasing demand for a minimally invasive spinal approach, the following criteria for percutaneous nucleotomy were set: (1) age less than 45 years, (2) no perforation of the posterior longitudinal ligament, (3) no preexisting of degenerative spinal canal stenosis, (4) no malformation of the neural structures, (5) at least 6 months conservative treatment without a response. In addition, the goal was a removal of disc from posterior part of herniation, preserving the central nuclear material.

In 1995, percutaneous radiofrequency thermocoagulation was introduced by Troussier [9]. Using a bipolar radiofrequency electrode and a radiofrequency alternating current could coagulate and necrose the nucleus polposus, decompressing the nerve root. The current state of the art in minimally invasive spinal surgery is quite interesting, enabling skilled spinal surgeons to make an accurate diagnosis and to perform more effective operations with lower morbidity.

Percutaneous Procedures for Lumbar Disc Herniation Treatment

Chemonucleolysis

Chemonucleolysis is the term used to denote chemical destruction of nucleus polposus (chemo–nucleo–lysis). The history of chemonucleolysis is related to Lyman Smith's studies [10]. Intradiscal injection of chymopapain, an enzyme derived from papyrus, causes hydrolysis of the cementing proteins of the nucleus polposus, without any damage on the annulus. The enzyme works in about 2 or 3 weeks, reducing the symptomatic bulging or protruded disc. Nucleus polposus is soft, gelatinous material in the center of the disc, surrounded by a tough fibrous coating (annulus). In disc herniation, weakened or torn annulus allows nucleus polposus to ooze out. A protruded disc is intact, but bulging. In an extruded disc the fibrous coating has torn, but it is still connected to the disc. In a sequestered disc, a fragment of nucleus polposus has broken loose from the disc and is free in the spinal canal. Chemonucleolysis is not effective in sequestered discs.

Indications

1. 18–50-year-old patient with contained disc herniation
2. No neurological deficits
3. Leg pain worse than lower back pain
4. Conservative treatment failure
5. Patient wishes to avoid surgery

The procedure is performed in the operating room, generally under local anesthesia. A small-gauge needle is placed under C-arm control in the center of the affected disc. Once needle placement is confirmed, discography is advisable. Next, only a small test dose of chymopapain is injected, following by a 10–15 min waiting period in order to observe signs of an allergic reaction. If no allergic reaction is noted, the procedure is completed. Patient is discharged in 24 h with absolute rest of 1 week. Because chymopapain is derived from papaya, about 0.3 % of patients are allergic to chymopapain and go into life-threatening shock when exposed to the enzyme. Symptoms of anaphylactic shock usually develop immediately, but can also occur up 2 h after procedure. Other signs of less severe allergic reaction such as rash, urticarial, could take place immediately or up to 15 days after the procedure. Neurological complications included acute transverse myelitis/myelopathy (ATM), paralysis, leg pain or weakness, foot drop, and numbness [11, 12]. The rate of good/excellent results is generally about 70–80 %, but about 30 % of patients require 6 weeks for relief of pain [11, 12]. In the United States, the procedure is accepted only on lumbar discs. The complication rate reported is about 0.2–0.5 %. The mortality rate is less than 0.2 % [11, 12].

Automated Percutaneous Nucleotomy

Automated percutaneous nucleotomy was introduced by Onik in 1985 [13].

In 1975, Hijikata [14] introduced the percutaneous manual nucleotomy, which was expanded by Onik, a radiologist, who developed an automated device (the nucleotome), consisting of a modified 2.5 mm probe. The probe contains a cutter and a suction mechanism. The first nucleotome aspiration probe had an attached needle 8 in. (20.3 cm) long, 2 mm diameter. It involved a rounded closed end with a single side port close to the distal end (Fig. 4.1). The nuclear material is cut and suctioned to an outside reservoir. The exact mechanism of action of the probe is not clear, and in 65–70 % of cases postoperative CT scan performed at 6 and 11 months after the procedure does not show significant change in the intervertebral disc [15]. Since 1985, more than 200,000 procedures have been performed with a recorded success rate of about 70–80 % [16]. Biomechanical studies suggest a reduction of the height of the disc with a reduction of the intradiscal pressure, in order to decompress the corresponding nerve root with a resolution of the symptoms.

Fig. 4.1 Onik's nucleotome

Indications

1. Patients under 45 years of age with leg pain greater than back pain
2. Contained disc herniation on CT scan and/or MRI
3. Failure after 6 weeks conservative treatment
4. No spondilosis
5. No central or lateral spinal stenosis

Provocative discography is advisable. When there is doubt about disc extrusion, discography could investigate annulus integrity and posterior longitudinal ligament. A free flow of contrast into the epidural space could confirm a complete tear, while flow into the area of herniation shows a communication with the nucleus polposus. In the presence of multiple levels of disc disease on CT or MRI, provocative discography revealed the levels requiring the surgical procedure. The procedure is performed in the operating room under local anesthesia and/or EVS (endovenous sedation). Under antero-posterior and lateral C-arm control, the 2.5 mm probe is positioned into the nucleus polposus via a standard posterolateral approach. The opening at the tip of the nucleotome in combination with the cutting blade allows the nuclear material to be pulled into the opening cut, and transferred to the suction section. The probe takes about 15–20 min to permit the cut and suction of about 2–5 g of intervertebral disc.

Many patients feel immediate relief from pain following the procedure, and most of them are able to perform daily living activities within 24 h. A hospitalization of 24 h may be advisable because, in some cases, low back spasms last a few days. Postoperatively, a physical therapy program is recommended.

The reported success rates of this operation by itself vary from 29 % [17] to 75 % [18]. From the above considerations, the best candidates for the procedure are those with small contained disc herniation; the disc should have a minimal amount of degeneration and should not be decreased in height too much. Noncontained disc herniation or sequestered disc are serious contraindications. Several days of postoperative low back pain have been described. The overall complications rate is very low.

Percutaneous Manual and Endoscopic Nucleotomy

The first report of percutaneous nucleotomy was in 1975 [14], through a posterolateral approach to the disc. In the first series, the approach to the disc was both unilateral that bilateral, using progressive dilators (3.5–4.5 mm) in which relative forceps, under C-arm control, were introduced for disc removal. The instrumentation used for the procedure involved an annulus cutter, forceps, and graspers to cut and remove nucleus polposus from the center of the disc. One drawback of the procedure was the repeated in-and-out movement of the probe through the disc, which is not good for the annulus. The technique resected the nuclear substance of the disc, and not the herniated portion, in order to reduce the intradiscal pressure, which in turn retracted the contained herniation back into the disc, relieving compression on the nerve root. Initial results of the procedure were satisfactory, with a 72 % success rate [19]. Because of vascular injuries and discitis, the need for further innovation was recognized.

In the early 1990s, Kambin [20] introduced the use of endoscope in the spine through an anatomic landmark called "Kambin's triangle" (Fig. 4.2a, b), in order to permit the direct surgical visualization of the nerve root and the disc herniation. Kambin's triangle is the site of surgical access for posterolateral endoscopic discectomy. It is defined as a right triangle over the dorsolateral disc. The hypotenuse is the exiting nerve, the base (width) is the superior border of the caudal vertebra, and the height is the traversing nerve root. Kambin initially emphasized avoiding the spinal canal and staying within the confines of the triangular zone. The endoscope and instruments are introduced through a cannula between the traversing and exiting nerves in the area known as Kambin's triangle (Fig. 4.2a, b).

Indications

- Patients with radicular pain persisting more than 3 months, relieving at rest
- Radicular pain radiating in standing position
- Contained disc herniation on CT scan and/or MRI
- Up to 50 % reduction of the spinal canal without central or lateral spinal stenosis
- Foraminal disc herniation

The equipment for the endoscopic discectomy is dedicated. A specially designed multichannel discoscope (Fig. 4.3a) with a large working channel provides the quality imaging needed to target disc pathology. The flow integrated system permits keeping the surgical field clear, even in case of bleeding. A pressure and volume controlled pump, coupled with a bipolar radiofrequency, helps to control the bleeding. Evocative discography is performed before the procedure, under fluoroscopic control, and following the discography, a guidewire is inserted into a 18-gauge (1.1 mm) spinal needle used for discography, followed by an incision with a no. 11 scalpel. An obturator dilates the muscles up the annulus, then a blunt technique is used to fenestrate the annulus and a cannula is inserted around the obturator as the tubular access to the disc. A beveled or open slotted cannula with a tang is employed to anchor the ventral portion of the cannula onto the annulus, leaving the dorsal window open towards the epidural space. The disc, posterior annulus, and the epidural space are in the field of vision of a 20° wide-angle endoscope (Fig. 4.3b). Special instruments, such as pituitary forceps and flexible shavers permit one to remove the disc, under direct endoscopic visualization.

a

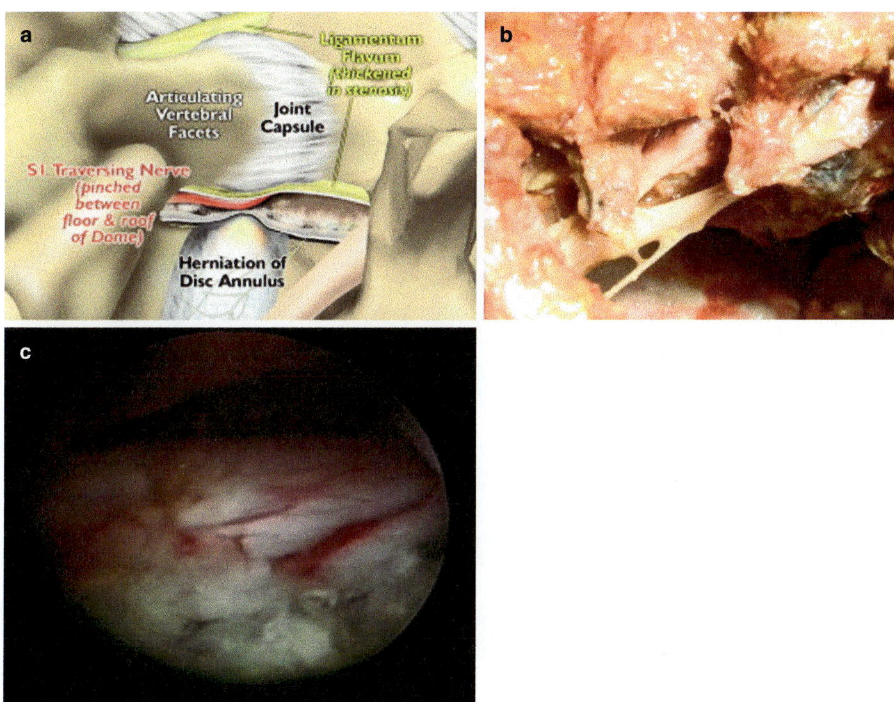

b

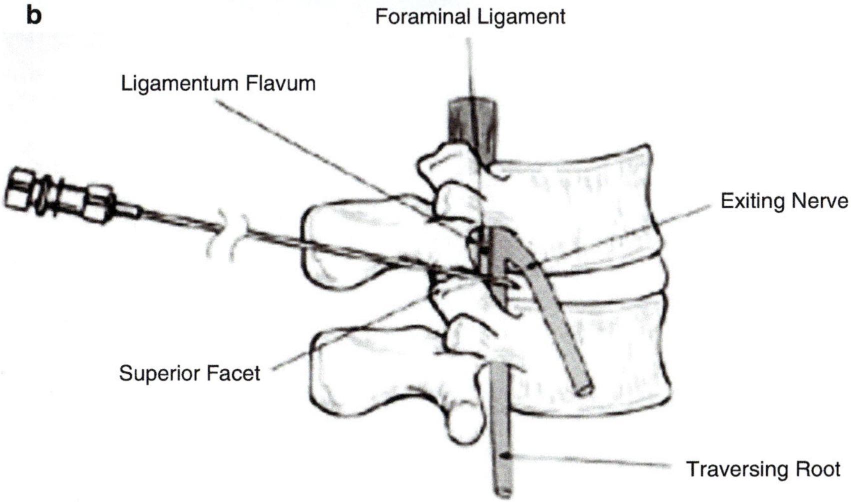

Fig. 4.2 (**a**) Kambin's triangle, a *right triangle* over the dorsolateral disc. The hypotenuse is the exiting nerve, the base (width) is the superior border of the caudal vertebra, and the height is the traversing nerve root. (**b**) Kambin's triangle anatomical landmarks on specimen spine. (**c**) intraoperative endoscopic view of disc herniation (at 6 'o clock) and nerve root (between 3 'o clock and 9 'o clock)

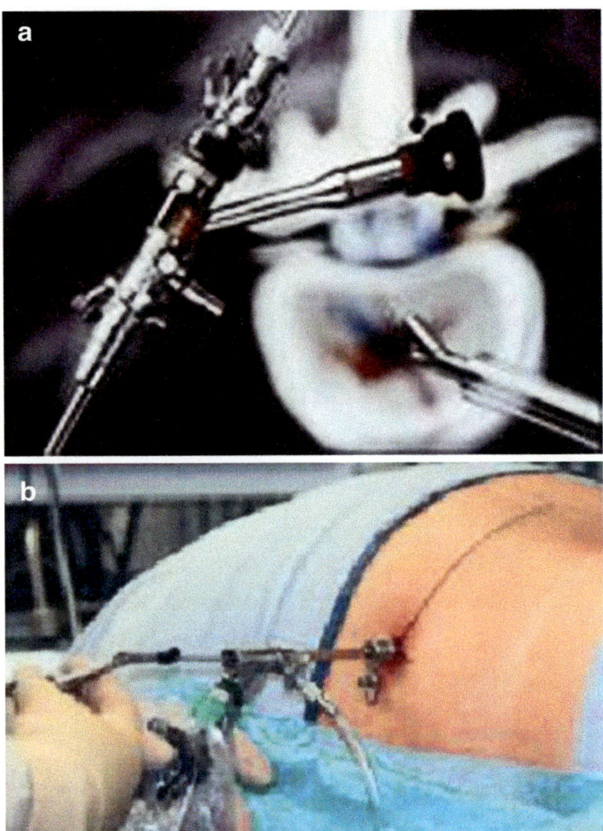

Fig. 4.3 (**a**) YESS® Spine Endoscope (Richard Wolf, Germany): Original Wolf spine endoscope, dual irrigation channels for a clearer field, rod lens optics for pristine images, 2.7 mm working channel accepts a wide range of instrumentation, including spine endoscopy forceps, trigger-flex bipolar probe, shaver blades and burrs, laser and water-jet cutter. (**b**) Transforaminal approach for lumbar discectomy

A strict selection of the surgical cases with a growing knowledge of the endoscopic techniques may give excellent/good results up to 72–88 %. Clinical outcome in over 2,500 patients evaluated both retrospectively and using an SF-36 questionnaire stated excellent/good results in more than 70 % of patients. No infection or nerve injury was found, but we must advance along the learning curve of the procedure in order to safely use the endoscope [21]. An interesting study [22] comparing microdiscectomy and percutaneous endoscopic discectomy showed, after 2 years, a success rate of 80 % using endoscopy, versus 65 % using microdiscectomy; after endoscopic discectomy, neurological deficits disappeared in 90 % of cases, versus 70 % after microdiscectomy. The return to daily activities was faster and at a higher percentage (95 %) after endoscopy compared to microsurgery (72 %).

From the above considerations, it appears that percutaneous discectomy (manual or endoscopically assisted) reduces postoperative complications and hyatrogenic damage due to open surgical approach for the following reasons:

- Posterolateral approach does not enter the spinal canal
- No periradicular/peridural scar formation (reported in 6–8 % after open surgery)
- Reduction of infection rate
- Does not give postoperative hyatrogenic instability
- Day surgery hospitalization
- Avoidance of general anesthesia
- Faster return to daily activities

In 1993, Destandau [23] designed a specially modified endoscopic instrumentation, the Destandau Endospine® System, Karl Storz (Fig. 4.4a, b), in order to realize an "endoscopically assisted lumbar microdiscectomy." The instrumentation was designed to resolve two main difficulties presented by endoscopic disc removal. First, the working space was created mechanically and not by fluid pressure. Second, the angle between the working channel and the optics channel provided the triangulation necessary to keep the distal ends of the instruments constantly in view.

In 1998, complete standard instrumentation was available (Karl Storz, Tuttlingen, Germany). Under general anesthesia and fluoroscopic control, in prone position, a 15 mm paramedian incision was performed, a 12 mm osteotome was inserted down to the lamina, and the ENDOSPINE™ tube with obturator was inserted down to the lamina. The device housed three access tubes, respectively for endoscope, suction cannula (4 mm diameter), and the largest (9 mm diameter) for surgical instruments. The first two were parallel, and the third was with an angle of 12° with the tubes converging into the plane of the posterior longitudinal ligaments. The angulation enabled the surgeon to keep the distal ends of the instruments in view at all times and to use the suction cannula as a second dissecting instrument. The system included also a nerve root retractor. Part of superior lamina and articular process was resected to expose the nerve root. Dissection of the nerve root and disc herniation removal proceeded only after adequate nerve root visualization under endoscopic illumination and magnification. Epidural veins and any bleeding points were cauterized if necessary. The total time for the procedure, after an adequately long learning curve, could vary from 60 to 120 min. Patient satisfaction was over 85 %. Low complication rates, less than 2 %, have been reported. The endoscope allowed the same access port and the same surgical technique to be used classically on the spinal canal and disc, reducing the skin incision and the overall tissue dissection. The advantages of this technique were the same as open microdiscectomy, but the immediate postoperative effects were reduced, providing a more rapid rehabilitation and return to daily activities. The method allowed a paramedial approach by partial bony resection of the isthmus, regardless of the location of the herniation and the level involved. The appropriate endoscopic view of the nerve root and ganglion reduced the risk for neural damage to a minimum.

In summary, the Destandau procedure, transporting the surgeon's field of vision directly into the operative site, enhances the visualization of structures and more than compensates for the absence of three-dimensional perception. The relatively wide angle of vision permits also a good approach to foraminal disc herniation.

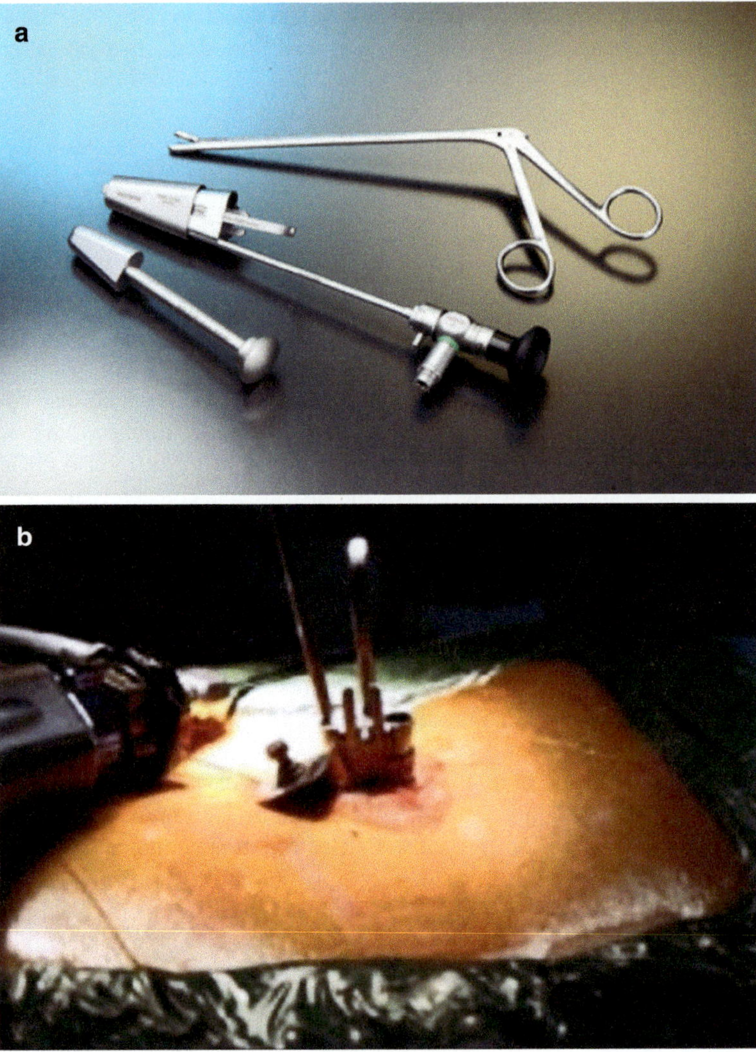

Fig. 4.4 (**a**) Destandau Endospine® System (Karl Storz). (**b**) Destandau Endospine® System (Karl Storz), patient positioning and operative setup

The paramedial endoscopic technique can also be applied for decompressing segmental stenosis and the wide field of view permits decompression of both sides through unilateral access.

Over the years, percutaneous discectomy, since its introduction, has experienced several innovations, due not only to the minimally invasive approach to the spinal canal with smaller instrumentations but also to the availability of several physical systems in order to decompress the compressed nerve root through a reduction of the volume of the herniated disc. Because the intervertebral disc could be considered a closed hydraulic space, from a physilas point of view, a small reduction of volume will give a great reduction of the intradiscal pressure.

For these reasons, since 1990, several physical energies have been used for percutaneous discectomy: monopolar radiofrequency, bipolar radiofrequency, and laser.

IDET (Intra Discal Electro Thermal) Therapy

Intra discal electro thermal therapy (IDET) has been introduced in latter the half of 1990s for the treatment of chronic discogenic low back pain due to ruptured annulus and/or small contained disc herniation. In 1997, Saal [24] proposed repairing the torn annulus with heat from a thermal resistive coil. Previous application in arthroscopy of radiofrequency current used for stabilizing a joint capsule by shrinkage of collagen and granulation tissue cauterization, followed by peripheral nerve tissue damage, lead to the understanding that intradiscal thermal resistive heating can increase annular temperatures to levels sufficient to obtain pain relief due to nociceptor neutralization. Original instrumentation involved the percutaneous threading of a flexible catheter into the disc under fluoroscopic control (Fig. 4.5a, b). The catheter, composed of thermal resistive coil, heats the posterior annulus of the disc, causing contraction of collagen fibers and destruction of afferent nociceptors. IDET is thought to decrease discogenic pain by two different mechanisms:

- Thermal modification of collagen fibers
- Destruction of disc nociceptors

Thermal modification of collagen fibers is the result of breakage of heat-sensitive hydrogen bonds of collagen, causing collagen contraction up to 35 % of its original size. The tightening of annular tissue may enhance the structural integrity of degenerated disc and repair the annular fissures. Destruction of nociceptors in the annulus is believed to contribute to pain relief. A particular thermal catheter is used for the procedure (SpineCATH System, Oratec Interventions, Inc., Menlo Park, CA). IDET is usually performed under local anesthesia or endovenous sedation. The catheter of 1.3 mm of diameter should be placed circumferentially around the inner surface of the posterior annulus (Fig. 4.5a, b), and after right positioning, it is heated from 37 to 65 °C. After temperature remains for 1 min without referred pain, the temperature is increased by 1 °C every 30 s until 80 and 90 °C. A maximum temperature of 72 °C was found in the disc, with a 46 °C in the outer annulus with catheter tip at 90 °C. It is important to understand that tissue temperature is highly dependent on the distance from the thermal source. An interesting study [25] formulated a predictive temperature map relative to the distance from the tip of the catheter. Using human specimen discs, multiple sensors were placed along the anterior annulus, posterior annulus, and endplates. Temperatures greater than 65 °C were reached at distances up to 2 mm from the SpineCATH. Temperatures of more than 60 °C were reached at distances between 2 and 4 mm from the SpineCATH in all discs. More than 45 °C was reached in all discs at distances of 9–14 mm from the catheter. Because collagen

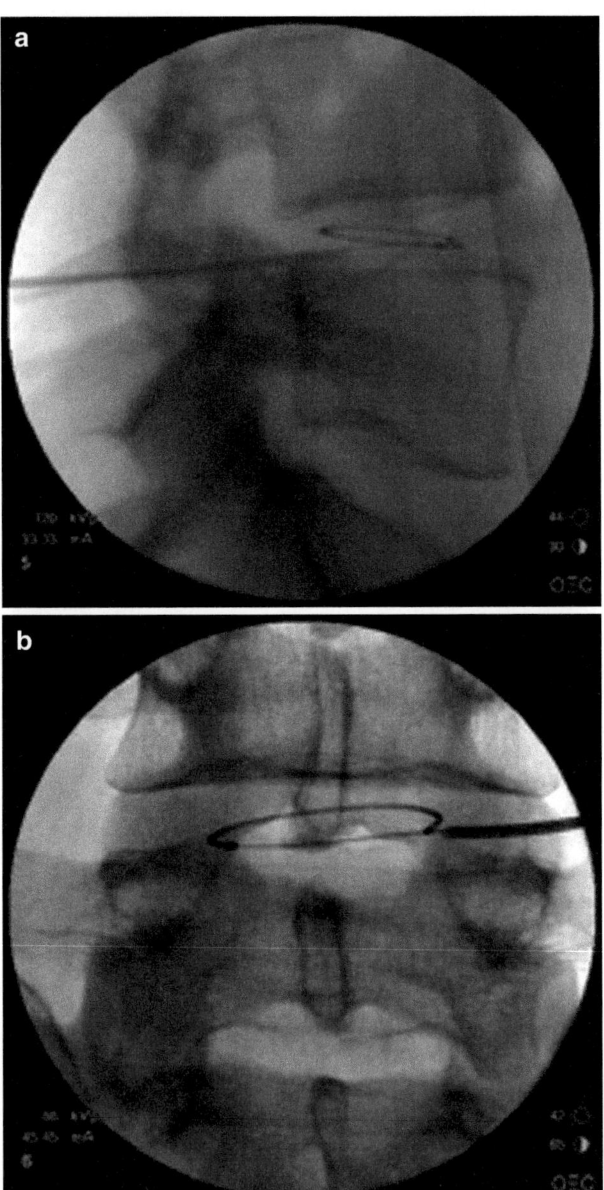

Fig. 4.5 (**a**) SpineCATH System inserted into the disc under fluoroscopic control (lateral view). (**b**) SpineCATH System inserted into the disc under fluoroscopic control (anteroposterior view)

denaturation it is considered to take place between 60 and 65 °C, sufficient denaturation thresholds are achieved within 2 and 4 mm from the SpineCATH.

Indications

- Age of patients 18–50 years
- Chronic low back pain that does not respond to at least 6 months of conservative therapy

- Prevalence of low back pain compared to leg pain
- Increasing of low back pain in standing or sitting position
- Normal disc height on lateral X-ray
- Contained disc herniation on MRI or CT scan not obliterating more than 30 % of spinal canal

After the operation, the patient might experience a significant increase in pain. Significant pain relief may take 8–12 weeks, with healing process reaching its peak 4 months after the procedure. In general, patients can return to heavy physical works after 4 months. A gradual increase in daily activities is recommended and a lumbar brace should be worn in the first 6 weeks. Results, in case of proper indication and appropriate selection of cases, are satisfied in 70 % of cases [24]. In summary, IDET is a safe procedure for patients with chronic lumbar discogenic back pain and with proper cases selection could be considered prior to the more aggressive surgical option such as fusion or disc replacement.

It must be stressed that IDET should be used in chronic low back pain treatment and not for relief of leg pain.

Nucleoplasty (Coblation)

Introduced in 2000, nucleoplasty seems to be the natural evolution of IDET. Because of the strict indications related to the prevalence of chronic low back pain and the surgical difficulties in the management of the catheter, there has not been a large diffusion of IDET. Coblation (controlled ablation) technology involves transmitting radio waves through a specially dedicated catheter called PercDCWand™ (ArthroCare® Spine, Sunnyvale, CA) (Fig. 4.6). The procedure generates a unique low-temperature plasma field in order to obtain a controlled ablation, avoiding the risks of thermal injury to vertebral end plates and surrounding tissues. By using bipolar radiofrequency, the instrument creates a series of channels into the disc by tissue ablation and coagulation, with a temperature between 40 and 70 °C. The tissue is broken down to low molecular weight gases that exit through the 17-gauge introducer needle. The plasma zone has approximately 1 mm radius, and about 1 cc of disc material is removed after creating six channels. Bipolar radiofrequency coagulation during withdrawal of the SpineWand™ denatured the adjacent collagen and proteoglycan within the nucleus for volume and pressure reduction. In the outer part of the channel there were viable cells. A total energy of 120 V is generated at the tip of the wand with a tip temperature of 50–70 °C. In this manner, a plasma field is created at the tip of highly energized particles resulting in molecular dissociation of the disc material directly in front of the tip. During the procedure, a channel is created from the posterolateral to the anterolateral annulus. On withdrawal, the coagulation mode is 60 V energy and a tip temperature of 70 °C. One millimeter from the catheter tip are 50 °C for coagulation and 40° for ablation. The nuclear tissue is ablated using bipolar radiofrequency energy with high voltage (100–300 V) and with a frequency of 120 KHz. This current creates a plasmatic field thickness of

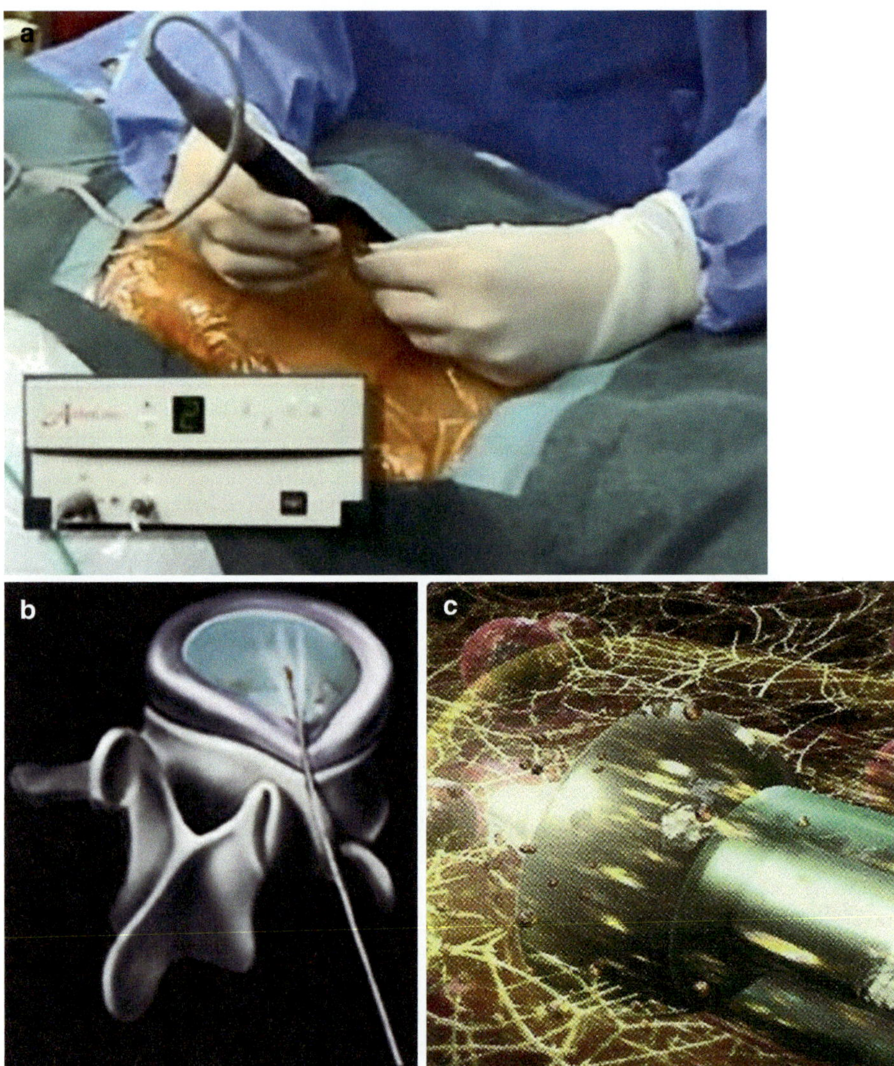

Fig. 4.6 (**a**) PercDCWand ™ (ArthroCare® Spine) inserted into 19 G needle. (**b**, **c**) Plasma field action created by PercDCWand™

approximately 75 μm, composed of ionized particles that have sufficient energy to break the organic molecular connections in the disk nucleus tissue and to vaporize thus this tissue.

Biochemical modification after the procedure has been found in the disc, with a reduction of interleukin-1 (associated with disc degeneration) and an increase of interleukin-8 (associated with tissue vascularization). Bipolar radiofrequency coagulation during withdrawal of the SpineWand™ denatured the adjacent collagen and proteoglycan within the nucleus for additional volume and pressure reduction.

On either side of the channel created, viable cells have been found on histologic studies, and any chance of structural damage to the endplates was minimal [26].

The procedure is performed under local anesthesia and/or endovenous sedation. Under fluoroscopic control, a 17-gauge needle is introduced into the disc through a posterolateral access. The needle is used as cannula for the Spine Wand™. For disc decompression, usually six channels are created at 2, 4, 6, 8, 10 and 12 o'clock, all extending in an anteromedial direction from the posterolateral annulus. The six channels decompress a cone-shaped area of nucleus. Potential complications include dysesthesia (worsening pain temporarily on the needle entry side in 10 %), nerve damage (rare), bleeding, and infection. Patients usually are discharged the same day of the procedure and allowed unlimited walking, standing, or sitting, but are not to perform any bending, lifting, or stooping. Return to work is allowed after 7 days, and usually physical therapy for lumbar stabilization is started 3 weeks after the procedure. To ensure a successful outcome, a proper preoperative evaluation combined with clinical history and imaging is mandatory. Physical examination has to show nerve root irritation with a positive straight leg raising, but a positive cross straight leg raising indicating an extruded disc or a non-contained disc herniation does not indicate coblation. MRI should demonstrate that the nuclear material is less than 50 % of the anteroposterior diameter of the thecal sac space and a narrowing of the disc does not exist.

Indications

- Patients age 20–55 years
- Prevalence of radicular pain on low back pain, nonresponding to at least 8 weeks conservative therapy
- Contained disc herniation on MRI and/or CT scan
- Disc height on lateral X-ray ≥75 %

Exclusion criteria included noncontained disc herniation, massive rupture of the annulus on MRI, disc height on lateral X-ray ≤50 %, and spinal canal stenosis. Excellent or good results are reported in about 70 % of cases [27]. However, in the most of cases the evaluation included only VAS (visual analogue scale), and it could be advisable to perform other investigations. From the above considerations, lumbar nucleoplasty becomes an alternative to conventional disc surgery. It is essential that the procedure is performed by experienced doctors with proper indications. In conclusion, there have been no major blood vessel injuries or permanent damage to the disc and supporting structures resulting in significant possible narrowing of the disc space or spinal instability following nucleoplasty.

Percutaneous Laser Discectomy

The word *laser* is an acronym for Light Amplification (by) Stimulated Emission (of) Radiation. In 1958, Schawlow and Townes published *Infrared and Optical Masers*, in the attempt to create a device for studying molecular structure, and extending their research from microwaves to infrared spectrum, they focused the shorter wavelengths. In 1960, a patent was granted for the laser. The Stimulated Emission of Radiation can be obtained by external stimulation of gas (CO_2 – carbon dioxide laser, CO – carbon monoxide laser, excited dimer – employed in ophthalmology), of solid (Nd:YAG – neodimium:YAG laser, Ho:YAG – holmium:YAG laser, Er:YAG – erbium:YAG laser, KTP – titanium and potassium phosphate) or a semiconductor (diode laser). Each laser has a respective specific wavelength in the emission of the energy, depending on the stimulated medium (gas, solid, semiconductor). Since 1960, laser has been used in ophthalmology, urology, vascular surgery, plastic surgery, and neurosurgery. Because of the characteristics of laser energy – high intensity, monochromatic, coherence, focusing – the high-intensity energy can be concentrated in a tissue with minimal leakage. The interaction between laser and the biologic tissue is determined both from the physical property of laser energy, such as wavelength, the mode of energy emission (continuous or pulsed), the time of energy emission, power energy, and the physiologic characteristics of the tissue, such as absorption, dispersion, and energy conduction in the treated tissue. From the above considerations, using the same laser energy and depending on the parameters employed, several effects can be obtained in the treated tissue – coagulation, vaporization, and thermal ablation.

Asher [28] was among the first investigators to use the carbon dioxide (CO_2) and ND:YAG – neodimium YAG laser in neurosurgery. He applied to lumbar discs, the laser experience in the treatment of the tumors in the brain with hemostasis and vaporization. Using different lasers (CO_2, Nd:YAG, KTP), a vaporization of the treated tissue was obtained, with a decompression of the herniated nucleus polposus [29]. Absorption of nucleus polposus is overlapping to avascularized biological tissues, with a peak absorption in the ultraviolet spectrum (wavelength 200–300 nm) and in the infrared (wavelength 750–10,000 nm). Peak absorption is the water absorption of the water contained in the intervertebral disc. Considering the above-mentioned evaluations, the most commonly used lasers for disc decompression and vaporization were Nd:YAG (neodimium:YAG) and Ho:YAG (holmium:YAG). The Nd:YAG laser wavelength is 1,064 nm, and by applying 1,000 J energy on the intervertebral disc, intradiscal pressure decreases by more than 50 % [30]. The Ho:YAG laser wavelength is 2,100 nm and the high water disc content peak absorption, increasing the temperatures in the adjacent tissues, needs to be applied under endoscopic irrigation control. The action of Ho:YAG laser in the disc is due to both vaporization and shrinkage (like a pneumatic mallet).

At the end of 1990, diode laser (wavelength 940–980 nm) was introduced in order to have the same Nd:YAG effects, but with improved handling and emission stability. Moreover, peak water disc content at 980 nm is five times more than at 1,064 nm (Nd:YAG laser wavelength), permitting application of energy with less dispersion on surrounding tissues and reducing the complication rate. The diode 980 nm laser contact fibers (400 μm) can be inserted into the disc through a 21-gauge needle (0.7 mm diameter) and the emission mode (pulsed) is able to concentrate linear energy on a few square millimeters with no damage to surrounding tissues. Percutaneous laser disc decompression and nucleotomy is based on a reduction of volume in a closed hydraulic space, resulting in a great drop in pressure. Because

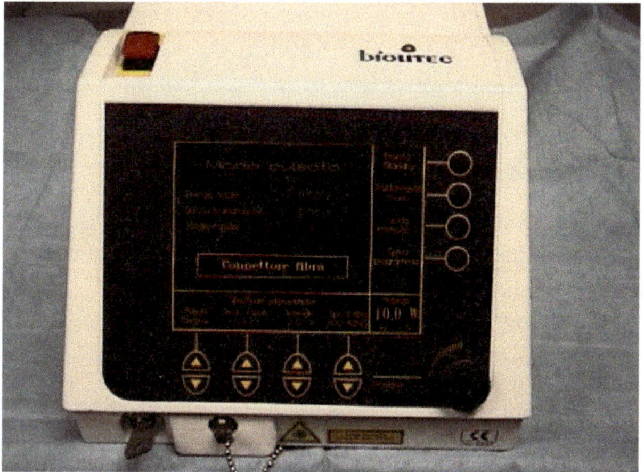

Fig. 4.7 Diode laser 980 nm (Biolitec, Germany)

water is the major component of the intervertebral disc and in disc herniation pain is caused by the disc protrusion pressing against the nerve root, vaporizing and shrinking the nucleus pulposus leads to immediate decompression of the nerve root [31, 32]. Since its first application [33], several types of lasers (Nd:YAG 1,064 nm, 1,320 nm; KTP 532 nm; CO_2 10.6 mm; Ho:YAG 2,100 nm; diode 940 nm, 810 nm) have been employed over the years.

We believe that 980 nm is the optimal wavelength for laser disc decompression and nucleotomy because 980 nm is ten times more absorbent than 810 nm and five times more absorbent than 1,064 nm, requiring less laser energy, which implies less heat diffusion in surrounding tissues. Moreover 980 nm is easier to handle (Fig. 4.7), permitting a better use in different surgical cases.

Percutaneous laser disc decompression and nucleotomy have been performed worldwide on more than 40,000 patients. The most commonly used lasers were KTP 532 nm, Ho:YAG 2,100 nm, and Nd: YAG 1,064 nm. Their combined success rate (excellent/good to fair) according to the Macnab and Oswestry score was more than 80 %, with a complication rate of less than 1.5 % [34–36]. In order to obtain a good result it is important not only to properly select patients but also to carefully choose the laser. We believe the diode 980 nm to be the best and most advanced laser in the treatment of disc herniation with optimal water absorption. Because 980 nm is ten times more absorbent than 810 nm and five times more absorbent than 1,064 nm, requiring less laser energy, it implies less heat diffusion in surrounding tissues and no undesirable side effects. A first introduction of diode 940 nm in disc herniation treatment was performed in 1998 by Hellinger [37] in a prospective randomized study versus Nd: YAG 1,064 nm. The overall success rate (90 %) confirmed the proper use of diode in order to decompress the nerve root in disc herniation. Nakai et al. [38] also confirmed, in an experimental study with a diode 810 nm, that diode is less aggressive in the surrounding tissue, preserving the end plate and the vertebral body from any damage. No secondary changes on the intervertebral disc and adjacent vertebral body after diode laser disc irradiation were detected. Experimental studies performed both on human and specimen lumbar discs using the diode laser 980 nm showed an absorption of laser light of 90.27 % in the disc and a retraction of about 55 % on 2.7 mm of the tissue after laser treatment [39].

Indications

1. Radicular pain persisting more than 6 months (even associated with paresthesia and reduced muscular strength), resistant to conservative therapy (rest, antiinflammatory medicine, physical therapy)
2. Contained disc herniation on CT-Scan or MRI
3. Disc height >30 %.

Absolute contraindications include noncontained disc herniation, sequestration, mild lumbar spinal stenosis, and periradicular scar following previous surgery.

The procedure is normally performed under local anesthesia and endovenous sedation. Under C-arm control or CT scan guidance, a 21 G needle (0.8 mm) is inserted into the disc and the disposable fiber optic (360 μm) advances into the disc. Under CT scan guidance it is possible to visualize both the nerve root and the needle (Fig. 4.8). Few complications have been reported in literature:

- Problems following puncture of the disc: nerve root damage has been reported in 0.46 % [40], compared to nerve root damage following microdiscectomy – up to 8 %.
- Hematoma: after repeated puncture attempts, psoas hematoma has been recorded in 1.7 % [41] versus 1 % reported in open spinal surgery.
- Intraabdominal injuries: the incidence of abdominal injuries, including vessels and ureter, was 1 in 3,000 cases [42].
- Infections: an intradiscal abscess was observed after percutaneous laser disc decompression and nucleotomy [43] in more than 3,000 lumbar cases, corresponding to previous reported incidence [28, 44, 45].
- Neurological complications: in lumbar cases, four cases of deteriorations have been detected of preexisting footdrops and in six cases a temporary weakness of muscles was observed. Other authors [40] reported five nerve root injuries in more than 3,000 patients. In open procedures of lumbar spine, neurological complications have been reported at 2 % [46].
- Damage to endplates: as a result of heat damage, there have been described lesions to the endplates following the Nd:YAG laser [47, 48], but no instabilities were found [43, 44].

In conclusion, the introduction of nonendoscopic percutaneous laser disc decompression and nucleotomy with Nd:YAG laser and diode laser 940–980 nm [47] has brought the contained disc herniation treatment to a new level of quality. The published advantages of intradiscal laser treatment include percutaneous minimally invasive option, small caliber of instruments (less than 1 mm), documented reduction of intradiscal pressure, low rate of complications of less than 1 %, and no spinal instability.

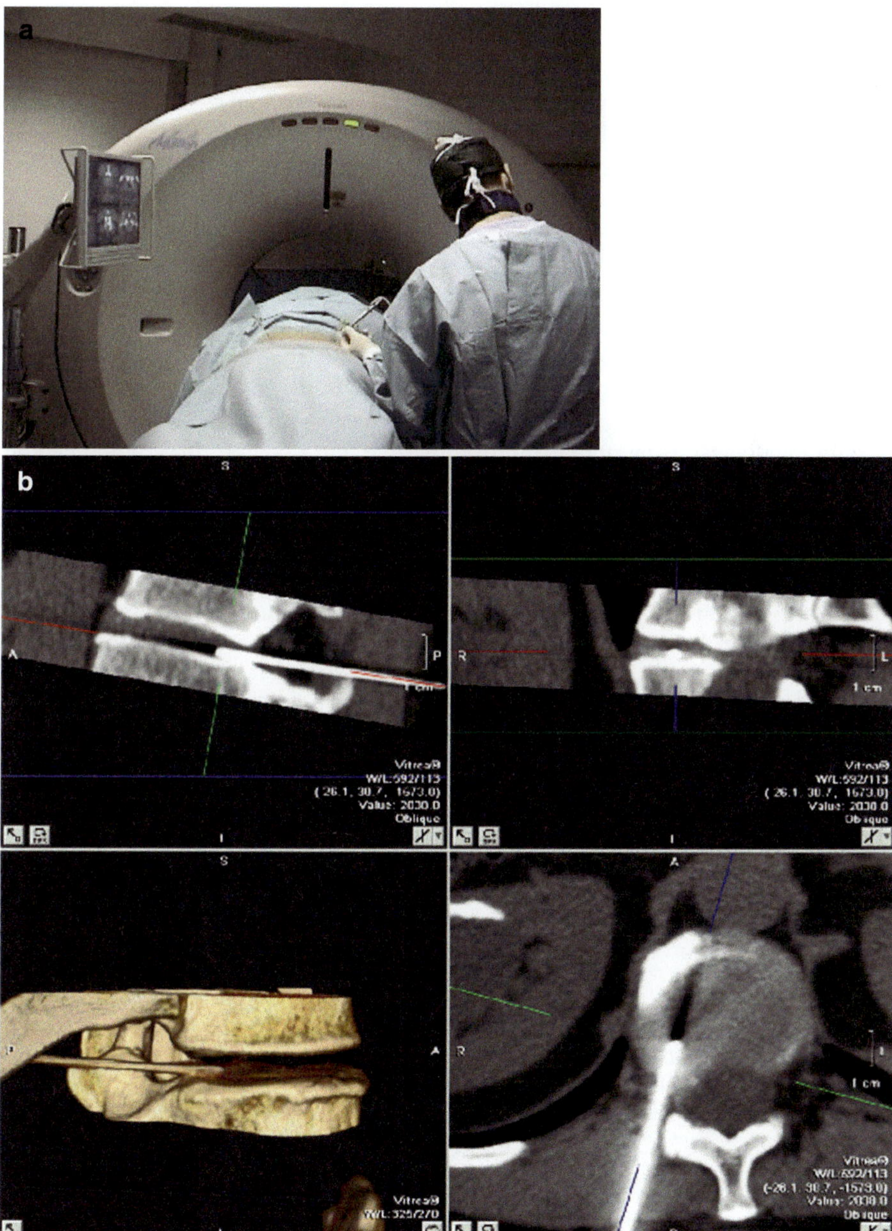

Fig. 4.8 (**a**, **b**) Percutaneous laser disc decompression and nucleotomy under CT scan guidance

Hydrodiscectomy

In 2003, a percutaneous procedure was developed using a high-speed water stream to remove herniated disc. This technique generates a power equivalent to energy procedures (radiofrequency, laser) without heating the surrounding tissues. The SpineJet® Hydrosurgery System (HydroCision, Inc., Billerica, MA, USA) (Fig. 4.9), using high-pressure fluidjet technology, has been adapted for percutaneous disc herniation removal. The SpineJet® System jets saline fluid with high velocity (900 km/h) to cut, ablate, and evacuate the disrupted disc materials safely, quickly, and efficiently. Using a cadaver model, it has been demonstrated that the SpineJet® XL (a similar disposable handpiece with SpineJet® MicroResector) removed nearly 96 % more nucleus pulposus from the posterior contralateral region compared to conventional instruments.

With local anesthesia, under fluoroscopic A-P and L-L control, a guide needle is inserted into the disc, then a dilator is inserted over the needle, and finally the introducer cannula is advanced over the dilator to the correct level. After the removal of the dilator and needle, the SpineJet Micro-Resector® is inserted through the access cannula to remove the protruded disc materials and decompress the nerve root. During the procedure the surgeon must constantly evaluate the exact position of each instrument under continuous fluoroscopic control, in order to avoid penetrating the ALL (anterior longitudinal ligament) and avoiding a dangerous bleeding. The procedure is indicated in contained disc herniation, with radicular pain more severe than low back pain, resisting to at least 6 months of conservative therapy, without spondilolysthesis and spinal stenosis. Preliminary results [49, 50] are interesting and it could be considered an alternative to percutaneous surgical techniques using energy, permitting avoidance of the potential complication resulting from heat damage to intradiscal structures and surrounding tissues.

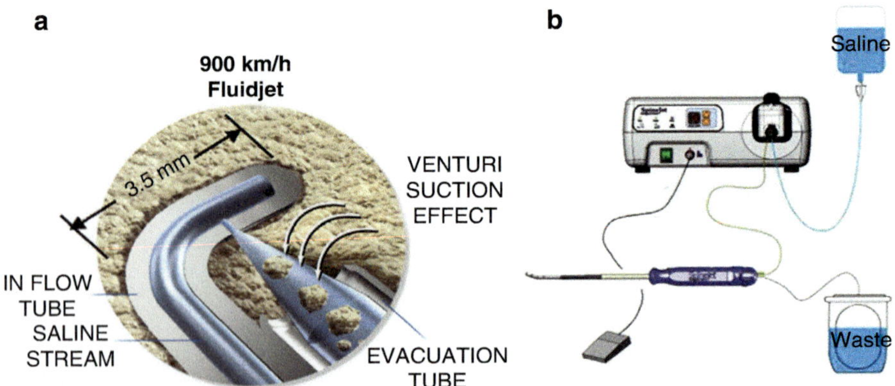

Fig. 4.9 The SpineJet® Hydrosurgery System (HydroCision, Inc.) (**a**) high velocity irrigation system and evacuation of disrupted disc (**b**) dedicated instrumentation for hydrodiscectomy

Conclusion

In conclusion, the history of minimalism in spinal medicine and surgery has moved forward in great leaps. In the last 30 years, magnetic resonance imaging has been able to investigate the spinal canal, opening the field to several advances in nonoperative pain management, including CT scan-guided treatments. Arthroscopic monitoring introduced by Kambin [20] advanced the percutaneous safety of minimally invasive surgery in disc herniation treatments. Ergonomics for spinal disorders, including restorative surgical care for intervertebral disc shock absorption, flexibility, and stability, permits management of the degenerative cascade in several steps, maintaining spinal segment motion and preserving the integrity of the vertebral joint.

Thus, today, minimally invasive spinal surgery often replaces open surgery. Procedures are safe, less traumatic, and well accepted by the patients because of day hospitalization, minimal blood loss, early mobilization, and fast recovery. Moreover, many elderly patients can be successfully treated avoiding general anesthesia and reducing postoperative complications related to surgical wounds, infection rate, and surgical pain. All the percutaneous procedures in disc herniation treatment and the relative results are strictly connected to the right indication. Only contained disc herniation without neurological deficits, resistant to at least 6 months of conservative therapy, should be managed and successfully treated.

Preserving spinal stability, tissue sparing, avoiding the spinal canal, and reducing bleeding, scar formation, and postoperative complications are the main benefits of the percutaneous treatments of disc herniation. In addition, the treatment does not preclude open surgery in case of failure.

References

1. Smith L. Enzyme dissolution of nucleus polposus in humans. JAMA. 1964;18:137–43.
2. Williams RW. Microlumbar discectomy: a conservative surgical approach to the virgin herniated disc. Spine. 1978;3:175–82.
3. Hijikata S, et al. Percutaneous nucleotomy. A new treatment method for lumbar disc herniation. J Toden Hosp. 1975;5:5–13.
4. Onik G, Helms CA, Ginsburg L, et al. Percutaneous lumbar discectomy using a new aspiration probe. Am J Neuroradiol. 1985;6:290–6.
5. Friedman WA. Percutaneous discectomy. An alternative to chemonucleolysys. J Neurosurg. 1983;13:542–7.
6. Sheppered J, James S, Leach B. Percutaneous disc surgery. Clin Orthop. 1989;238:43–8.
7. Asher PW. Application of the laser in neurosurgery. Lasers Surg Med. 1986;2:91–7.
8. Yonezawa T. Percutaneous nucleotomy: an anatomic study of the risk of root injury. Spine. 1990;15:1175–85.
9. Troussier B. Percutaneous intradiscal radio-frequency thermocoagulation. Spine. 1995;20:1713–8.
10. Smith L. Chemonucleolysis. Clin Orthop. 1969;67:72–80.
11. Shah NH, Dastgir N, Gilmore MFX. Medium to long-term functional outcome of patients after chemonucleolysis. Acta Orthop Belg. 2003;69(4):346–9.

12. Simmons JE, Nordby EJ, Hadjipavlou AG. Chemonucleolysys. The state of the art. Eur Spine J. 2001;10(3):192–202.
13. Onik G, Mooney V, Maroon JC, et al. Automated percutaneous discectomy: a prospective multi-institutional study. Neurosurgery. 1990;26:228–33.
14. Hijikata S, Yamagishi M, Nakayama T, et al. Percutaneous nucleotomy: a new treatment method for lumbar disc herniation. J Toden Hosp. 1975;5:39–42.
15. Dullerud R, et al. In: di Postacchini F, Percutaneous Treatments, Postacchini F, Mayer HM, editor. Lumbar disc herniation. New York: Springer Wien; 1999. p. 403–8.
16. Rezaian SM, Ghista DN. Percutaneous discectomy: technique, indications, and contraindications, 285 cases and results. J Neurol Orthop Med Surg. 1995;16:1–6.
17. Chatterjee S, Foy PM, Findlay GF. Report of a controlled clinical trial comparing automated percutaneous lumbar discectomy and microdiscectomy in the treatment of contained lumbar disc herniation. Spine. 1995;20(6):734–8.
18. Onik G, Mooney V, Helms C, et al. Automated percutaneous discectomy: a prospective multi-institutional study. Neurosurgery. 1990;28:226–32.
19. Hijikata S. Percutaneous nucleotomy. A new concept technique and 12 years' experience. Clin Orthop Relat Res. 1989;238:9–23.
20. Kambin PK. Posterolateral percutaneous lumbar discectomy and decompression: arthroscopic microdiscectomy. In: Kambin PK, editor. Arthroscopic microdiscectomy: minimal intervention in spinal surgery. Baltimore: Urban & Schwarzenberg; 1991. p. 67–100.
21. Yeung AT, Yeung CA. Advances in endoscopic disc and spine surgery: foraminal approach. Surg Technol Int. 2003;XI:253–61.
22. Mayer H, Brock M. Percutaneous endoscopic discectomy. Surgical technique and preliminary results compared to microsurgical discectomy. J Neurosurg. 1993;78:216–25.
23. Destandau J. A special device for endoscopic surgery of lumbar disc herniation. Neurol Res. 1999;21(1):39–42.
24. Saal JA, Saal JS. Intradiscal electrothermal treatment for chronic discogenic low back pain: a prospective outcome study with a minimum 2 year follow-up. Spine. 2002;27:966–74.
25. Bono CM, Iki K, Jalota A, et al. Temperatures within the lumbar disc and endplates during intradiscal electrothermal therapy: formulation of a predictive temperature map in relation to distance from the catheter. Spine. 2004;29:1124–31.
26. Singh V, Piryani C, Liao K, et al. Percutaneous disc decompression using coblation (nucleoplasty) in the treatment of chronic discogenic pain. Pain Physician. 2002;5:250–9.
27. Sharps L, Isaac Z. Percutaneous disc decompression using nucleoplasty. Pain Physician. 2002;5:121–6.
28. Asher PW. Perkutane Bandscheibengehandlung mit verschiedenen Lasern. In: Laser in medicine. Heidelberg: Springer; 1995. p. 165–9.
29. Danaila L, Pascu ML. Lasers in neurosurgery. Bucharest: Ed. Ac.Romane; 2001. p. 543–54.
30. Choy DSJ, Altman P. Fall of intradiscal pressure with laser ablation. Spine. 1993;7(1):23–9.
31. Case RBC, Choy DS, Altman P. Intervertebral disc pressure as a function of fluid volume infused. J Clin Laser Med Surg. 1985;13:143–7.
32. Choy DS, Ascher PW, Ranu HS, Alkaitis D, Leibler W, Altman P. Percutaneous laser disc decompression. A new therapeutic modality. Spine. 1993;18(7):939.
33. Asher PW. Application of the laser in neurosurgery. Lasers Surg Med. 1986;2:291–7.
34. Turgut A. Effect of Nd:YAG laser on experimental disc degeneration, part 2. Histological and MRI findings. Acta Neurochir. 1996;138:1355–61.
35. Tonami H, Yokota H, Nakagawa T, et al. Percutaneous laser discectomy: MRI findings within the first 24 hours after treatment and their relationship to clinical outcome. Clin Radiol. 1997;52(12):938–44.
36. Yonezawa T, Onomura T, et al. The system and procedures of percutaneous intradiscal laser nucleotomy. Spine. 1990;15(11):1175–85.
37. Hellinger J. Introduce of diode laser (940 nm) PLDN. Meziziert 2000;335–58

38. Nakai S, Naga K, Maehara K, Nishimoto S. Experimental study using diode laser in discs the healing processes in discs and adjacent vertebrae after laser irradiation. Lasers Med Sci. 2003;18–19.
39. Menchetti PPM, Longo L, Canero G, et al. Diode laser effect on intervertebral disc. PL3D Rationale Laser Med Sci. 2005;20:S17.
40. Mayer HM, Scheetlick G. Komplikationen der perkutanen Bandscheibenchirurgie. Orthop Mitteilungen. 1993;1:23–33.
41. Hilbert J, Braun A, Papp J, et al. Erfahrungen mit der perkutanen Laserdiskus-dekompression beim lumbalen Bandscheibenschaden. Orthop. Praxis. 1995;31:217–21.
42. Schwartz AM, Brodkey JS. Bowel perforation following microsurgical lumbar discectomy. Spine. 1989;4:104–6.
43. Hellinger J, Hellinger S. Complications of nonendoscopic percutaneous laser disc decompression and nucleotomy. J Min Inv Spinal Tech. 2002;2:66–9.
44. Siebert W. Percutaneous laser disc decompression: the European experience. Spine. 1993;7:103–33.
45. Choy DSJ. Percutaneous laser disc decompression (PLDD): 12 years' experience with 752 procedures in 518 patients. J Clin Laser Med Surg. 1998;16:325–31.
46. Messing–Jünger AM, Bock WJ. Lumbale Nerwenwurzel-kompression: Ein kooperatives Projekt zur Qualitätssicherung in der Neurochirurgie. Zentralbl Neurochir. 1995;56:19–26.
47. Simons P, Lensker E, von Wild K. Percutaneous nucleus polposus denaturation in treatment of lumbar disc protrusion. Eur Spine J. 1994;3:219–21.
48. Grasshoff TH, Mahlfeld K, Kayser R. Komplikationen nach perkutanen Laser-Diskus Dekompression (PLDD) mit dem Nd:YAG Laser. Lasermedizin. 1998;14:3–7.
49. Wang W, Yu X, Cui J, Wu D, et al. The treatment of lumbar disc herniation through percutaneous hydrodiscectomy. Chinese J Pain Med. 2010;16(2)71–5.
50. Han HJ, Kim WK, Park CK, et al. Minimally invasive percutaneous hydrodiscectomy: preliminary report. Kor J Spine. 2009;6(3):187–91.

Chapter 5
Assessment and Selection of the Appropriate Individualized Technique for Endoscopic Lumbar Disc Surgery

Clinical Outcome of 400 Patients

Rudolf Morgenstern and Christian Morgenstern

Key Points
- Endoscopic lumbar disc surgery is well established as safe and effective treatment for disc herniation but choosing and performing the most appropriate procedure for an individual patient is still a challenge for spine surgeons.
- Three different endoscopic techniques, transforaminal posterolateral or selective endoscopic discectomy (SED), transforaminal posterolateral with foraminoplasty (ITE), and posterior interlaminar endoscopy (ILE), were performed in a 400 consecutive patients with lumbar disc herniation.
- Based on preoperative imaging data, patients with extraforaminal, foraminal, lateral, and central herniations as well as low-grade migrations underwent lumbar discectomy with the SED technique; patients with high-migrated intracanal fragments underwent ITE technique; and patients with L5–S1 disc herniation and a high iliac crest had endoscopic discectomy via an ILE approach.

R. Morgenstern, MD, PhD (✉)
Orthopedic Spine Surgery Unit, Centro Médico Teknon, C/Vilana 12,
Barcelona E-08022, Spain
e-mail: rudolf@morgenstern.es

C. Morgenstern, MD, PhD
Centrum für Muskuloskeletale Chirurgie, Charité Universitätsmedizin Berlin,
Charitéplatz 1, 10117 Berlin, Germany

Centrum für Muskulo-skeletale Chirurgie, Charitè Hospital, Berlin, Germany

P.P.M. Menchetti (ed.), *Minimally Invasive Surgery of the Lumbar Spine*,
DOI 10.1007/978-1-4471-5280-4_5, © Springer-Verlag London 2014

- After a mean follow-up of 5.4 years, excellent/good results were obtained in 90.75 % of the patients. Outcomes were similar for the three procedures. The three study groups showed similar significant decreases in VAS and ODI scores as compared with preoperative values, but scores at 1, 3, 6, 12, and 24 months after surgery were similar.
- Individualized preoperative assessment allowed targeting lumbar disc excision using the most appropriate endoscopic technique. Only with careful planning of the surgical approach can an optimal targeted access be achieved.

Introduction

Lumbar disc surgery has evolved from open microdiscectomy to minimally invasive procedures. A broad range of different endoscopic techniques currently exist, each one covering a specific and limited range of indications, so that not only a high level of expertise is necessary, but also sufficient skills are required to choose and perform the most appropriate procedure for a given individual patient.

The transforaminal intradiscal technique, originally described by Kambin and Gellman [1], was later modified by Yeung and Tsou [2], who introduced a unique rigid rod-lens and a flow-integrated and multichannel operating endoscope with slotted and beveled cannulas that allowed a same-field viewing of the epidural space, the annular wall, and the intradiscal space. This posterolateral transforaminal approach, called "selective endoscopic discectomy" (SED), provides intradiscal access and excision of low-grade migrated intracanal herniations. Ruetten et al. [3] described lateral access for a full endoscopic transforaminal operation, but it was limited to the L4–L5 level due to anatomic restrictions like the iliac crest and the kidney. However, Lee et al. [4] found that SED could fail depending on the level of migration of the fragment, so that percutaneous endoscopic lumbar discectomy can be considered to be a surgical option in nonmigrated herniations and low-grade migrations. Choi et al. [5] described percutaneous endoscopic foraminoplasty as an effective procedure for highly migrated intracanal disc herniations. Ahn et al. [6] and Hoogland [7] introduced an alternative endoscopic technique, usually referred to as "intracanal transforaminal endoscopy" (ITE) that also permits reaching high-migrated intracanal fragments. This technique uses a transforaminal posterolateral approach that requires a mandatory drilled foraminoplasty to access the canal with an endoscope [8]. Finally, Ruetten et al. [9] described an "interlaminar endoscopy" (ILE) technique that uses a posterior approach through the yellow ligament into the epidural space for the solution of intracanal herniations, especially at the L5–S1 level. This ILE approach is performed under direct endoscopic vision with minimal dissection of the yellow ligament under general anesthesia.

The use of the most suitable technique for the individual patient facilitates the access to the target area and reduces the intrinsic anatomic difficulties for the spine surgeon. This prospective study presents the clinical outcome of 400 consecutive nonrandomized patients with lumbar disc herniation undergoing SED, ITE, or ILE. The selection of the endoscopic approach was based on the location of the herniation, the degree of migration, and the bony access conditions (e.g., the height of the iliac crest and a minimal width of the interlaminar gap).

Materials and Methods

Patient Population

Between January 2001 and January 2010, patients with symptomatic lumbar disc herniation from L1–L2 to L5–S1 who were candidates for one of the three endoscopic techniques (SED, ITE, or ILE) were eligible to participate in a prospective study. These patients were consecutively diagnosed and treated at Centro Medico Teknon in Barcelona, Spain. All patients were preoperatively informed about the type of operation, technical difficulties, and potential complications. Written informed consent was obtained from all patients.

Inclusion criteria for all three endoscopic procedures required clinical evidence of lumbar disc herniation and findings from a physical examination consistent with the magnetic resonance imaging (MRI) findings. Every patient had had at least 3 months of failed nonsurgical treatment and clinical signs of radiculopathy that included intractable leg or buttock pain with or without leg pain. Lumbar sagittal and frontal X-rays and MRI were the standard minimal images used to correlate symptoms of back and neuropathic pain.

Imaging Parameters

All patients underwent preoperative MRI and anterior-posterior (A/P) and lateral lumbar spine X-ray studies. A careful preoperative planning was performed by superimposing the MRI image of the herniated mass fragment on the A/P and lateral X-ray images (Figs. 5.1, 5.2 and 5.3). This allowed demonstration of the precise virtual location of the herniated mass in the A/P and lateral views and correlation during surgery with the C-arm fluoroscopic images (A/P and lateral projections), which was important for the surgeon to be able to orient the endoscopic instruments in the operative field (Figs. 5.4 and 5.5).

Based on preoperative imaging data, patients with extraforaminal, foraminal, lateral, and central herniations as well as low-grade migrations underwent lumbar discectomy with the SED technique, patients with high-migrated intracanal fragments with ITE technique, and patients with L5–S1 disc herniation and a high iliac crest had endoscopic discectomy via an ILE approach.

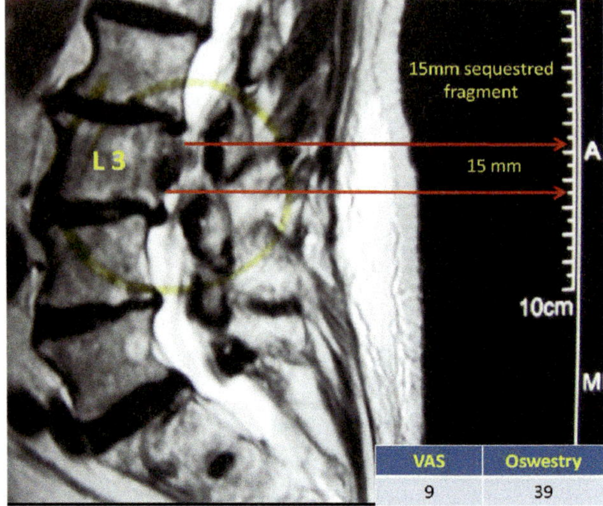

Fig. 5.1 MRI sagittal view of a L2–L3 intracanal caudal sequestered 15 mm herniation. Size and fragment measurement on the MRI scale

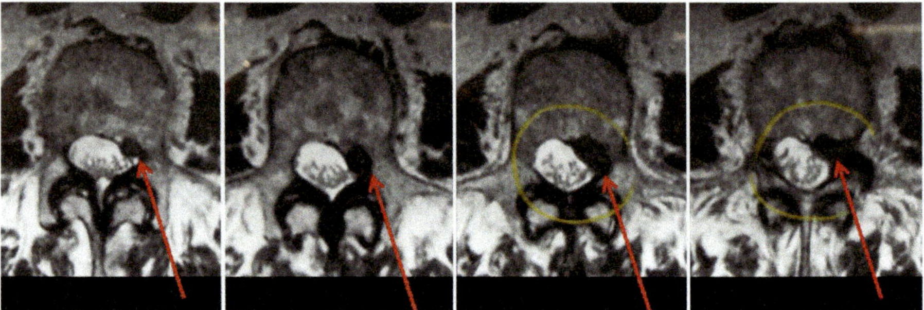

Fig. 5.2 MRI axial view of the same 15 mm intracanal fragment from Fig. 5.1 in four consecutive L3 serial cuts, (*red arrow*) extruded herniation, (*yellow circle*) herniation level

Surgical Procedures

Endoscopic transforaminal lumbar discectomies (SED, ITE) were performed under local anesthesia and light sedation, whereas the endoscopic ILE approach was performed under general anesthesia. A contrast discography with indigo carmine (Taylor Pharmaceuticals, Decatur, IL, USA) diluted with iopamidol 300 1:10 was performed in all patients to blue-stain abnormal nucleus pulposus.

The SED procedure was performed as described by Yeung and Tsou [2] using a 20° rigid endoscope (Joimax GmbH, Karlsruhe, Germany) with a working channel of 3.7 mm of diameter and radiofrequency coagulation system probes (Ellman International Inc., Hewlett, NY, USA). To perform this approach, it is necessary to first insert a needle into the disc, and a dilator is passed using the needle central guide wire. This central guide wire is then extracted and a 30° beveled cannula is passed over the dilator and the dilator extracted. The fluoroscopy X-ray arch is used

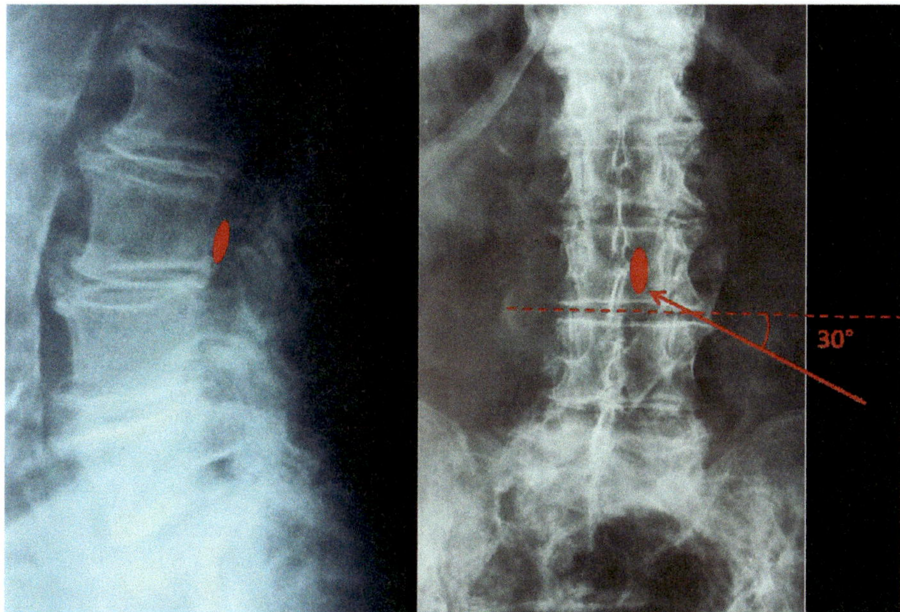

Fig. 5.3 Virtual transposition of the herniated intracanal fragment on the preoperative lateral and A/P lumbar X-ray image with preoperative planning of the access trajectory of the endoscopic instruments

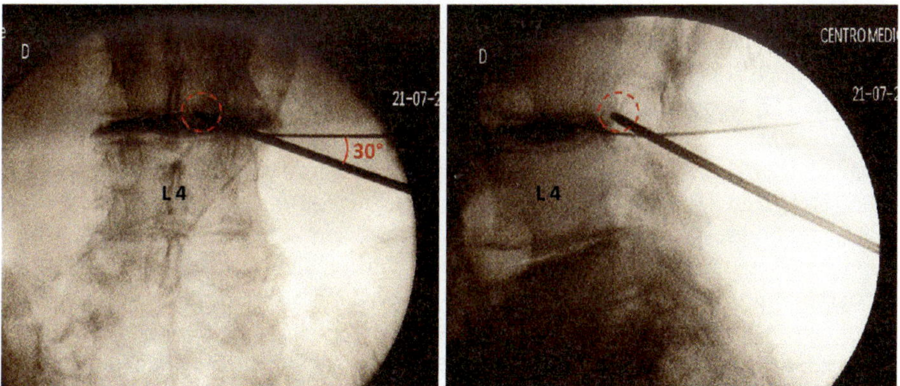

Fig. 5.4 Intraoperative fluoroscopic images in A/P and lateral with the 3 mm small dilator in the access trajectory to the intracanal herniation. See the L3–L4 discography with the intradiscal needle in position and the access from the level below the herniation, (*dotted circle*) endoscopic target

to control in A/P and lateral view the proper position of the dilator and cannula into the disc through this foraminal approach. The endoscope is passed through the cannula and under saline irrigation the disc structures are visible on the camera monitor. The careful dissection of the posterior longitudinal ligament and disc tissues with single-action baskets allows the surgeon to see the blue-stained nucleus

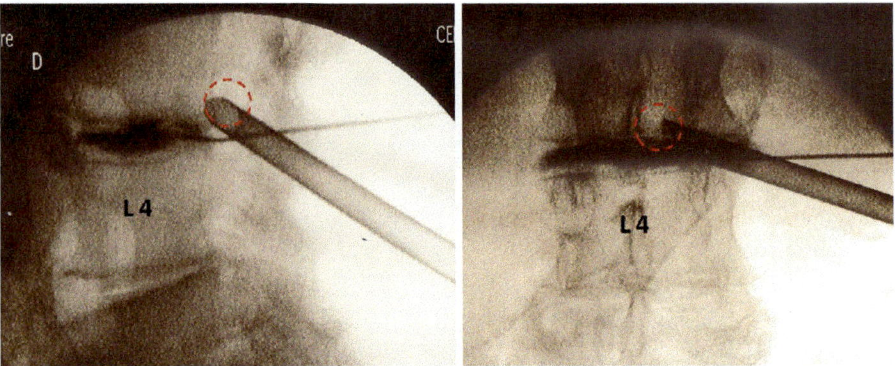

Fig. 5.5 Intraoperative fluoroscopic images in A/P and lateral with the 7.5 mm beveled cannula in the access trajectory to the intracanal herniation. See the L3–L4 discography with the intradiscal needle in position and the access from the level below the herniation (*dotted circle*) endoscopic target

pulposus and the herniation and, with careful identification, the neural structures. A foraminoplasty can optionally be performed to ablate the upper part of the superior facet and the articular capsule. Sometimes, foraminoplasty is essential to approach herniations, especially at the L5–S1 level, and also caudal migrated herniations [2, 5, 6, 8]. The reamed foraminoplasty is performed under direct endoscopic vision [8] through the endoscope's working channel employing an endoscopic chisel, high-speed burrs, or manual reamers, all with 3.5 mm outer diameter (Joimax GmbH). In order to further widen the foramen, a 5 mm trephine [2, 6] can additionally be employed through the same beveled cannula. After the herniation removal, disc curettage is usually performed.

In the ITE technique, it is mandatory to perform previously a foraminoplasty in order to remove sequestrated disc fragments [5, 7]. The manually drilled foraminoplasty was performed only under X-ray fluoroscopic control using progressive manual drills (Hoogland Spine Systems GmbH, Munich, Germany). Drill diameter starts with 6 mm and progresses to 7, 8, and 9 mm. The drills are always directed to the target through the caudal part of the foramen. Once the drilling has reached the canal, a dilator of 6.5 mm is passed through the drilled hole and a beveled cannula is passed over the dilator. After the dilator is retrieved, the endoscope can be placed through the beveled cannula, the canal and the epidural space can be visually inspected, and the herniated fragment removed. The ILE approach was performed as described by Ruetten et al. [3] under direct endoscopic vision through the yellow ligament [5, 9].

In all procedures after retrieving the endoscope, the skin was sutured. A corticoid such as depomedrol 125 mg was locally injected before the skin suture. During the endoscopic procedure and 16 h later, a third-generation cephalosporin (1 g every 8 h) was administered intravenously. All procedures were video-recorded for subsequent analysis. Discography images were printed for the patient's documentation.

Early deambulation was usually resumed 4 h after surgery. Most patients were discharged in less than 24 h after surgery.

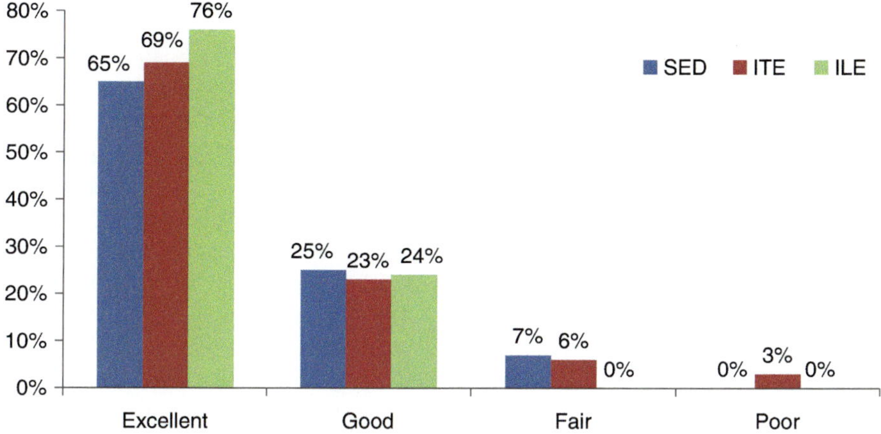

Fig. 5.6 Comparative outcome like Macnab (11) in % for three different endoscopic techniques

Outcome Evaluation

Clinical and neurological examination was performed at 1 h after operation and repeated at 12 h and 30 days after the procedure. Patients with neurological symptoms (paresis, dysesthesia, hypoesthesia, etc.) underwent electromyographic evaluation. Total pain and pain in the back and the lower extremity was scored on a visual analog scale (VAS) (0=no pain, 10=most severe pain) and the disability was evaluated with the Oswestry Disability Index (ODI) [10] for every patient. Assessments were performed pre- and postoperatively for the VAS and the ODI score at 1, 3, and 6 months after surgery, and every 6 months thereafter to achieve a minimal follow-up of 24 months for every case. VAS and ODI scores were determined blindly by independent physiotherapists who routinely participated in the physical rehabilitation of surgical patients. Patient outcomes were graded as excellent, good, fair, and poor using modified Macnab criteria [11] (see Fig. 5.6).

Statistical Analyses

Differences in VAS and ODI scores between the three intervention groups were assessed with the Wilcoxon rank-sum test. Moreover, differences in VAS and ODI scores between the groups with excellent/good results (threshold at a VAS score ≤ 4 and an ODI score ≤ 15) and fair/poor results (threshold at a VAS score ≥ 5 and an ODI score ≥ 16) were also analyzed. The Statistical Package for Social Sciences (SPSS) (version 15.0) for Windows was used for the analysis of data. Statistical significance was set at $P < 0.05$.

Results

A total of 400 patients met the inclusion criteria and underwent endoscopic lumbar discectomy. There were 245 men and 155 women, with a mean (standard deviation, SD) age of 46 (13.9) years (range 17–87 years). The mean age of male (45.3 years) and female (47.2 years) patients was similar. The SED technique was performed in 344 patients, the ITE in 35, and the ILE in 21. A total of 480 discs were operated on, with an average of 1.2 discs per patient. The type of herniation and the operated disc distribution in the three study groups are shown in Table 5.1. Patients were followed for a mean (SDS) of 5.4 (2.5) years (range 0.5–10 years). The overall follow-up rate was 97.5 %.

Clinical outcome was considered excellent in 264 (66 %) patients, good in 99 (24.75 %), fair in 27 (6.75 %), and poor in 10 (2.5 %) (Table 5.2). Overall, excellent and good results were obtained in 90.75 % of the patients. As shown in Table 5.2, results were similar for the three endoscopic techniques, with outcomes rated as excellent/good in 90.1 % of cases for the SED group, 91.4 % for the ITE group, and 100 % for the ILE group. The rates of fair/poor results were 9.9 % in the SED group and 8.6 % in the ITE group.

At follow-up, the mean VAS and ODI scores decreased significantly as compared with preoperative values ($P < 0.05$) (Table 5.3). Statistically significant

Table 5.1 Type of hernia and distribution of the operated discs in the three study groups

	Transforaminal endoscopy (SED)	Intracanal transforaminal endoscopy (ITE)	Interlaminar endoscopy (ILE)	Total
Herniation				
Central	48	5	2	55
Lateral	131	27	19	177
Foraminal	160	3		163
Extraforaminal	5			5
Total	344	35	21	400
Disc level				
L1–L2	4			4
L2–L3	12	1		13
L3–L4	46	2		48
L4–L5	206	10	4	220
L5–S1	156	22	17	195
Total	424	35	21	480

Table 5.2 Results by endoscopic technique in 400 patients

Outcome	Transforaminal endoscopy (SED)	Intracanal transforaminal endoscopy (ITE)	Interlaminar endoscopy (ILE)	Total
Excellent	224 (65.1 %)	24 (68.5 %)	16 (76.2 %)	264 (66 %)
Good	86 (25 %)	8 (22.9 %)	5 (23.8 %)	99 (24.75 %)
Fair	25 (7.3 %)	2 (5.7 %)	0	27 (6.75 %)
Poor	9 (2.6 %)	1 (2.9 %)	0	10 (2.5 %)
Total	344	35	21	400

differences between preoperative and postoperative VAS and ODI scores for each endoscopic technique were also observed; however, differences between the three study groups in VAS and ODI scores after 1, 3, 6, 12, and 24 months of surgery were not found (Table 5.4). On the other hand, postoperative VAS and ODI scores were significantly lower in patients in the excellent/good group than in those in the fair/poor group ($P < 0.05$) (Table 5.5).

Sterile discitis of unknown cause was reported in four patients in the SED. Postoperative neuropathic pain was reported in ten patients in the SED group. Nine of these cases were classified as transient dysesthesias and were treated with corticosteroids (2 mg every 8 h), gabapentine (75 mg every 8 h), and benzodiazepines (5 mg every 8 h) for 2–3 weeks. In one of these patients, a drop foot syndrome with residual partial paresis of the L5 nerve root was found. No dural tears or wound infections were reported.

Table 5.3 Results of clinical assessments for pain and functional disability in 400 patients

	VAS score, mean (SD)		ODI score, mean (SD)
	Back pain	Leg pain	
Preoperative	6.6 (2.1)	7 (2.1)	31.3 (7.1)
Follow-up			
1 month	2.8 (2.8)[a]	3.8 (2.8)[a]	16.5 (13)[a]
3 months	2.1 (0.2)[a]	2.3 (0.2)[a]	11.6 (7.1)[a]
6 months	1.6 (2.1)[a]	1.5 (2.1)[a]	7.8 (13)[a]
12 months	1.5 (0.1)[a]	1.4 (1.4)[a]	7 (7.1)[a]
>24 months	1.8 (0.1)[a]	1.2 (1.4)[a]	6.6 (2.1)[a]

[a]$P < 0.05$ as compared with preoperative values

Table 5.4 Results of clinical assessments for pain and functional disability according to the endoscopic technique

		Follow-up				
	Preoperative	1 month	3 months	6 months	12 months	>24 months
VAS back, mean (SD)						
SED	6.4 (2.2)	2.8 (2.5)[a]	2.1 (2.2)[a]	1.6 (1.9)[a]	1.6 (2.0)[a]	2.2 (2.4)[a]
ITE	6.8 (1.9)	2.4 (2.3)[a]	1.5 (1.9)[a]	0.9 (1.2)[a]	0.6 (1.3)[a]	0.6 (1.1)[a]
ILE	6.2 (1.6)	2.0 (2.1)[a]	1.4 (1.9)[a]	1.5 (1.2)[a]	1.3 (1.3)[a]	1.3 (1.1)[a]
VAS leg, mean (SD)						
SED	6.2 (2.5)	3.5 (2.5)[a]	2.1 (2.0)[a]	1.4 (1.9)[a]	1.4 (2.4)[a]	1.3 (2.2)[a]
ITE	8.0 (1.1)	3.9 (2.4)[a]	2.2 (2.6)[a]	1.2 (1.7)[a]	1.0 (1.5)[a]	0.7 (1.3)[a]
ILE	8.4 (1.4)	1.9 (2.0)[a]	1.2 (1.8)[a]	1.2 (1.7)[a]	1.2 (1.5)[a]	1.2 (1.3)[a]
ODI score, mean (SD)						
SED	28.1 (8.4)	15.7 (10.1)[a]	11.4 (9.1)[a]	7.4 (7.0)[a]	7.1 (7.4)[a]	7.3 (8.1)[a]
ITE	34.6 (8.4)	15.7 (9.8)[a]	8.6 (8.1)[a]	5.8 (6.0)[a]	4.4 (4.8)[a]	4.1 (4.8)[a]
ILE	35.6 (8.8)	10.8 (6.8)[a]	6.6 (2.1)[a]	3.8 (2.0)[a]	3.4 (1.8)[a]	3.1 (1.8)[a]

SED transforaminal endoscopy, *ITE* intracanal transforaminal endoscopy, *ILE* interlaminar endoscopy

[a]$P < 0.05$ as compared with preoperative values

Table 5.5 Results of clinical assessments for pain and functional disability according to outcome

Outcome	Follow-up				
	1 month	3 months	6 months	12 months	>24 months
Excellent/good					
VAS back, mean (SD)	2.1 (2.8)	1.6 (0.3)	1.2 (2.1)	0.9 (0.1)	1.0 (0.1)
VAS leg, mean (SD)	3.0 (2.8)	1.9 (0.3)	1.1 (2.1)	0.7 (1.4)	0.5 (1.4)
ODI score, mean (SD)	13.1 (13)	9.0 (7.1)	6 (13)	4.5 (7.1)	3.6 (2.1)
Fair/poor					
VAS back, mean (SD)	5.2 (3.1)[a]	3.3 (2.6)[a]	4.0 (2.4)[a]	4.7 (2.1)[a]	4.9 (2.2)[a]
VAS leg, mean (SD)	5.4 (2.9)[a]	2.8 (2.3)[a]	3.7 (2.3)[a]	4.8 (2.4)[a]	5.0 (2.3)[a]
ODI score, mean (SD)	23.4 (13.3)[a]	15.6 (13)[a]	18.3 (10.6)[a]	20.8 (8.4)[a]	19.7 (7.4)[a]

[a]$P<0.05$ as compared with the corresponding values in the excellent/good outcome group for each follow-up interval

In 18 patients, reoperation was required because of persistent postoperative pain, usually due to the presence of small disc fragments that have been missed during the initial SED operation. In 8 patients, residual intracanal fragments were removed by ITE with drilled foraminoplasty under local anesthesia. Four patients with re-herniation at the same disc level and side underwent a second SED procedure. In four patients in whom the transforaminal approach with foraminoplasty had been too difficult because of a high iliac crest, reoperation with the ILE approach under general anesthesia was carried out. In the remaining two patients in whom the interlaminar gap was too small for an ILE approach, an open microdiscectomy under general anesthesia was performed. In all patients, satisfactory results were obtained.

Discussion

This study presents the outcome of 400 consecutive patients with lumbar disc herniation treated with endoscopic discectomy. Three different endoscopic techniques were presented and for each specific case only one approach was selected and applied, depending on the patient's specific anatomic and pathological characteristics. The selection criteria of the most convenient endoscopic procedure were primarily based on the anatomic location of the herniation and the level of migration (high or low level migration). The outcome was graded as excellent or good in 90.75 % of the patients. These results are similar to data reported in other clinical series [2, 7, 9] in which only one endoscopic approach was used and usually including a small range of migrated herniations and level distributions. In our opinion, the key point in obtaining optimal and consistent results is the technical ability to access all lumbar disc levels (especially L5–S1) by selecting the ideal needle trajectory, performing a drilled facetectomy [7, 8, 12] when required, and choosing the most appropriate instrument angle depending on the location of the herniation with a selective and direct targeted approach (Fig. 5.7). The angle in degrees of the needle's direction and the distance in centimeters to the midline depend on the anatomy

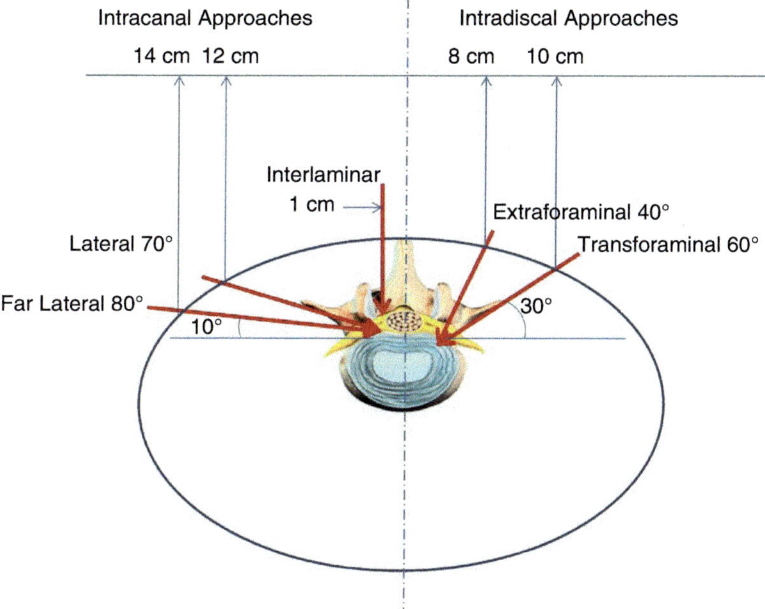

Fig. 5.7 Axial representation of the intradiscal and intracanal access trajectories with approximated angles and midline distances. Central or lateral herniation in L5–S1 with a high iliac crest: interlaminar (1 cm) lateral from the midline and 0° needle direction; extraforaminal herniation: distance to the midline 5–8 cm, use a more steep 40° needle direction; foraminal herniation: distance to the midline 8–12 cm, use a more medial entry and 60° needle direction; lateral herniation: distance to the midline 12 cm, use a more lateral entry and slight horizontal 70° needle direction; and central herniation: distance to the midline ≥14 cm, use an extreme far lateral entry and a horizontal 70°–80° needle direction

of the patient and can vary in each particular case. However, some technical specifications are also shown in Fig. 5.7.

The SED technique was convenient for removing intradiscal material and to extract all types of herniations that can be reached from the operated disc level (Fig. 5.8). In cases of low-grade intracanal migration, this procedure allowed extraction of fragments that were migrated less than the distance of one disc space height when measured from the adjacent endplate [4]. The extreme far lateral approach [3] was not considered in this study as a separate technique and was included into the group of SED. In our case, a lateral shallow access with an angle between 70° and 80° was applied (Fig. 5.7). We consider that this approach should be limited to treat herniations at the L4–L5 level, given that the iliac crest may prevent a far lateral access to the levels below, while the kidney could become a dangerous obstacle when accessing the levels above it.

The ITE approach was especially indicated for high-grade intracanal migration (see Fig. 5.9) and was suitable for fragments that were migrated more than the distance of one disc space height measured from the adjacent endplate [12]. The ILE approach was only employed in cases where the height of the iliac

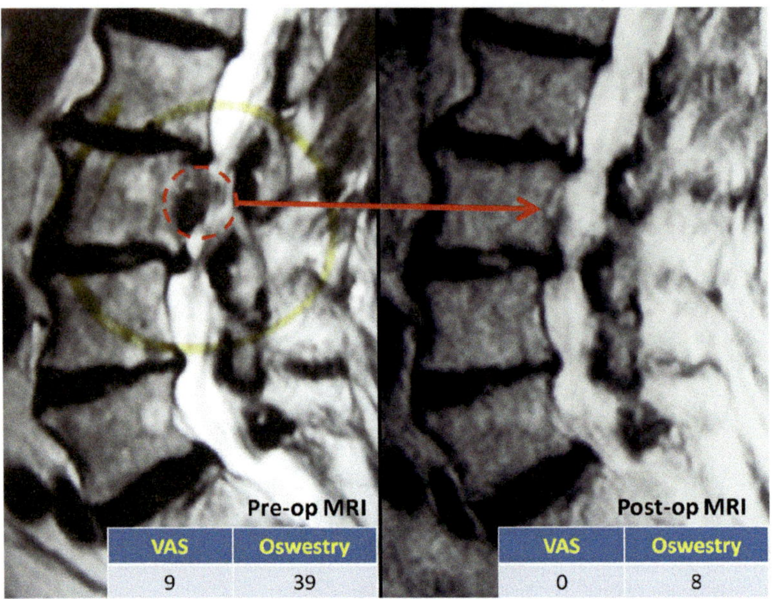

Fig. 5.8 Comparative pre-op and post-op MRI sagittal view showing the complete removal of the L3 intracanal migrated fragment

crest did not allow a direct transforaminal access even if a drilled foramino-plasty was performed. In these cases, the access angle in the A/P frontal plane becomes too steep and difficult, reaching the intracanal space especially in cases with cranially migrated fragments. The ILE approach was only employed if the interlaminar gap was wider than 2 cm, allowing the access through the yellow ligament into the vertebral canal.

In the group of operated ILE cases, men accounted for 71.4 % of the cases, prob-ably due to the gender-specific anatomic characteristic of a higher iliac crest. In comparison, men accounted only for 62 and 60 % of cases in the SED and ITE groups, respectively. In these circumstances, the selection criteria of the degree of migration of the herniated fragment prevailed over gender-related anatomic condi-tions. Choi et al. [5] introduced an interlaminar approach that can be performed under local anesthesia by employing direct needle intracanal puncture and tissue dilatation only under fluoroscopic control. However, we preferred the approach described by Ruetten et al. [9] because, according to this technique, the yellow liga-ment dissection and epidural access are performed under direct endoscopic vision and additionally fluoroscopic control. This is an important advantage of the tech-nique as it facilitates better intraoperative identification of anatomic structures despite the use of general anesthesia. A schematic overview of the advantages and limitations of the three endoscopic techniques is provided in Table 5.6.

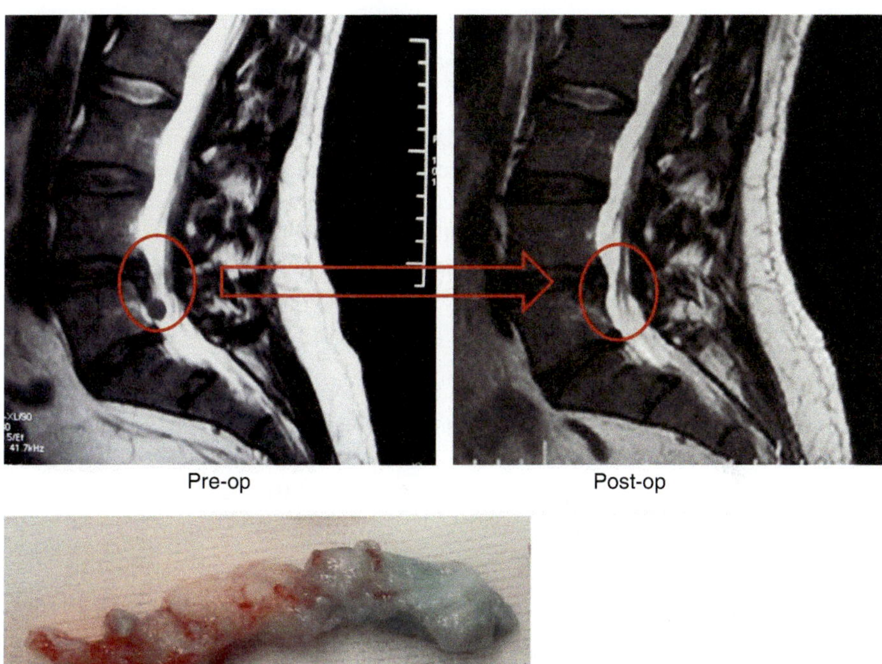

Fig. 5.9 Comparative pre-op and post-op MRI sagittal view showing the complete removal of the L4-L5 intracanal migrated herniation and the 5 cm blue stained extracted fragment, (*red circle*) fragment location

Table 5.6 Indications and limitations of different endoscopic approaches for reaching lumbar disc herniated fragments at various anatomic sites

Approach	Intradiscal	Intracanal	Limitations
Transforaminal posterolateral (SED)	Foraminal herniations [2]	Low-grade migration [2, 4]	High-grade migration
Transforaminal posterolateral with foraminoplasty (ITE)	Lateral herniations [2]	High-grade migration [6, 7]	Too high iliac crest, high-grade canal compromise
Transforaminal far lateral	Intradiscal limited access	Lateral and central herniations [3, 9]	Only for L4–L5
Posterior interlaminar (ILE)	Intradiscal limited access	Lateral and central herniations [3, 5, 9]	Mostly for L5–S1 if enough interlaminar gap

SED selective endoscopic discectomy, *ITE* intracanal transforaminal endoscopy, *ILE* interlaminar endoscopy

Conclusion

Endoscopic lumbar disc surgery can be performed using different intradiscal or intracanal approaches. In this study, three different endoscopic procedures were combined to target most of the typical spectrum of herniations. The selection of different endoscopic techniques helps to overcome natural anatomic obstacles. The approach and the needle position must be carefully chosen depending on multiple factors, including location of the herniation, herniation size, disc level, and other anatomic conditions such as height of the iliac crest and width of the interlaminar gap. Only after a careful planning of the approach can optimal targeted access be achieved.

Acknowledgment The authors thank Marta Pulido, MD, for editing the manuscript.

References

1. Kambin P, Gellman H. Percutaneous lateral discectomy of the lumbar spine: a preliminary report. Clin Orthop Relat Res. 1983;174:127–32.
2. Yeung AT, Tsou PM. Posterolateral endoscopic excision for lumbar disc herniation: surgical technique, outcome, and complications in 307 consecutive cases. Spine. 2002;27:722–31.
3. Ruetten S, Komp M, Godolias G. An extreme lateral access for the surgery of lumbar disc herniations inside the spinal canal using the full-endoscopic uniportal transforaminal approach-technique and prospective results of 463 patients. Spine. 2005;30:2570–8.
4. Lee SH, Kang BU, Ahn Y, et al. Operative failure of percutaneous endoscopic lumbar discectomy: a radiologic analysis of 55 cases. Spine. 2006;31:E285–90.
5. Choi G, Lee SH, Raiturker PP, et al. Percutaneous endoscopic interlaminar discectomy for intracanalicular disc herniations at L5-S1 using a rigid working channel endoscope. Neurosurgery. 2006;58(1 Suppl):ONS59–68.
6. Ahn Y, Lee SH, Park WM, et al. Posterolateral percutaneous endoscopic lumbar foraminotomy for L5-S1 foraminal or lateral exit zone stenosis. Technical note. J Neurosurg. 2003;99(3 Suppl):320–3.
7. Hoogland T. Transforaminal endoscopic discectomy with foraminoplasty for lumbar disc herniation. Surg Tech Orthop Traumatol. 2003;C40:55–120.
8. Morgenstern R. Transforaminal endoscopic stenosis surgery: a comparative study of laser and reamed foraminoplasty. Eur Musculoskelet Rev. 2009;4:1–6.
9. Ruetten S, Komp M, Merk H, et al. Full-endoscopic interlaminar and transforaminal lumbar discectomy versus conventional microsurgical technique: a prospective, randomized, controlled study. Spine. 2008;33:931–9.
10. Fairbank JC, Pynsent PB. The Oswestry disability index. Spine. 2000;25:2940–52.
11. Macnab I. Negative disc exploration. An analysis of the causes of nerve-root involvement in sixty-eight patients. J Bone Joint Surg Am. 1971;53:891–903.
12. Choi G, Lee SH, Lokhande P, et al. Percutaneous endoscopic approach for highly migrated intracanal disc herniations by foraminoplastic technique using rigid working channel endoscope. Spine. 2008;33:E508–15.

Chapter 6
Interspinous Devices: State of the Art

Christian Giannetti, Rapahel Bartalesi, Miria Tenucci, Matteo Galgani, and Giuseppe Calvosa

Biomechanics

Introduction

Interspinous devices are in the class of medical devices that can be implanted in the lumbosacral spine using a minimal and often mini-invasive approach. Because their use has boomed over the last decade, we can state with confidence that this techno-logical sector attracts a great deal of interest in a quest for techniques and materials able to reduce the invasiveness of the surgical procedure and increase its general bio-compatibility. An initial classification of interspinous devices from a biome-chanical viewpoint may be carried out by assessing the rigidity of the distraction element. This identifies devices that are inaccurately categorized as nondeformable, involving the insertion of material with high mechanical rigidity into the space between the spinous process, where the distraction between the spinous processes may be considered constant. In other devices, a material with a shock-absorbing function is inserted between the spinous processes, which then undergoes appre-ciable elastic or visco-elastic deformation under physiological loads to increase bone implant compliance. In parallel with this sub-category, there are also devices that work by rigid stabilization of the interspinous space where stable posterior interspinous fusion is brought about by applying autologous or homologous bone and cruentation of the spinous processes. Clinical trials on interspinous devices available in the literature show a good relationship between the benefits for the patient and the use of resources in the disease treatment. Nevertheless, there is still

C. Giannetti, MD • M. Tenucci, MD • M. Galgani, MD • G. Calvosa, MD (✉)
Department of Orthopaedics and Traumatology, Santa Maria Maddalena Hospital,
Volterra, Italy
e-mail: giucalvosa@virgilio.it

R. Bartalesi, PhD
Department of Bioengineering, University of Pisa, Pisa, Italy

P.P.M. Menchetti (ed.), *Minimally Invasive Surgery of the Lumbar Spine*,
DOI 10.1007/978-1-4471-5280-4_6, © Springer-Verlag London 2014

margin for clinical investigation and for the establishment of verification and validation procedures of these devices in order to clearly define the relationship between the effects on the biomechanics of the functional unit and the clinical indications of such devices.

Notes on Biomechanics

The spinal column is a multi-segmented structure made up of 33 vertebrae, 24 of which are mobile while the remaining 9 are fused to one another. It is attached to the pelvis, stabilized and controlled in three-dimensional space due to its specific structure and to the muscle bands inserted into it. These muscles constitute, for all intents and purposes, a system of stays similar to those that stabilize the main mast of a ship against the actions of outside elements [1] (Fig. 6.1). Each mobile vertebra is connected, that is, kinematically constrained to the others by means of intervertebral ligaments, an intervertebral disc, a synovial joint between the facets, and lastly by the intervertebral muscles. The set of two successive jointed vertebrae and their associated connective tissue (excluding the muscles) takes the name of a functional unit (Functional Spinal Unit, FSU). The FSU, known also as a mobile segment, requires in-depth kinematic study in order to assess the effect of an interspinous device. The biomechanics of such devices are studied with the aim of determining their performance together with the mechanical properties of the spinal column, which guarantee their main functions, including that of maintaining an overall compromise between stability and mobility under the action of loads transmitted to the column via the tissues to which it is connected.

Functional Spinal Unit

The FSU contains two types of joint: an intervertebral joint between vertebral bodies and the intervertebral disc, and also a joint between the facets of adjacent vertebral joint processes. The first is a synarthrosis, made up of two bone segments, joined in this case by the intervertebral disc. The second is a synovial joint, where the joint faces are separated from one another by a cavity and are able to slide over one another because of the cartilage that covers them and the interposed meniscus. The muscles are generally inserted into the spinous processes and transverse processes and, together with the numerous ligaments present, guarantee two types of stability:

- Mechanical (or elastic) stability, that is, the ability of any structure placed under a load to return to its original position when it is perturbed;
- Clinical stability, that is, the ability of an anatomical structure under the action of physiological loads to limit trajectories or movements in such a way as to give rise to pain, functional uncoupling, or deformity. When studying the kinematics

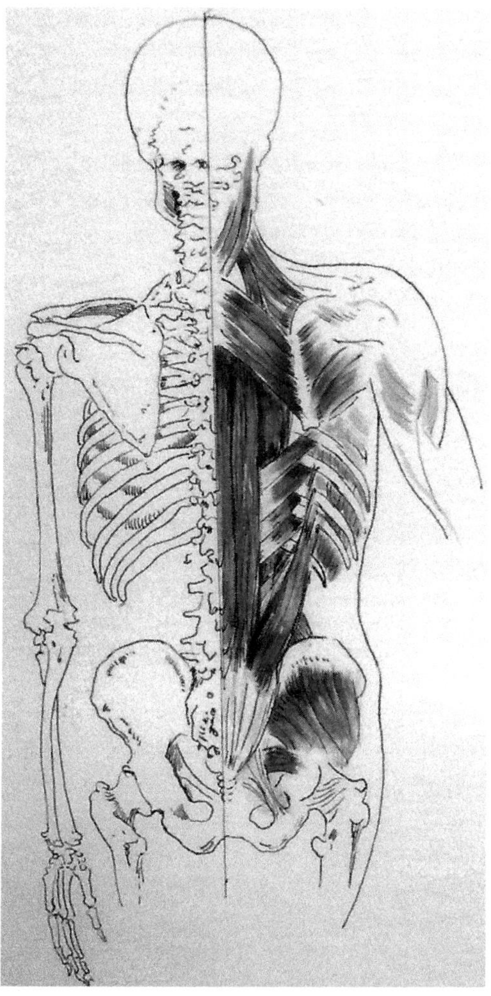

Fig. 6.1 Rear view of the human spine with partial overlapping of muscle layers involved in functional units' stabilization and mobility

of the FSU, it is normal to refer to the kinematics of rigid bodies, often overlooking deformations in the intervertebral disc and defining an instantaneous axis of rotation (IAR) to describe the rotation of the centroid of one vertebra in relation to another. Six degrees of freedom in a three-dimensional space are attributed to each FSU: three rotational and three translational.

The following terminology is used to define segment movements:

- Range of motion (ROM): range of movement arising out of the application of physiological loads as the sum of two areas defined, respectively, as the neutral area and the elastic area. The former corresponds to movements delimited by muscle action, the latter corresponds to movements where the ligaments exercise a stabilizing action;

- Pattern of motion (POM): the trajectory described by the vertebral body centroid in movements within its ROM;
- Coupling: because movement about one axis is often associated with movement about another axis.

The most mobile segments are the cervical spine segments. Movements of the thoracic vertebrae are relatively limited because the thoracic cage, the fine intervertebral discs, the configuration of the vertebral joint faces, and the opposition of extending spinous processes contribute to the limited mobility of this section of the spine during flexo-extension and lateral bending. In lumbar lordosis, the intervertebral discs are relatively thick and allow great freedom of movement, while axial rotation in the lumbar region is limited by the facet joints [2]. Table 6.1 shows the approximate ROMs for normal uncoupled movements of a healthy spine.

Effects of Distraction on Biomechanical Properties of Vertebral Tissues

Implications for Structure, Kinematic and ROM

Inserting a device between the spinous processes gives rise to a distractive effect at the affected site, while adjacent levels that are unaffected by the device do not generally undergo appreciable influences. The following effects occur:

1. Increase in the size of the spinal canal and foraminal canals. For example, during an in vitro study on cadavers [3] and an in vivo study with a pMRI examination [4], both based on the X-STOP device, increases of 18–23 % were recorded for the spinal canal area and 20–25 for the foraminal canal area in the extended position achieved for levels treated with the device as compared to intact levels. These values decline when changing from an extended to a neutral position until no changes are demonstrated in the flexion movements.
2. Increase in the thickness of the posterior part of the annulus fibrosus. This result is difficult to quantify due to issues of accuracy and resolution of the diagnostic imaging instruments. Although it has been reported in some in vivo studies with MRI investigation, there is no overall consensus [5, 6].

Table 6.1 Approximate ROM of an healty spine

Vertebrae	Flexo-extension (°)	Lateral flexion (°)	Rotation (°)
Cervical	10–20	4–11	2–7
Thoracic	4–12	5–9	2–9
Lumbar	9–12	3–8	1–2

3. Limitation of ROM: in a comparative in vitro study between different interspinous devices [7], the ROM for each implanted device was found to be particularly limited in extension, while the effects on flexion were less evident or absent (Fig. 6.2). Lateral flexion is only slightly or not at all affected by a reduction in ROM, while rotation remains essentially unchanged, as shown in Table 6.1. These findings agree with previous in vitro studies on cadavers [8] and in vivo postural MRI studies [6].
4. Movement of the instantaneous axis of rotation [9]: this effect occurs during extension when the device shows a tendency to act as a fulcrum, moving the normal IAR closer to itself with a consequent loading of the facet joints and the posterior pan of the fibrous ring.

Mineral Density and Tensile Strength of the Vertebral Bone

A fine shell of variable thickness that, in addition to distributing load, is also a semi-permeable membrane to nutrient agents, encloses a spongy trabecular structure whose branches are oriented in directions that offer appropriate resistance to compressive loads. Tried and tested equations establish the relationship between BMD (Bone Mineral Density) and the compression strength S_c and elastic modulus E_b of trabecular bone [10], respectively:

$$S_c \text{ oc } BMD^2$$
$$E_b \text{ oc } BMD^{2 \div 3}$$

This result shows that a reduction in mineral density of 30 % (e.g., in the case of osteoporosis) can halve the compression strength of bone. It is known that a lumbar vertebra body is able to support an external compression load of approximately 8 kN on average and the typical load exercised during walking on the same vertebra is in the order of approximately 3 times body weight. In other words, approximately 2 kN for an average 70 kg person, and up to five to six times body weight (=4 kN) when lifting a heavy object [11]. A safety factor of approximately 2 therefore seems to be present in the compression strength of the vertebrae of a young, healthy subject but the process of osteoporosis can drastically reduce the strength properties.

The tensile strength of spinous processes subject to compression forces in a craniocaudal direction therefore depends on the load itself and its distance of application from the peduncles, and also on the bone mineral density. The results of in vitro experiments on cadavers to measure the strength of the spinous processes by means of forces applied with hooks in a craniocaudal direction are given in the literature [12] and show that an average value of 339 N is affected by a strong BMD-dependent standard deviation and also reveal that fracture mechanisms may take place in three areas: in the vertebral body, in the peduncles, and in the spinous processes themselves. In a subsequent systematic in vitro study [13], the loads transmitted to the vertebrae during the process of inserting an X-STOP interspinous device (Fig. 6.2b) were measured and the ultimate tensile strength was related to the BMD. The load transmitted

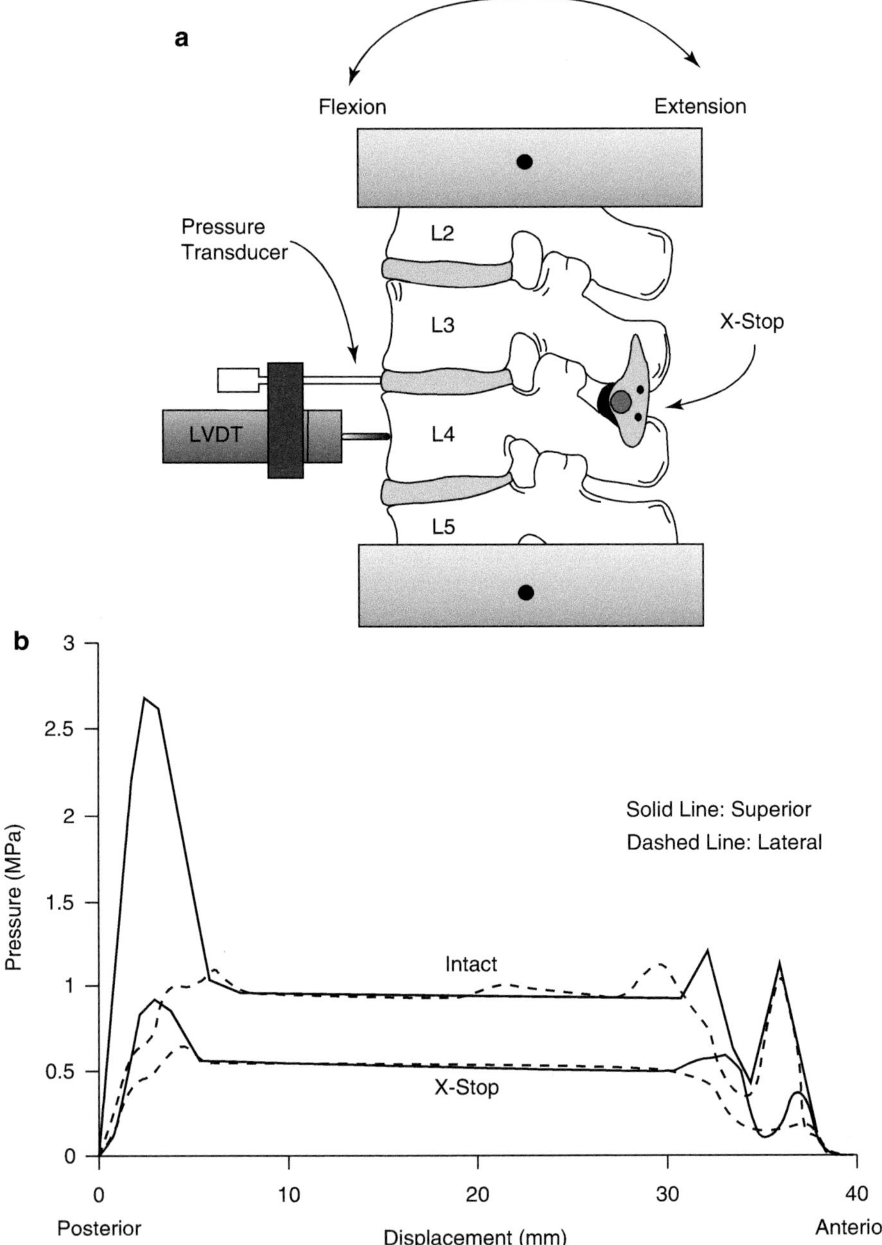

Fig. 6.2 (**a**) A schematic of the testing configuration for measuring intradiscal pressure with the X-STOP device inserted; (**b**) a representative plot of data collected at L3–L4 in extension with and without the X-STOP implant [18], courtesy of the author and with permission from Wolters Kluwer Health

in a craniocaudal direction during insertion was compared with the ultimate tensile strength of spinous processes subjected to loading in a lateral direction, when values of 65.6±46.2 and 316.9±195.5 N were obtained, respectively. These results agree with previous studies and the results discussed above for the relationship between ultimate tensile strength and BMD. The risk of the spinous processes breaking during insertion of an interspinous device is therefore low for subjects with good mineral density, but extreme caution is required in subjects with low mineral density.

Effect on Intradiscal Pressure and on the Facet Joints

An intervertebral disc consists of a nucleus pulposus and an annulus fibrosus. Loads transmitted by compression from the vertebral bodies are evenly distributed via hydrostatic pressure in the nucleus pulposus, which is in turn constrained by circumferential stresses set up in the layers of the fibrous ring, within which alternately oriented collagen fibers ensure the necessary mechanical strength. In degenerative processes, partial rehydration of the nucleus pulposus prevents the build-up of the necessary hydrostatic pressure, with consequent transfer of the load to the annulus fibrosus. This phenomenon is accentuated by combining compression with lateral and sagittal flexion movements [14, 15].

The function of the posterior elements is to determine the kinematics of the functional unit and implement motion. The transverse processes and spinous processes are an anchorage site for muscles and ligaments, while the three-dimensional configuration of the synovial joint of the facet joints determines segment mobility, particularly by limiting twisting movements of the lumbar vertebrae.

The configuration formed from the intervertebral disc and facet joints acts as a tripod to support vertebral loads, and we know from the literature that the contribution of the facet joints varies from 30 % during hyperextension to 10–20 % when standing erect and up to 50 % of the shear load in flexion [16]. The posterior thickness of the intervertebral discs also affects pressure in the synovial joint, exacerbating the negative effects of degenerative processes [17].

In some in vitro studies on cadavers with X-STOP devices [7, 8], it has been shown that intra-discal pressure is greatly reduced in a neutral position and during extension in a sagittal plane, while no significant differences are noted in other directions of motion. Information was subsequently added on spatial dependency of the pressure measurement probe position and the affected level, revealing that the biggest pressure drops occur at level L3–L4 (from 46 to 63 % in extension) and that the parts mainly involved are the anterior and posterior parts of the intervertebral disc [18] (Fig. 6.4a, b). It should be noted that the studies mentioned are based on hydrostatic pressure measurements in the nucleus pulposus and that this should be considered informative for cases of mild degeneration (up to grade I). As already mentioned, advanced processes of degeneration prevent the generation of intradiscal hydrostatic pressure, the measurement being strongly influenced by the position in which it is taken.

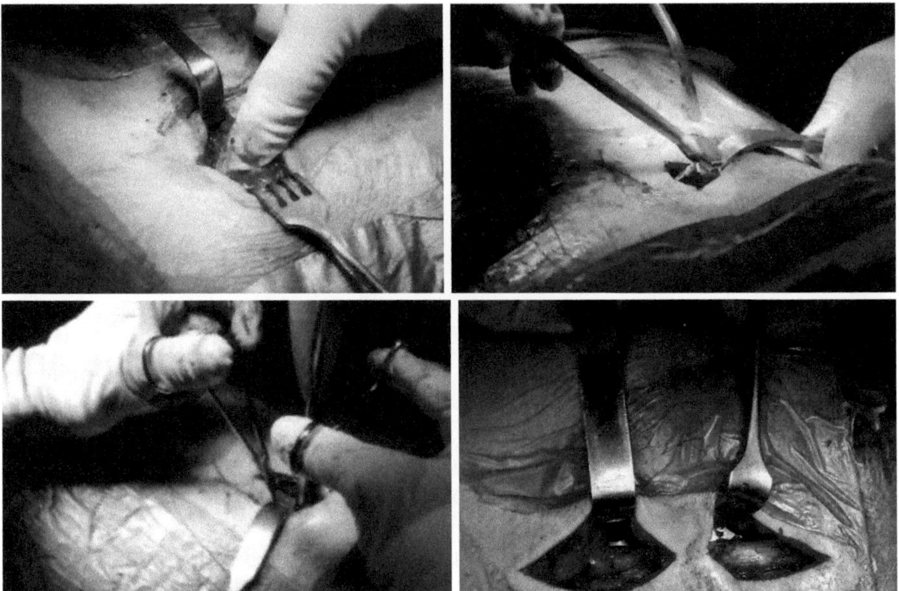

Figs. 6.3, 6.4, 6.5, and 6.6 Surgical exposure after performing a midline incision and preserving the caudal part of multifidus permits correct positioning of device

In an in vitro study with the X-STOP [19], it was shown that the device acts by reducing pressure in the synovial joint. It may therefore be said that the facet joints are directly affected by the presence of an interspinous device. The same study showed no changes in facet joint kinematics, while a pressure discharge of up to 55 % was recorded without affecting adjacent segment parameters (Fig. 6.5). The presence of a rigid element also acts as a fulcrum in extension movements by attracting toward itself the axis of instantaneous rotation that is normally located in an anterior position near the facet joints (Fig. 6.6a) during such movements, thus helping to relieve the load on the latter and on the rear part of the intervertebral disc.

Effects on the Spinal Ligament System

The ligaments are subdivided into intrasegmental (joining adjacent vertebrae) and intersegmental (connecting several vertebrae together). Each of these plays an important role in the stability of the functional unit [20], and the set of spinal ligaments provides a response to loads within the ROM subdivided into two areas: neutral and elastic.

All interspinous devices sacrifice part or all of these ligaments, particularly the interspinous ligament. Despite the considerable tissue damage suffered, the interspinous ligament is nevertheless able to offer residual rigidity; this outcome is assumed to be attributed to the fact that the collagen fibers are not really removed, although they are moved from their axial direction. Many authors consider that the supraspinous ligament performs a crucial role in functional unit stabilization processes [5]: as we can see from Fig. 6.6b, the posterior ligaments are put under tension in flexion movements and their distance from the axis of rotation guarantees a strong stabilizing moment (particularly of the supraspinous ligament), meaning that they constitute, for all intents and purposes, a system of tension bands. The presence of receptors in the above ligaments enables activation of the vertebral muscles to prevent excessive flexion [21]; it is therefore necessary to take into account the consequent loss of function when using devices that require complete sacrifice of the supraspinous ligament within the affected level.

Design of Interspinous Devices

Materials Used

The parts of the device that interface with the bone in the spinous processes are made using materials and configurations that guarantee the device has different biomechanical properties. PEEK (poly ether ether ketone) is commonly used in many devices because of its good elastic compliance with the spinous process cortical bone layer (which displays an elastic modulus of approximately 18 GPa) and due to the fact that it does not generate debris and is radiotransparent [22]. Some devices use visco-elastic materials such as silicone or titanium alloys in elastic configurations. The latter is widely used in the manufacture of prosthetic components because of its excellent biomechanical properties, and it is generally recommended in spinal implant protocols [23], particularly the alloy Ti–6Al–4 V ELI (extra-low interstitial), which offers good properties of mechanical strength, elasticity, lightness, workability, and corrosion resistance.

Advanced materials such as shape memory metal alloys are beginning to appear on the market. It is also possible to exploit other properties of these materials in addition to their thermo-plastic properties. For example, in the case of Ni-Ti alloys (Nitinol), the hyperelasticity considerably extends the range of applicability compared to conventional materials, without running the risk of elasto-plastic deformation [24, 25].

Testing and Simulation Instruments *(Table 6.2)*

The theoretical instruments available for investigating forces, moments, rigidity, strength, pressure, stress, and deformation are those typically used in the mechanics of continuums, statics and classic dynamics, poroelasticity, and fracture mechanics.

Table 6.2 Spinal tissues mechanical properties

Component	Young's modulus (MPa)	Poisson's modulus
Cortical bone	$3-20 \times 10^3$	0.3
Trabecular bone	300	0.2
Fibrous ring	450	0.3
Nucleus pulposus	1	0.499
PEEK	3.5×10^3	0.3
Ti–6Al–4V	120×10^3	0.3

These methods are often implemented in tried and tested software tools, particularly finite element (FE) analysis software, used to simulate the mechanical response of bodies with complex geometry and to optimize device design [25–28]. It is therefore possible to study the distribution of stresses and deformations under the action of complex external loads, and computer-aided engineering (CAE) software is helping the rapid development of computational biomechanical software by making it possible to implement optimization algorithms to resolve muscle recruitment issues. The FE method may also be reamed with bone remodeling algorithms for accurate distraction body design. The possibility that the distraction function of an over-rigid device or a device of inappropriate design may become ineffective over the long term must also be ruled out. Table 6.2 shows values commonly used to characterize the properties of spinal tissues and components analyzed using linear finite elements.

As far as interspinous distractors are concerned, simple FE simulations with linear elements are sufficient to calculate the forces at play in and around bone-implant interface, and the results agree with those available in the literature. More accurate studies with nonlinear elements have been carried out to examine the effect on a particular level of varying the distraction thickness. These revealed the advantages and limitations of FE simulations: according to the studies, distraction is the discriminating factor for the onset of forces and moments caused by implant insertion, while the elastic modulus of the device only minimally affects system response [29]. The same data only partly agree with the experimental results on intradiscal pressure [18], showing changes in relation to the level not fitted with a device only in the extension movements.

Verification Methods

Theories and premises adopted when designing an interspinous device are often validated by means of in vitro tests and experiments on cadavers, while it is rare to use instruments for the in vivo analysis of the above parameters because of their relatively invasive nature. In the latter case, the use of tried and tested diagnostic imaging tools to evaluate the anatomy and kinematics generally takes precedence over the use of instruments for the analysis of movement, in which it is sought to make inferences about internal kinematics through external measurement parameters [6].

The tests and validations required to obtain marketing authorization for spinal implants mainly refer to standards issued by international bodies, such as ISO and ASTM, which establish the tests required to check device strength, fatigue, and wear.

Interspinous device load patterns and failure modes have not yet been clearly delineated because of the complexity determined by the many factors at play [23, 30]. In the case of these devices, particular attention must also be paid to risks of migration and expulsion from their position between the spinous processes. To conclude, in order to analyze the risk of interspinous devices, rational adaptation of the above standards is required, together with further research and clinical evaluation studies.

Guidelines and Experience

Indications and Experience

According to Louis Breck and Compere Basom in 1943, conservative flexion treatment of the lumbosacral spine improved recurrent low back pain attacks. Positioning the lumbosacral spine in permanent flexion by in situ fusion of the interspinous space through distraction brought about permanent increasing of the intervertebral space and prevented recurrences in cases of disc bulging and also in canal stenosis with subluxation of the facet joints.

The same authors claimed that this surgical treatment was excellent, easier, and less dangerous, and that its approach was more biological than the invasive hemi-laminectomy surgery that was beginning to gain popularity at the time [31].

In his 1954 patent application, Knowles claimed that the indications for his metal interspinous device were lumbar spine instability, laxity of the facet joints, and disc bulging. The purpose of this surgical technique was therefore to support the spinous processes and to unload the rear part of the disc and the facet joints to slow down the degenerative process.

Knowles specified that a laminectomy operation with fusion costs the patient approximately 6 months of disability and emphasized that the advantages of this new surgical technique were simplicity of implementation, absence of complications, as well as short surgery times and post-operative recovery periods [32].

Although these claims were clear and up-to-date, Knowles unfortunately only mentioned them in the notes to his patent. This meant that they were not acknowledged and this surgery did not become common for many years.

The advent of Bronsard and his 'ligamentoplastie inter-épineuse' in 1987 brought a resurgence of interest in surgery performed in the interspinous space, and in 1988 Sénégas finally set out the scientific bases for the technique with a decidedly innovative approach. Sénégas himself was responsible for writing articles theorizing about a surgical strategy for early treatment of degenerative discal disease (DDD) that would reduce but not eliminate movements of the functional spinal unit (FSU), paving the way for biological effects to take place in the disc, which would be encouraged to regenerate by the cushioning effect of the device [33–35].

Sénégas suggested the following indications: Pfirrmann's grade 2, 3, 4 DDD [36], massive herniated disc in young patients, recurring disc hernias, conservation of segments adjacent to the fusion area, Modic's grade I disc space damage, and canal stenosis in combination with recalibrage.

The contraindications were as follows: Pfirrmann's grade 5 DDD, spondylolisthesis, osteoporosis, non-specific low back pain without a diagnosis, malformation of the spinous processes and treatment of the L5-S1 space.

Sénégas began experimenting with a titanium interspinous blocker and then moved on to a more flexible Wallis device in PEEK to avoid stress fractures of the spinous processes. Sénégas also emphasized that this method was fully reversible and did not affect the possibility of other future surgery in the treated space.

During the same period, another Frenchman brought about a significant advance in interspinous space surgery, clearly stating his indications: his name was Jean Taylor. He also believed that ligamentoplasty with DIAM, a technical precursor to the no-fusion technique, was a viable technical surgical alternative to joint fusion. His approach was subtle: his interspinous device aimed to distract and compress in synchrony, thus restoring space to the FSU by exploiting the ligamentotaxis of the supraspinous ligament. In effect, this "soft" ligamentoplasty changed the local conditions, reduced venous congestion, and brought about a decompressant effect on the spinal ganglia.

The indications were black disc, functional lumbar stenoses with retrolisthesis, lumbar hyperlordosis, discal rift, facet syndrome, and topping off of areas adjacent to areas of joint fusion. The contraindications were spondylolisthesis, instability, tumors, fractures, isthmic spondylolysis, and idiopathic scoliosis.

Taylor always maintained that particular care was required when positioning his DIAM interspinous device [37]. His first design did not envisage saving the supraspinous ligament, but his second version allowed the ligament to be saved in its entirety and laid the basis for a mini-invasive approach. He always stressed that, in spinal surgery, if the normal segmentation of the musculature is damaged, the intrinsic stability of the spine is impaired and the outcome is affected. He therefore describes a minimal approach that aims to safeguard the robust lumbar back aponeurosis insertion at the level of the spinous processes.

Taylor recommends that the fascia incision should be made approximately 1 cm from the spinous process and also suggests saving the powerful caudal and dorsal insertions of the multifidus muscle. The neurovascular connection to the multifidus muscle from the medial offshoot of the spinal dorsal branch can only be salvaged in interspinous device positioning operations that do not involve additional neurological time for lateral laminectomy.

The indications established for the use of interspinous spacers by the first designers have therefore not changed over the years.

Our experience in the use of interspinous devices began in 2004 with the DIAM in patients over 50 years of age who presented symptoms of neurogenic intermittent claudication (NIC) resulting from the presence of foramina (stenosis, selected cases of first-degree degenerative spondylolisthesis, and massive disc herniation).

NIC is defined as a specific set of symptoms, namely pain, heaviness, and sluggishness of the lower limbs that the patient reports while standing upright or walking and that regress completely when the patient assumes a seated position [38, 39].

Case Studies

Between 2006 and 2009, the Pisa University 1st Orthopaedic Clinic treated 40 patients with an interspinous device, 13 males and 27 females, with a mean age of 64 (range 34–89). The cases treated included 20 cases of foraminal stenosis with NIC, 4 of grade 1 degenerative spondylolisthesis, 14 herniated discs, and 2 cases of herniated disc recurrence.

In our case studies, the device was implanted at a single level in 14 cases and at two levels in 21 cases. In 4 selected cases requiring treatment at several levels, only three adjacent levels were treated because the patients' poor clinical condition meant that they were not suitable candidates for major surgery.

As far as the levels treated were concerned, the two levels where the interspinous device were positioned were L4–L5 and L3–L4 with 32 and 19 devices being inserted, respectively.

We also positioned the interspinous device at level L5–S1 in nine cases after carefully assessing, at the pre-operative and intra-operative stages, the presence of a sufficient support on the S1 spinous process.

Patients with macroinstability of the lumbar spine, degenerative scoliosis with a Cobb angle >25°, spondylolisthesis of a grade greater than 1, severe osteoporosis, Paget's disease, severe obesity, or systemic inflammatory diseases were not considered suitable candidates for treatment with an interspinous device.

The clinical diagnosis was confirmed in all patients by carrying out a static and dynamic X-ray examination and second-level exploration such as CT and MRI scans. For the purposes of careful pre-operative planning, we consider it essential to carry out a dynamic X-ray examination of the lumbar spine (maximum flexion and maximum extension) because this allows us to identify situations of segmental instability that would not otherwise be detected by static examination alone.

When choosing an "ideal" device to be implanted, we considered certain characteristics [5, 40]:

- Materials: to optimize the absorption of load forces and to prevent the periprosthetic fibrosis effects that have occurred with the use of certain Dacron devices [41].
- Invasiveness: meaning with respect to the bone and ligament structures of the spine and, in particular, the supraspinous ligament, which is sacrificed with the use of certain devices [5].

- Surgical technique: one that would allow the surgery to be carried out under local anesthetic and sedation.
- Short learning curve.
- Low potential for complications.

For this reason, we chose the X-STOP device because we consider it currently ideal for the treatment of patients with the conditions mentioned above [44–45].

The technique typically involves quick post-operative recovery by patients, who are able to stand from the first day with the aid of a rigid fabric corset, which we advise them to wear for the next 3 weeks. The patient is generally discharged on the day 3 after surgery. Clinical and X-ray checks are carried out 1 month after the operation and then every 3 months for 1 year.

Patients are assessed before surgery by means of the Visual Analog Scale (VAS) and the Oswestry Disability Index for the lumbar spine [42, 43]. The average preoperative VAS score was 8 out of a maximum of 10, while the average preoperative Oswestry Disability Index (ODI) was greater than 62.32 %, which is the mark of a high level of disability. Postoperatively, the VAS was 2 and the ODI was 19.1 %.

In the cases discussed here, we did not encounter intraoperative or postoperative complications and blood loss was always minimal. In follow-up X-rays, the implanted devices were always correctly positioned and we can report that no movement or migration occurred in any of the cases we followed up.

Our results allow us to confirm that, strictly for the above indications, the X-STOP device currently represents one of the most reliable interspinous devices for the treatment of degenerative diseases of the lumbosacral spine.

Surgical Technique and Clinical Cases

The surgical technique we used is mini-invasive and requires a median cutaneous incision a few centimeters long in proximity of the interspinous space to be created.

The patient is positioned in prone position with a support for abdominal decompression and under fluoroscopic control. We require the patient to be in a prone position with limbs bent in order to open the interspinous space, but we do not agree with extreme positions such as a genupectoral position, which would open the FSU excessively, making the measurement of the device to be implanted less accurate to gauge. In selected cases, the surgery may be carried out under local anesthesia (2 % lidocaine and 6 % naropine) and sedation.

We make the incision in the dorsolumbar fascia at a distance of approximately 1 cm from the median line, initially only in the right recess, cutting into the dorsoventral cephalic part of the multifidus muscle, and perform a "soft" spread with a finger that just reaches the joint process of the pertinent level (Fig. 6.3).

To preserve the caudal part of the multifidus muscle in its entirety, we maintain the opening with a deep hook on the muscle plane (Fig. 6.4).

We then introduce various probes into the interspinous space to penetrate the interspinous ligament, always with full preservation of the supraspinous ligament.

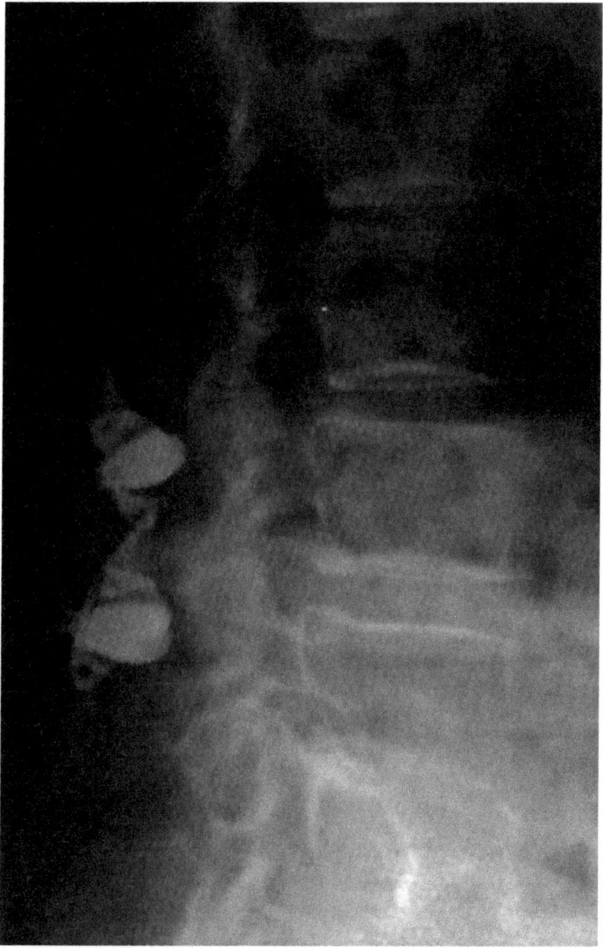

Fig. 6.7 Lateral X-ray showing two levels of implants

When choosing the size of the device, we consider it important to assess the tension of this ligament by carrying out various tests. Authors agree on the need to avoid excessive humping of the level [46]. The X-STOP may be inserted using the appropriate tool in the required size. At this point, we make an incision in the left recess and spread the multifidus muscle in the same way described for the contralateral recess to expose the screw entry hole for the stabilizing wings.

After positioning the screw and before tightening it with a torque screwdriver, we slide the wings toward the spinous processes along the appropriate guide with the aid of two Kocher clamps to prevent unwanted dislocations (Fig. 6.5).

The surgical technique is therefore quick and allows maximum preservation of the soft tissue. Without additional time for disc or radicular review, implantation of the X-STOP allows quick functional recovery by the patient, who is able to walk again on the first day after surgery (Figs. 6.6 and 6.7).

136 C. Giannetti et al.

Clinical case 1: Male aged 35. Bulging L4–L5 with discogenic low back pain and radicular irritation. Case resolved using a standalone L4–L5 interspinous device (Figs. 6.8 and 6.9).

Clinical case 2: Male aged 40. L4–L5 herniated disc with sacralization of L5. Hemilaminectomy, discectomy and L4–L5 interspinous device (Figs. 6.10 and 6.11).

Clinical case 3: Female aged 40. Right lombosciatic pain L4–L5 L5–S1 due to foraminal disk protrusion at two levels. Standalone L4–L5 and L5–S1 interspinous device (Figs. 6.12 and 6.13).

Clinical case 4: Diabetic and cardiopatic patient aged 73, affected by intermittent spinal claudication due to lumbar stenosis and left radicular pain. Positioning of two L3–L4 and L4–L5 standalone X-Stop interspinous device. After surgery, the left sciatic pain remained, and a post-operative MRI scan revealed the presence of a left foraminal and extra-foraminal hernia at L4–L5 level. The case was resolved after repeating the surgery with a left L4–L5 hemilaminectomy, disk cleanout at L4–S1 fusion stabilization, removal of the L4–L5 device, and maintenance of the L3–L4 interspinous device (Figs. 6.14, 6.15, and 6.16).

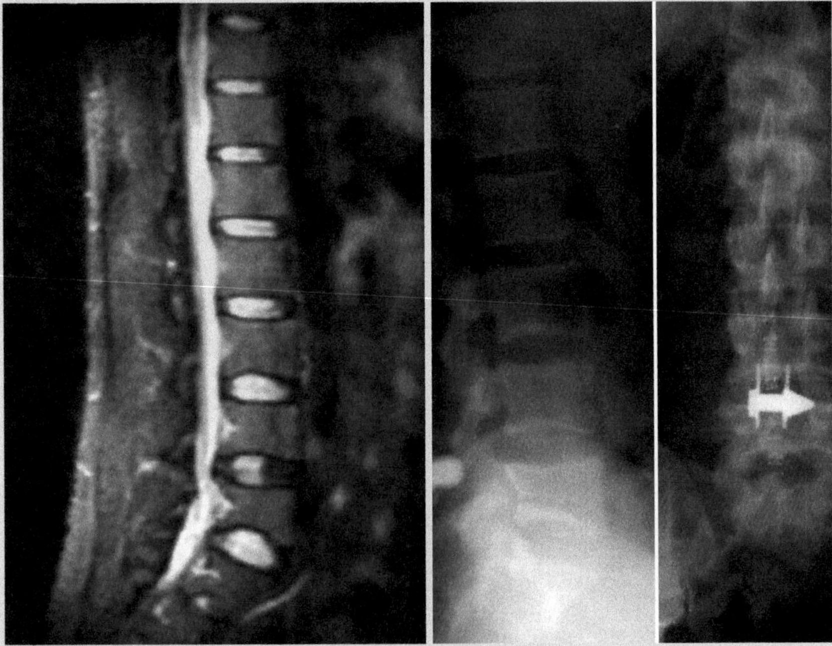

Figs. 6.8 and 6.9 Standalone L4–L5 interspinous device

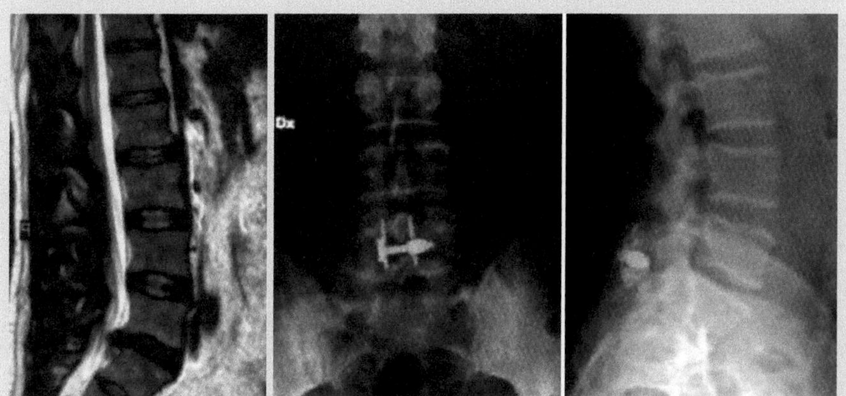

Figs. 6.10 and 6.11 Disc herniation treatment, interspinous device augmented after hemilaminectomy

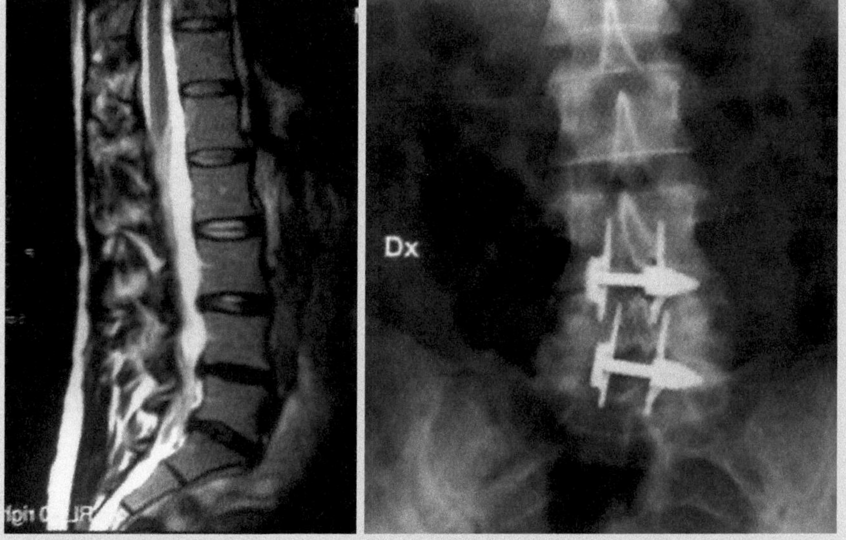

Figs. 6.12 and 6.13 Two levels disc protrusion, treated with interspinous device standalone

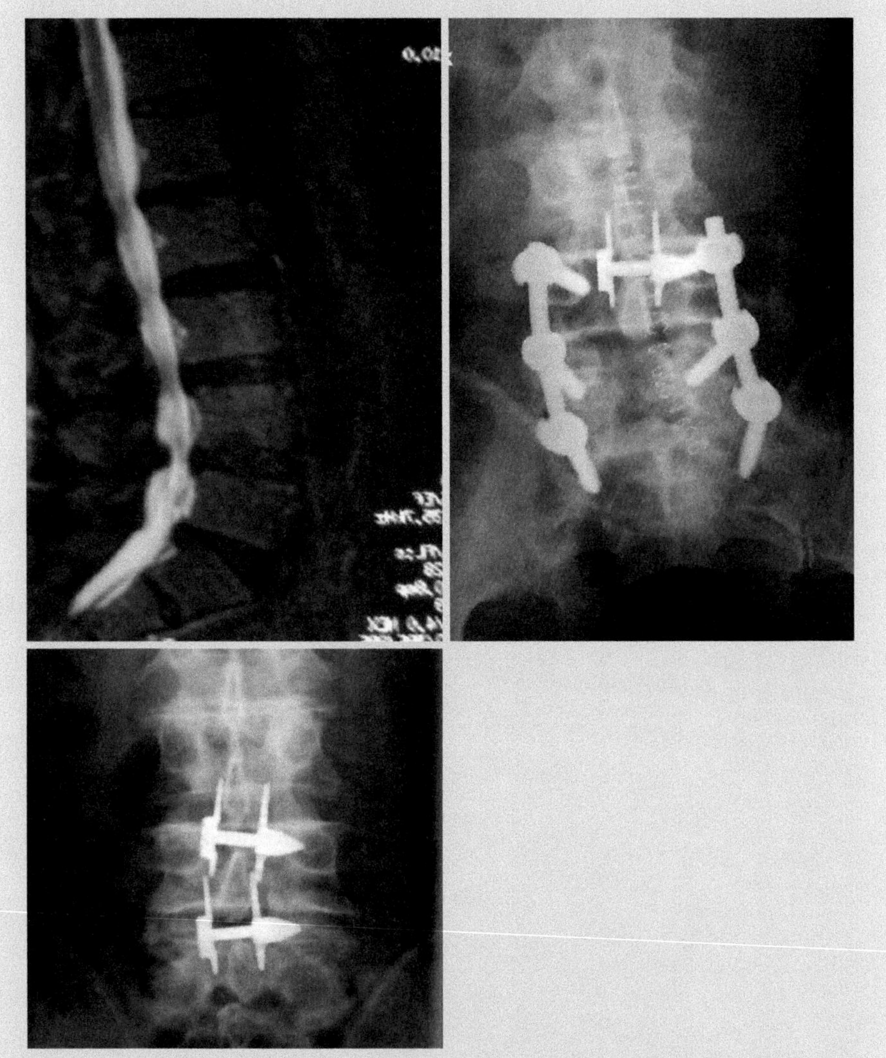

Figs. 6.14, 6.15, and 6.16 L3–L4, L4–L5 interspinous device implant, converted on L4–L5 in rod and screw

Complications Related to and Failure of Interspinous Devices

Interspinous distraction devices are a barely invasive treatment method, and in some cases the procedure may be carried out under local anesthesia. This reduces major complications, such as the neurological damage that is certainly more frequent in conventional open surgery. The main intra-operative complication that may occur is fracture of the spinous processes, which means that the implant will not hold.

We should remember, as described in Chap. 4, the force necessary to implant the X-STOP device on cadavers varies considerably according to bone density and is on average 66 N (range 11–150 N) [46]. Because the lateral force that must be applied to fracture the spinous processes is on average 317 N, there is an area of overlap between the maximum force applied to insert the device (150 N) and the minimum strength at which the spinous processes may fracture if weakened (95 N). Stress fractures are also described, particularly for titanium devices in osteoporotic and decompensated patients.

Jerosch et al. [42] described a foreign body reaction due to material debridement following the use of polythene interspinous spacers. We should also emphasize that the significant biological reaction of releasing polythene particles causes the onset of periprosthetic fibrosis, which renders revision surgery more complex.

We note that Verhooff et al. described a high rate of failure with the X-STOP in the treatment of first-degree degenerative spondylolisthesis with a high percentage of repeat surgery [47]. Little data is available in the literature on long-term mechanical failure, breakage and dislocation. The incidence varies according to the case studies considered and currently stands at about 3.8 % [48–51].

We should also mention that Floman et al. raised doubts over the efficacy of the Wallis device in reducing the rate of recurrence of herniated discs in patients who have undergone discectomy [52]. In our own experience with the X-STOP, the interspinous device was positioned at the incorrect level in two cases. Despite fluoroscopic monitoring, it is sometimes difficult to identify the exact level preselected for implantation, particularly in patients with lumbosacral hyperlordosis. We therefore always advise intraoperative and postoperative monitoring in order to avoid unpleasant medical and legal consequences.

Most cases of device failure are, therefore, the result of incorrect positioning or an error in the surgical indication.

We can nevertheless draw some points for further reflection from a review of our case studies. Although surgery with interspinous devices improves or resolves irradiated radicular symptoms of the lower limbs, the response of low back pain is variable and we did not find total and long-lasting resolution of this symptom, although a significant reduction in pain was achieved in some cases. This is probably due to the fact that these devices have an effect on the radicular conflict in the sense that they increase the foraminal area and decongest the root but that they can have no effect on the etiology of the low back pain, which is multi-factorial.

Regression of peripheral pain and rapid functional recovery often prompts more active patients to take up sports or activities that put the lumbosacral spine under excessive load. This causes the reappearance of the pain and functional limitation that regresses with medical treatment and rest.

References

1. Kapandji I. The physiology of the joints. In: The trunk and the vertebral column, vol. 3. Edinburgh: Churchill Livingstone; 1998.

2. Wnek G, Bowlin G. Encyclopedia of biomaterials and biomedical engineering. New York: Informa Healthcare; 2008.
3. Richards J, Majumdar S, Lindsey D, Beaupre G, Yerby S. The treatment mechanism of an interspinous process implant for lumbar neurogenic intermittent claudication. Spine. 2005;30(7):744.
4. Siddiqui M, Karadimas E, Nicol M, Smith F, Wardlaw D. Influence of X-STOP on neural foramina and spinal canal area in spinal stenosis. Spine. 2006;31(25):2958.
5. Bono C, Vaccaro A. Interspinous process devices in the lumbar spine. J Spinal Disord Tech. 2007;20(3):255.
6. Siddiqui M, Karadimas E, Nicol M. Effects of X-STOP device on sagittal lumbar spine kinematics in spinal stenosis. J Spinal Disord Tech. 2006;19(5):328–33.
7. Wilke H, Drumm J, Haussler K, Mack C, Steudel W, Kettler A. Biomechanical effect of different lumbar interspinous implants on flexibility and intradiscal pressure. Eur Spine J. 2008;17(8):1049–56.
8. Lindsey D, Swanson K, Fuchs P, Hsu K, Zucherman J, Yerby S. The effects of an interspinous implant on the kinematics of the instrumented and adjacent levels in the lumbar spine. Spine. 2003;28(19):2192.
9. Kim D, Cammisa F, Fessler R. Dynamic reconstruction of the spine. New York: Thieme Medical Pub; 2006.
10. Wittenberg R, Shea M, Swartz D, Lee K, White III A, Hayes W. Importance of bone mineral density in instrumented spine fusions. Spine. 1991;16(6):647.
11. Callaghan J, Pada A, McGill S. Low back three-dimensional joint forces, kinematics, and kinetics during walking. Clin Biomech. 1999;14(3):203–16.
12. Shepherd D, Leahy J, Mathias K, Wilkinson S, Hukins D. Spinous process strength. Spine. 2000;25(3):319.
13. Tal war V, Lindsey D, Fredrick A, Hsu K, Zucherman J, Yerby S. Insertion loads of the X-STOP interspinous process distraction system designed to treat neurogenic intermittent claudication. Eur Spine J. 2006;15(6):908–12.
14. Adams M, Dolan P. Recent advances in lumbar spinal mechanics and their clinical significance. Clin Biomech. 1995;10(I):3–19.
15. Adams M, McNally D, Dolan P. Stress distributions inside intervertebral discs. J Bone Joint Surg Br. 1996;78:965–72.
16. Boos N, Aebi M. Spinal disorders: fundamentals of diagnosis and treatment. Berlin/New York: Springer; 2007.
17. Dunlop R, Adams M, Hutton W. Disc space narrowing and the lumbar facet joints. J Bone Joint Surg Br. 1984;66(5):706–10.
18. Swanson K, Lindsey D, Hsu K, Zucherman J, Yerby S. The effects of an interspinous implant on intervertebral disc pressures. Spine. 2003;28(I):26.
19. Wiseman C, Lindsey D, Fredrick A, Yerby S. The effect of an interspinous process implant on facer loading during extension. Spine. 2005;30(8):903.
20. Sharma M, Langrana N, Rodriguez J. Role of ligaments and facets in lumbar spinal stability. Spine. 1995;20(8):887–900.
21. Adams M, Dolan P. Spine biomechanics. J Biomech. 2005;38(10):1972–83.
22. Kurtz S, Devine J. PEEK biomarerials in trauma, orthopedic, and spinal implants. Biomaterials. 2007;28(32):4845–69.
23. Goel VK, Panjabi MM, Patwardhan AG, Dooris AP, Serhan H. American Society for Testing and Materials. J Bone Joint Surg Am. 2006;88 Suppl 2:103–9.
24. Duerig T, Pelton A, Stockel D. An overview of nitinol medical applications. Mater Sci Eng A. 1999;A273–275:149–160.
25. Vena P, Franzoso G, Gastaldi D, Contra R, Dallolio V. A finite element model of rhe L4-L5 spinal motion segment: biomechanical compatibility of an interspinous device. Comput Methods Biomech Biomed Engin. 2005;8(1):7–16.
26. Zhang Q, Teo E. Finite element application in implant research for treatment of lumbar degenerative disc disease. Med Eng Phys. 2008;30(10):1246–56.

27. Lafage V, Gangner N, Senegas J, Lavasre F, Skalli W. New interspinous implant evaluation using an in vitro biomechanical study combined with a finite-element analysis. Spine. 2007;32(16):1706.
28. Minns R, Walsh W. Preliminary design and experimental studies of a novel soft implant for correcting sagittal plane instability in rhe lumbar spine. Spine. 1997;22(16):1819.
29. Rohlmann A, Zander T, Burra N, Bergmann G. Effect of an interspinous implant on loads in the lumbar spine/Einuss eines interspinosen Implantars auf die Belasrungen der Lendenwirbelsaule. Biomed Tech (Berl). 2005;50(10):343–7.
30. Kurtz S, Edidin A. Spine technology handbook. Amsterdam/Boston: Academic; 2006.
31. Louis W, Breck LW, Basom WC. The flexion treatment for low-back pain: indications, outline of conservative management, and a new spine-fusion procedure. J Bone Joint Surg Am. 1943;25:58–64.
32. Knowles FL. Apparatus for treatment of the spinal column. Patented I954 n.2677369.
33. Sénégas J. La ligamentoplastie intervertébrale, alternative à l'arthrodèse dans le traitement des instabilitiés dégénératives. Acta Orthop Belg. 1991;57 Suppl 1:221–6.
34. Sénégas J, Etchevers JP, Baulny D, Grenier F. Widening of the lumbar vertebral canal as an alter-native to laminectomy, in the treatment of lumbar stenosis. Fr J Orthop Surg. 1988;2:93–9.
35. Sénégas J, Vital JM, Guérin J, Bernard P, M'Barek M, Loreiro M, Bouvet R. Stabilisation lombaire souple. In: Gastambide D, editor. GlEDA: instabilités vertébrales lombaires. Paris: Expansion Scientifique Française; 1995. p. 122–32.
36. Pfirrman CWA, Metzdorf A, Zanetti M, Hadler J, Boos N. Magnetic resonance classification of lumbar intervertebral disc degeneration. Spine. 2001;26:4873–8.
37. Taylor J, Ritland S. Technical and Anatomical Consideration fot the Placement of a Posterior Interspinous Stabilizer. H.M.Mayer (ed.) Minimally Invasive Spine Surgery Second Edition 2006:466–75.
38. Katz JN. Lumbar spinal fusion. Surgical rates, costs, and complications. Spine. 1995;20(24 Suppl):78S–83.
39. Sengupta OK. Dynamic stabilization devices in the treatment of low back pain. Orthop Clin North Am. 2004;35(1):43–56.
40. Christie SD, Song JK, Fessler RG. Dynamic interspinous process technology. Spine. 2005;30(16 Suppl):S73–8.
41. Jerosch J, Moursi MG. Foreign body reaction due to polyethylene's wear after implantation of an interspinal segment. Arch Orthop Trauma Surg. 2008;128(1):1–4.
42. Fairbank JC, Pynsent PB. The Oswestry disability index. Spine. 2000;25(22):2940–52.
43. Zucherman JF, Hsu KY, Hartjen CA, Mehalic TF, lmplicito DA, Martin MJ, Johnson 2nd DR, Skidmore GA, Vessa PP, Dwyer JW, Puccio S, Cauthen JC, Ozuna RM. A prospective randomized multi-center study for the treatment of lumbar spinal stenosis with the X-STOP interspinous implant: 1-year results. Eur Spine J. 2004;13(1):22–31.
44. Zucherman JF, Hsu KY, Hartjen CA, Mehalic TF, lmplicito DA, Martin MJ, Johnson 2nd DR, Skidmore GA, Vessa PP, Dwyer JW, Puccio ST, Cauthen JC, Ozuna RM. A multicenter, prospective, randomized trial evaluating the X-STOP interspinous process decompression system for the treatment of neurogenic intermittent claudication: two-year follow-up results. Spine. 2005;30(12):1351–8.
45. Schönström N, Lindahl S, Willen J, Hansson T. Dynamic changes in the dimension of the lumbar spinal canal: an experimental study in vitro. J Orthop Res. 1989;7(1):115–21.
46. Inufusa A, An HS, Lim TH, Hasegawa T, Haughton VM, Nowicki BH. Anatomic changes of the spinal canal and intervertebral foramen associated with flexion-extension movement. Spine. 1996;21(21):2412–20.
47. Verhoof OJ, Bron JL, Wapstra FH, van Royen BJ. High failure rate of the interspinous distraction device (X-STOP) for the treatment of lumbar spinal stenosis caused by degenerative spondylolisthesis. Eur Spine J. 2008;17(2):188–92.
48. Schwarzenbach O, Berlemann U, Stoll TM, Dubois G. Posterior dynamic stabilization systems: DYNESYS. Orthop Clin North Am. 2005;36(3):363–72.

49. Serkan I. Posterior dynamic stabilization of the lumbar spine. WSJ. 2007;1(2):62–7.
50. Khoueir P, Kim K, Wang M. Classification of posterior dynamic stabilization devices. Neurosurg Focus. 2007;22(1):E3.
51. Whitesides TE. The effect of an interspinous implant on vertebral disc pressures (letter). Spine. 2003;28:1906–8.
52. Chiu JC. Interspinous process decompression (IPD) system (X-STOP) for the treatment of lumbar spinal stenosis. Surg Technol Int. 2006;15:265–75.

Chapter 7
Less Invasive Decompression and Posterolateral Fusion Using Interlaminar Lumbar Instrumented Fusion (ILIF) with or Without Supplemental Transforaminal Lumbar Interbody Fusion (TLIF)

Anton A. Thompkins

Introduction

In the United States, lumbar spinal stenosis (LSS) is the most common indication for lumbar spine surgery in those over 65 years of age [1]. The prevalence of LSS in the population is estimated at 8–11 % and disproportionately affects the elderly [2]. The rapidly expanding elderly population brought on by maturation of "baby boomers" (59 % increase expected from 2010 to 2025 to 64 million people) confluences with extended life expectancy to bring about cubic growth curve in the incidence of LSS when factoring in the increases in both the population rate (per 100,000 people) and absolute number of those afflicted [2, 3]. This results in a growing need to manage this disease with efficient, appropriate, and cost-effective treatment.

Medical management of LSS can, as can most spine-related diagnoses, be performed with a continuum of methodologies and interventions ranging from physical therapy to complex spinal fusion. Unfortunately, inconsistency within the literature detailing the best course of treatment for LSS complicates evidence-based practice. Nonoperative care in those with severe symptoms has been largely shown to be an ineffective permanent solution [4–8], while simple decompressions provide early (1 year) relief that is not always maintained in longer follow-up [9–11]. Arthrodesis in the treatment of LSS, while being a definitive and largely successful procedure with maintenance of outcome [4, 6, 7], is considered by some to be controversial in patients without concomitant instability or disc pathology. Additionally, and possibly more importantly, advanced age and the resultantly more frequent presence of medical comorbidities have led some surgeons to avoid surgical intervention [12], at least when using conventional open-exposure surgical approaches and procedures.

A.A. Thompkins, MD
Department of Orthopaedic, Lakeshore Bone and Joint Institute,
Chesterton, IN, USA
e-mail: kmalone@nuvasive.com

P.P.M. Menchetti (ed.), *Minimally Invasive Surgery of the Lumbar Spine,*
DOI 10.1007/978-1-4471-5280-4_7, © Springer-Verlag London 2014

Modern, minimally disruptive surgical approaches have more recently been introduced into the surgical armamentarium that enable treatment in patients previously contraindicated or considered higher risk for surgery (i.e., those with advanced age or significant medical comorbidity), with significantly lower morbidity [13–15]. Interlaminar lumbar instrumented fusion (ILIF®, NuVasive, Inc., San Diego, CA), and a modification of the procedure to incorporate a specialized transforaminal lumbar interbody fusion (TLIF), is one such procedure that has been developed to treat the continuum of the disease LSS and which will be the subject of the following chapter.

Background/Etiology

Lumbar spinal stenosis is a condition of later life, typically presenting in the fifth or sixth decades. [16]. It can be a complex disease process and is often one part of a multifactorial degenerative cascade, though congenital factors (such as vertebral malformations) may also contribute to LSS [3, 9]. LSS is defined as a narrowing of the central spinal canal or neuroforamen [3, 6, 9]. LSS is most often the result of soft tissue or bony degeneration encroaching upon the neural elements. Intervertebral disc bulging herniation, facet arthropathy, ligamentum flavum hypertrophy or buckling, degenerative spondylolisthesis, and degenerative scoliosis is regularly associated with this condition [3, 9, 17]. As previously mentioned, prevalence of symptomatic stenosis in the general population is estimated to be between 8 % and 11 %, though as many as 20 % of the population may exhibit a radiographic diagnosis of stenosis asymptomatically [2, 12]. The most common level for LSS is L4–5, followed by L3–4, L2–3, and then L5–S1 [16, 18, 19].

Three main classifications of LSS exist: central stenosis, lateral or lateral recess stenosis, and neuroforaminal stenosis [9]. Central stenosis represents a decrease in the cross-sectional area of the spinal canal and is often associated with ligamentum flavum thickening, intervertebral disc bulging, or with bony abnormalities affecting the canal area (e.g., osteophytes, congenitally short pedicles). Congenital stenosis, however, is a relatively rare diagnosis, seen in only approximately 9 % of LSS patient population [16]. Lateral stenosis commonly accompanies central narrowing and is notably different from neuroforaminal stenosis, though both lateral and neuroforaminal stenosis affect existing nerve roots/spinal nerves rather than the cauda equina. Exiting lumbar nerve roots immediately travel through the lateral recess, a relatively small bony passageway bordered by the pedicle laterally, the superior articular facet posteriorly, and anteriorly by the posterior aspect of the vertebral body. Lateral recess stenosis is more common than neuroforaminal stenosis as this passageway is substantially smaller than the neuroforamen and is more sensitive to encroachment by intervertebral disc bulging and facet arthropathy. Foraminal stenosis is most commonly seen with degenerative spondylisthesis or an intervertebral disc herniations and is rarely seen outside of these diagnosis.

There are multiple mechanisms by which LSS can cause neural impairment and a variety of clinical presentations. LSS symptoms are most commonly caused by direct mechanical compression of the nerve roots or spinal nerves [16]. However, venous congestion and reduced arterial flow, resulting in increased epidural pressure, are commonly associated with multilevel LSS and is directly related to neurogenic claudication [6, 17]. Additionally, local inflammatory processes in LSS can result in nerve root or spinal nerve Irritation.

Presentation/Investigation/Treatment Options

Presentation/Evaluation

As LSS is often one part of a multifaceted disease complex, a single definitive differential diagnosis does not exist. Instead, a detailed patient history, physical examination, and variety of imaging studies are needed to determine the presence, location, and severity of LSS as well as any accompanying pathology such as degenerative spondylolisthesis or scoliosis [2, 3, 12]. Clinically, LSS often presents as low back pain and/or leg pain with or without neurogenic claudication [16]. Severe cases of LSS may exhibit myelopathic symptoms or cauda equina syndrome, including lower extremity motor deficits, sensory loss, and/or loss of bowel or bladder function [6, 9, 16]. In such extreme cases, immediate surgical intervention is normally indicated.

Physical evaluation should include a detailed review of both neurological and mechanical symptoms [16]. Patients with primarily neurological symptoms will generally exhibit characteristics of neurogenic claudication and radiculopathies. Mechanical symptoms, conversely, will present mainly as back pain.

Neurogenic claudication has been described as a "constellation of symptoms," of which central stenosis may be only one contributing factor [17]. Neurogenic claudication secondary to stenosis more commonly affects women than men and generally presents as discomfort in the lower extremities, often brought on by walking or activity [17]. Symptoms of vascular claudication and neurogenic claudication are similar. Any evaluation of neurogenic claudication should begin with a detailed patient history to rule out peripheral vascular disease. Evaluation of symptoms should show a proximal to distal progression on onset during neurogenic claudication with distal to proximal progression in vascular claudication. A useful test to differentiate neurogenic claudication from peripheral vascular disease includes evaluating symptoms following a walk downhill as well as a bicycle ride. In neurogenic claudication, symptoms will often be exacerbated on the downhill walk and non-apparent in cycling [17]. Peripheral vascular disease symptoms are often exacerbated by cycling, while symptoms are attenuated on a treadmill [16].

Walking and stoop tests are common examination techniques for neurogenic claudication. A walking test includes a self-paced walk with recording of the distance walked prior to onset of symptoms, typically weakness, tiredness, or a heaviness of the lower extremities [20]. The threshold for walking is approximately twice the distance from when the patient first experiences discomfort [17]. A stoop test includes evaluation of symptom resolution following hitting the stop point on the walking test and instructing the patient to lean on a wall or stoop to tie a shoelace (flexion). In patients with neurogenic claudication, symptom resolution generally follows with this test or with lying supine or when sitting.

All history and physical evaluations for LSS should be accompanied by several modalities of imaging. Standing static and dynamic radiography should be obtained on all patients to evaluate any bony or gross abnormalities. Static films can be used to determine the presence of spondylolisthesis, deformity, or osteophytes, while dynamic films can be used to determine the presence of instability. Instability has been defined by Posner et al. [21] as horizontal translation on lateral dynamic films of at least 8 % anteriorly or 9 % posteriorly when evaluating single levels between L1–2 and L4–5 and of at least 6 and 9 % at L5–S1, respectively. Angular displacement is also defined as a measure of instability, with at least −9° displacement on flexion for levels L1–2 through L4–5 and of +1° at L5–S1 qualifying as instability.

Magnetic resonance imaging (MRI) is considered the "gold standard" imaging study for evaluating stenosis. On MRI, the intervertebral disc can be visualized to determine the extent and nature of any degenerative processes (e.g., bulging, prolapse, degeneration), and the quality of the disc can be evaluated on T2-weighted images, where healthy discs exhibit increased proton signal at the nucleus pulposus and a decreased signal in degenerative discs. Axial views are useful in determining the extent of central and lateral stenosis, while sagittal MRI reconstructions are the most useful imaging modality in evaluating neuroforaminal stenosis. A determining criterion in neuroforaminal stenosis is the absence of fat around the nerve roots in the foramen on MRI due to stenosis.

Myelography and CT myelography are also useful in determining the extent of central stenosis. In patients with stenosis, an "hourglass"-shaped dura at the level of the intervertebral disc is characteristic of central stenosis and is consistent in diagnosis of stenosis at multiple levels in a patient with neurogenic claudication symptoms. CT myelography provides additional detail, with an ability to evaluate stenosis in multiple planes as well as being able to evaluate the integrity of the nerve root sleeve.

As LSS impacts the elderly and females disproportionately, a dual-energy X-ray absorptiometry (DEXA) study can be performed to evaluate bone mineral density, especially in surgically indicated patients.

Treatment Options

Following a positive LSS diagnosis, a detailed medical treatment plan should be made with the patient. Considerations in determining a course of treatment should include the severity of symptoms and their effect on the patient, patient expectations from treatment, the ability for the patient to tolerate certain medical interventions, and the physician's preference and ability with such interventions. Except in extreme cases or in those patients with cauda equina syndrome, medical management of LSS typically begins with a course of nonoperative care. Common nonoperative treatments for patients with LSS include orthotics, bed rest, nonsteroidal anti-inflammatory drugs (NSAIDs), narcotic medication, oral corticosteroids, physical and rehabilitation therapy, or epidural steroid injections.

NSAIDs and/or glucocorticosteroids can be used as part of a "first-line" anti-inflammatory therapy, though care must be taken with their long-term use as NSAIDs may cause cardiovascular or gastrointestinal side effects. In long-term use, liver and kidney function should be monitored by a primary care physician. In addition to nonsteroidal anti-inflammatory drugs, oral steroids (e.g., prednisolone, methylprednisolone) may also be effective. If prescribed, care should be taken in patients with diabetes as oral steroids may elevate blood glucose.

Lumbar flexion and isometric core strengthening exercises are appropriate rehabilitation exercises in addition to low-impact aerobic conditioning. In any rehabilitation or physical therapy, evaluation of patient tolerance for certain activities which may exacerbate stenotic symptoms (i.e., walking) may be replaced with aquatic therapy or recumbent bicycle riding.

Epidural steroid injection therapy is an additional means of nonsurgical intervention in the treatment of LSS, further along the invasiveness continuum of medical treatment than other forms of nonoperative care. The role and efficacy of injection therapy has been debated in the literature for some time, though more recent studies have suggested a positive dose effect exists in some patients. Manchikanti et al. [22], in a randomized, double-blind, controlled trial of 120 patients receiving lumbar facet injections with either a local anesthetic alone or local anesthetic with steroids, found that between 85 and 90 % of patients (depending on treatment group) with chronic function-limiting low back improved with the administration of analgesic injections with or without steroids.

Most patients with mild symptoms associated with LSS are adequately managed with nonoperative care, often indefinitely [1, 6, 23]. In a study of Medicare patients with a first-time diagnosis of LSS, Chen et al. [24] found that only 21 % of patients subsequently went on to have surgery within 3 years of diagnosis. However, in patients with multiple degenerative processes, instability, myelopathy, and/or other progressing or moderate to severe LSS symptoms, surgical intervention is generally warranted and shows significant clinical gains compared to nonoperative care [3–8]. In a study of 49 patients treated nonoperatively for LSS and followed for an average of 3 years after their first LSS diagnosis, Simotas et al. [8] found that 19 % of patients had undergone surgical intervention. Of those remaining who did not subsequently undergo surgical treatment in the study timeframe, 5 % experienced significant motor function deterioration, 13 % had symptom worsening, 30 % experienced no change in symptoms, and 28 % reported a mild improvement in symptoms, while only 30 % reported a sustained improvement in symptoms.

Simple Decompressions

Laminectomy is considered to be the "gold standard" treatment for lumbar spinal stenosis [11, 16]. Such pedicle-to-pedicle decompressions are useful in treating central and lateral stenosis as the canal is obviously decompressed with the removal of the laminas, but access is also gained to the subarticular and neuroforaminal space facilitating direct nerve root decompression. Laminectomy, however, has largely been replaced with alternative decompression techniques for a variety of reasons. First, the wide decompression afforded by laminectomy (in those cases with >50 % resection of the facet joints) [10, 25] results in iatrogenic destabilization of the spine. This, paired with bony regrowth and epidural fibrosis development, has been associated with progressively increasing postoperative symptoms in some patients, known as failed back/back surgery syndrome or post-laminectomy syndrome/instability [9, 26–28]. A study by Martin et al. [29] found that surgically indicated recurrent stenosis following laminectomy occurred in nearly 20 % of patients. In study by Postacchini et al. [28] in 40 patients treated with a decompression for LSS (32 patients received laminectomy, 8 laminotomy), the authors found that 88 % of patients had radiographic evidence of posterior vertebral arch regrowth, and in those with "marked regrowth," only 40 % reported a satisfactory clinical results. This regrowth positively correlated with instability at the postoperative spinal level, due either to iatrogenic factors or to the presence of spondylolisthesis.

As a result of these challenges with laminectomy, bilateral laminotomy was increasingly adopted to provide a vehicle for similar, though slightly more limited, decompression while maintaining the central portion of the osteoligamentous arch and, thus, better preserving segmental stability. This largely remains a viable option for simple decompression in the treatment of LSS, though central stenosis has the potential to be inadequately addressed due to the maintenance of the central portion of the osteoligamentous arch.

Both laminectomy and laminotomy are primarily carried out using conventional surgical approaches and open exposures. This results in elevated associated surgical morbidity and has been described as a consideration against surgical intervention in medical decision making in elderly patients, potentially opting for less effective treatment protocols (nonoperative care) due to elevated risk of complication using conventional exposure procedures. Several examples of decompression morbidity include Deschuyffeler et al. [30] in 2012 reporting a 17.1 % complication rate in patients over 65 who underwent a unilateral laminotomy with bilateral decompression. A study by Kaymaz et al. [31] found similar results in laminectomy, with a complication rate of 19 % and incidence of failed back surgery syndrome of 8 % at between 6 and 12 months postoperatively.

Fusions

The addition of arthrodesis to decompressive procedures for LSS remains controversial, with a few exceptions. These exceptions include LSS accompanied by instability (iatrogenic or degenerative), degenerative spondylolisthesis, deformity (scoliosis or kyphosis), or cases of recurrent stenosis [10, 32]. Additionally, fusion is indicated in patients undergoing a decompression requiring removal of more than 50 % the facet, in those undergoing total laminectomy or laminotomy who are middle-aged and/or the intervertebral disc of the segment involved has normal or near-normal height (suggesting substantial anterior column mobility predisposing posterior decompressions to failed back syndrome), or in patients with segmental hypermobility, especially with back pain as the predominant symptom [9].

Despite the ongoing debate over fusion (and fusion type) for LSS alone, lumbar fusion has been found to be effective in more definitively treating LSS and has been shown to have incrementally superior outcomes than simple decompressions in some indications. Yone et al. [11] studied a series of patients treated with decompression with or without fusion for either LSS alone or LSS with instability. In the LSS with instability group, patients were treated with fusion procedures and realized an 80 % excellent or good clinical result. In those with LSS with instability who underwent a simple decompression, excellent or good outcomes were achieved in only 29 % of patients. Finally, in patients with LSS without instability who underwent simple decompression, patients fared similarly to fusion patients through 1 year postoperative, though their outcome precipitously deteriorated thereafter, settling on a 47 % excellent or good outcome rate at last follow-up. Many other high-quality studies have similarly found an incremental improvement in performing fusions for more advanced presentations of LSS (e.g., instability, spondylolisthesis, scoliosis) [4, 5, 7, 23]. In an analysis of fusion outcome by diagnosis, Glassman et al. [33] found that degenerative spondylolisthesis and scoliosis with concomitant LSS were two of the most responsive diagnoses to treatment with spinal fusion in terms of improvement in pain, disability, quality of life, and number of patients who met minimally clinically important difference.

Differences between uninstrumented and instrumented fusion mostly are related to patient and pathologic characteristics as well as surgeon preference. In patients with a likelihood for pseudoarthrosis (i.e., smoker, metabolic disease) or in spinal segments with normal anterior or hypermobile anterior segments or inherent instability (spondylolisthesis), instrumented fusions have been found to be superior to non-instrumented fusion [34–36]. In a comparative study of instrumented and non-instrumented fusion in the treatment of LSS with instability, Fischgrund et al. [34] found that 83 % of patients who underwent instrumented posterolateral fusion (PLF) went on to fuse, in contrast to fusion in only 45 % of those with uninstrumented fusions. Also, clinical outcomes were categorized as excellent or good in 86 % of those who were fused, while the same outcome was only achieved in 56 % of those who were not fused.

A Level I evidence literature review evaluating outcomes of LSS treatment with spinal fusion compared to nonoperative care found in all studies that operative care significantly improved pain, disability, and quality of life compared to nonoperative care. When taking into consideration the expanding elderly population and their extended life expectancy in connection to the relatively high incidence of subsequent reoperation in decompression, fusions may increasingly become more commonplace in order to treat LSS more definitively in an attempt to avoid reoperation when medical comorbidities are likely to be increased [3, 6].

One drawback to fusion is that conventional surgical approaches for fusion have been associated with higher complications rates when compared to those of simple decompressions [2, 33]. For example, single-level TLIF has been associated with complication rates as high as 46 % and early reoperation rates (many for infections) as high as 10 % [37]. The development of modern minimally disruptive approaches for fusion has led to the expanded availability of surgery to patients who were previously considered to be high-risk patients, namely, the elderly [15]. This host of newly developed approaches and instrumentation allow for more effective and expeditious treatment, minimizing the rate of complication and hastening postoperative recovery.

While several interspinous spacers are currently available for use in the USA, those which do not incorporate posterior fusion as part of their procedure have been challenged in adoption by elevated rates of complication, restenosis, and revision [38]. In a series of 13 patients treated with an interspinous, non-fusion device at the University of Utah, immediate postoperative clinical improvement deteriorated over the course of a 43-month follow-up, ultimately resulting in 77 % of patients experiencing return of preoperative symptoms, with a final "failure rate" of patients requiring reoperation of 85 %. A perioperative complication rate of 38 % was also realized.

Interspinous spacers paired with grafting and rigid fixation, making up a posterolateral fusion construct, have a long history in spinal surgery, and early results of newly designed procedures (ILIF) show promise in being able to provide adequate decompression with sufficient long-term segmental stability through a less invasive midline exposure in patients with LSS. In the early 1900s, Russell Hibbs and Fred Albee developed and published, independently of each other, procedures for fusion of the posterior lumbar spinal elements [39, 40]. These procedures were originally used primarily to treat Pott's disease and required autogenous bone graft harvested from the spinous processes or tibia and then laid along the interlaminar space to stop motion between the segments by fusing together posterior elements of the vertebrae. Following treatment, even using these rudimentary techniques (by today's standards), early positive clinical outcomes were reported. In most cases, disease progression was stopped following fusion and improvements in pain were realized. Further development of the procedure was outlined in a report by Howorth [41], in which he highlighted the advances made in spinal fusion procedures. These advancements include a more focused approach of harvesting autogenous graft material from other parts of the body (e.g., tibia) and stressing orientation of the graft material for solid fusion. More recently, focus has been to preserve as much of the posterior segment as possible while still decompressing the spinal canal in order to relieve pain [25].

ILIF uses some of the early principles of Hibbs' fusion, though with a medialized and less invasive surgical exposure, implementation of decompression laminoplasty [25] to adequately decompress the segment while not compromising endogenous stability, and has an option to perform a specialized interlaminar grafting and interspinous plating to perform and maintain the posterior decompression with posterolateral fusion.

Interlaminar lumbar instrumented fusion is indicated for a variety of thoracolumbar pathologies. Primarily, ILIF is indicated for stenosis with or without mild to

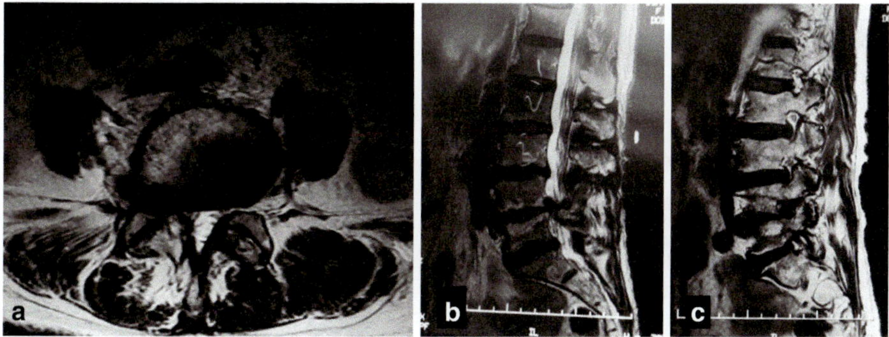

Fig. 7.1 (a–c) Magnetic resonance imaging (MRI) showing lumbar spinal stenosis primarily at the L4–5 disc space on axial view and sagittal reconstruction

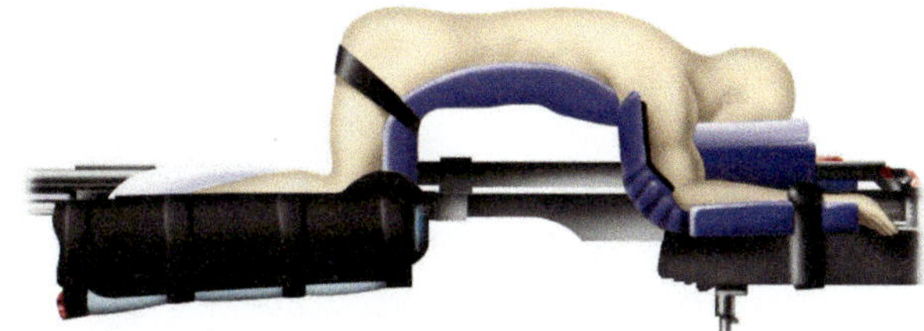

Fig. 7.2 Lateral view of a patient in the prone position in a Wilson frame, one possible patient positioning for the interlaminar lumbar instrumented fusion (ILIF®, NuVasive, Inc., San Diego, CA) procedure

moderate instability. It is also indicated for the treatment of degenerative disc disease, trauma, spondylolisthesis, and tumors. Potential limitations to use of the ILIF procedure include patients with inadequate bone stock or quality.

Surgical Technique and Rehabilitation

Standard preoperative planning should be conducted prior to surgery. Relevant imaging studies to review can include static and/or dynamic radiography, computed tomography (CT) scans, and magnetic resonance imaging (MRI), as available (Fig. 7.1). Confirmation of level being treated and presence of any anatomical variations should be noted and marked.

The ILIF procedure is performed under general endotracheal anesthesia, most commonly with the patient in the prone position with flexed hips. A Wilson frame or equivalent table will facilitate patient positioning (Figs. 7.2 and 7.3). Prior to incision, the surgical level is identified using guided fluoroscopy. Skin marking, preparation, and draping are performed using standard procedures. The spinous process and laminae of both adjacent vertebrae are exposed using a standard midline exposure, approximately 3–5 cm in length (Fig. 7.4). Self-retaining retractors are used to retract soft tissue and a Cobb elevator is used to elevate the paraspinal muscles and remove soft tissue on either side of the spinous processes. A scalpel or

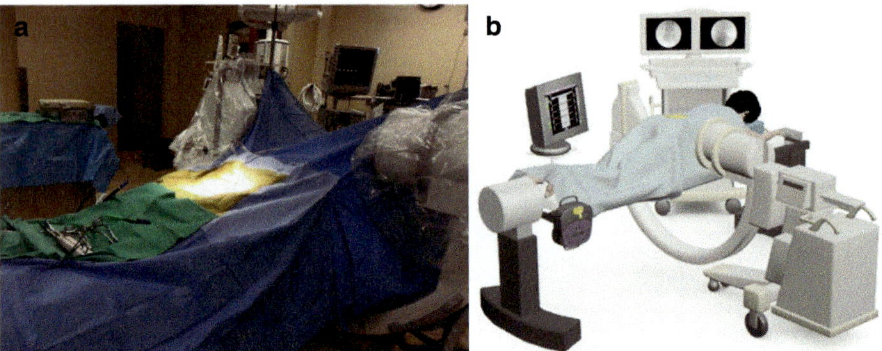

Fig. 7.3 Intraoperative photograph (**a**) and illustration (**b**) showing an alternative patient position, on a radiolucent Jackson table for interlaminar lumbar instrumented fusion (ILIF) with supplemental transforaminal interbody fusion (TLIF)

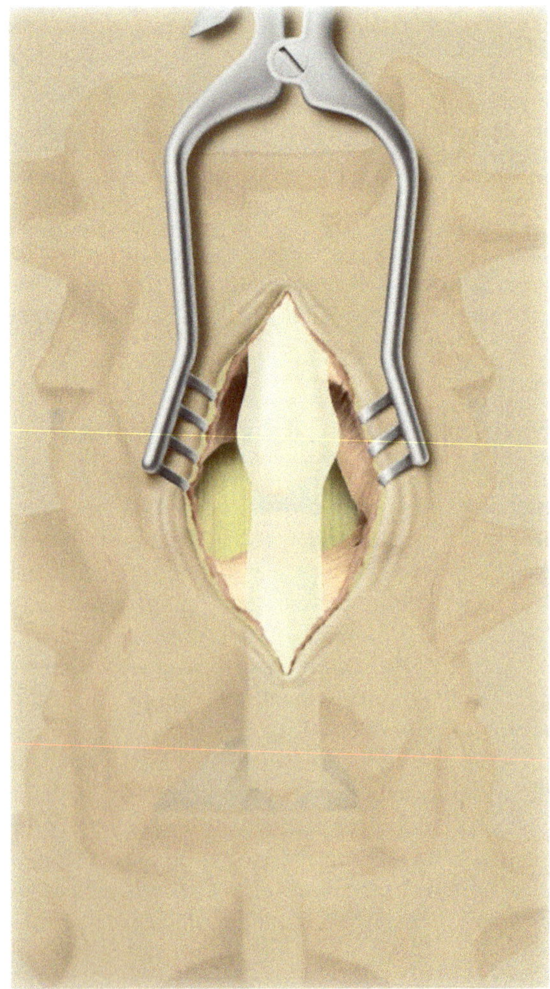

Fig. 7.4 Posterior view illustrating the midline posterior incision used in the ILIF procedure

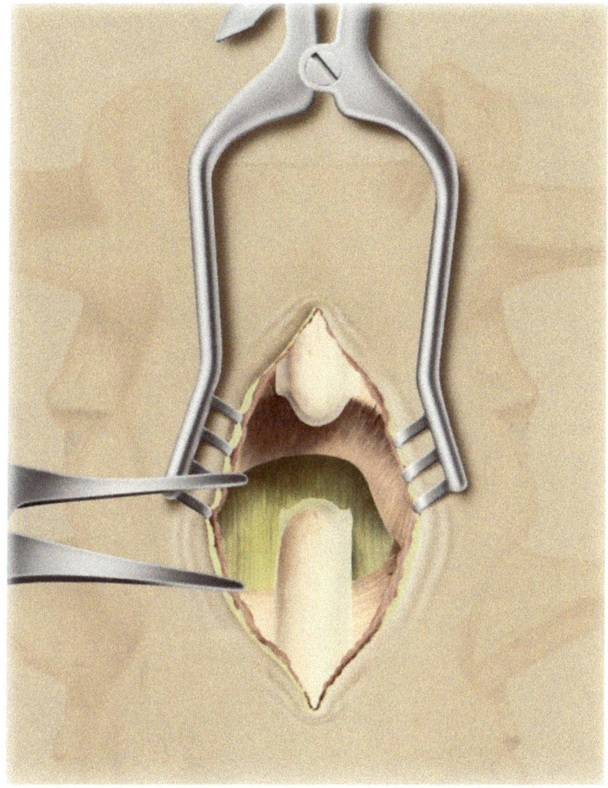

Fig. 7.5 Posterior view showing dissection of the intraspinous ligament at the index level, with the ligamentum flavum visualization facilitated by the laminar spreader

Leksell is used to remove the supraspinous ligament (Fig. 7.5). Distraction pins are placed into the spinous processes and a rack distractor is used to distract the spinous processes at the operative level. Bovie cautery is used to remove the interspinous ligament and expose the bony edges of the lamina. To open access to the spinal canal in preparation of the decompression procedure, a high-speed burr or Kerrison rongeur is used to remove portions of the inferior edge of the superior spinous process and lamina as well as the superior edge of the caudad spinous process that may limit access to the canal. To perform the decompression the ligamentum flavum is removed and the lamina may be thinned out or partially removed using the burr, with care to adequately decompress the space without compromising the integrity of the posterior bony arch. If necessary, rongeurs can be used to remove soft tissue from the medial aspect of the facet joints, taking only as much as it needed to adequately access and decompress the lateral space. This usually translates to between 10 and 20 %, though no more than 50 % of the facets should be taken in patients without plan for arthrodesis [25]. Partial facetectomy and proximal foraminotomies may be performed as needed. Throughout this section of the procedure, the rack distractor can be used to visualize all neural elements through targeted and, often temporary, changes in distraction amount.

After decompression, the interspinous space is carefully prepared using a rasp in a ventral/dorsal motion to lightly decorticate the inferior edge of the superior spinous

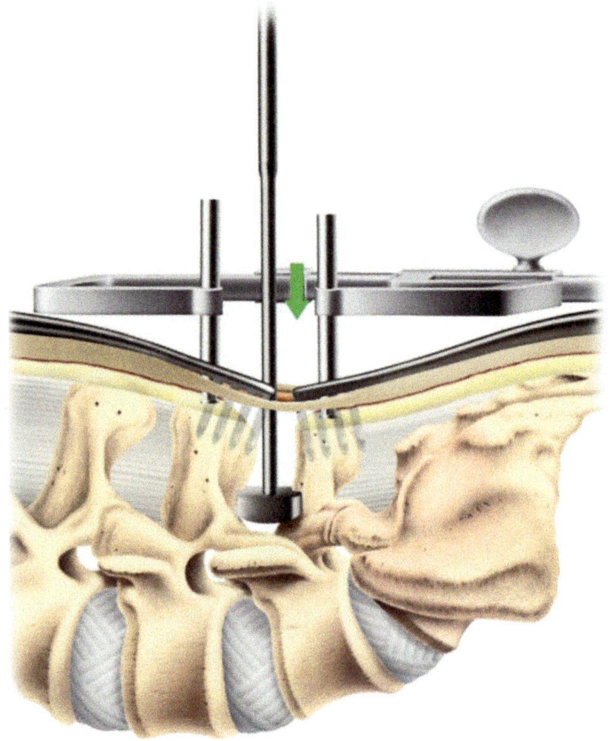

Fig. 7.6 Lateral illustration showing spinous process distraction and interlaminar graft sizing in the ILIF procedure

process and the superior edge of the inferior spinous process. After measuring the interspinous space an ExtenSure® H2™ (NuVasive, Inc.) trial is placed in the interspinous space (Fig. 7.6). Sizing can be assessed by releasing distraction on the rack distractor and toggling the trial ventral/dorsal and superior/inferior to confirm that the trail is snuggly secured between the laminae and spinous processes. To preserve sagittal balance, it is not advisable to oversize the trial but rather to use the smallest trial that fits snuggly within the anatomy. Once the appropriate allograft size has been identified, the ExtenSure H2 allograft can be inserted by attaching the allograft to the end of the inserter. The allograft is introduced into the interspinous space until it rests on the superior and inferior laminae (Fig. 7.7a, b). If necessary, the position of the allograft can be adjusted using a tamp. Once the allograft is in position the rack distractor is released and removed, and the rack and Caspar pins are removed.

The spinous process is prepared for plate insertion using a Cobb elevator and/or curette to remove any remaining soft tissue along both sides of the spinous processes. To identify the appropriate size for the spinous process plate, a sizing template is placed along the lateral aspect of the spinous processes and a lateral fluoroscopic image is taken. An appropriately sized plate should provide maximum surface area coverage of both spinous processes without extending beyond the cranial edge of the superior spinous process or beyond the caudal edge of the inferior spinous process (Fig. 7.8). Once the plate size has been selected, the

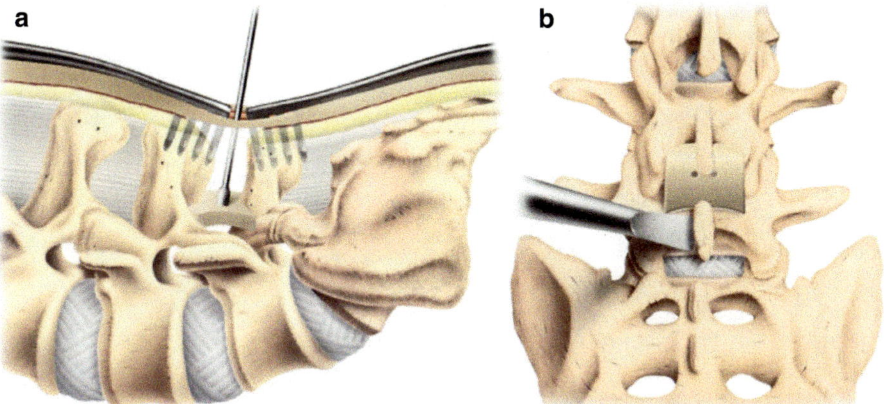

Fig. 7.7 Lateral view (**a**) of interlaminar spacer insertion and posterior view (**b**) of final placement of the interlaminar spacer

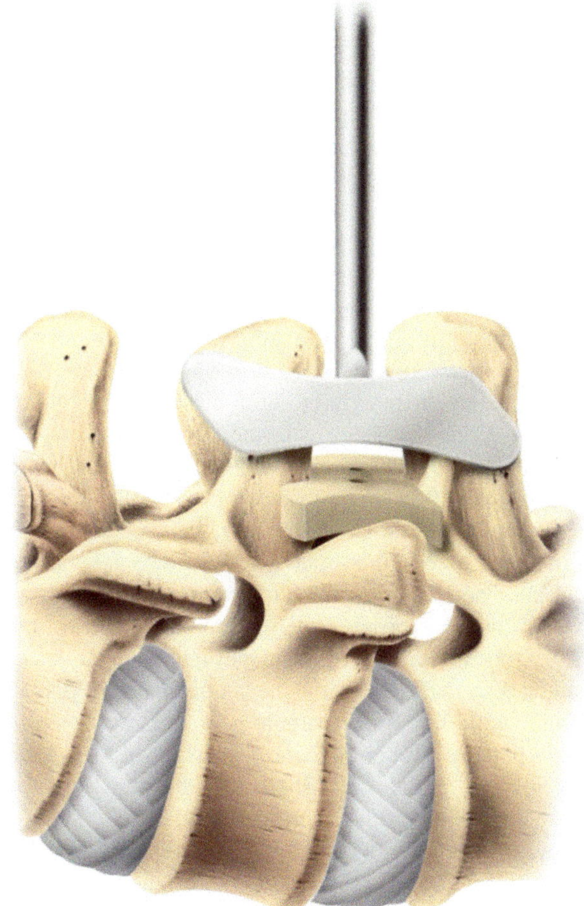

Fig. 7.8 Lateral view of the sizing of the spinous process plate

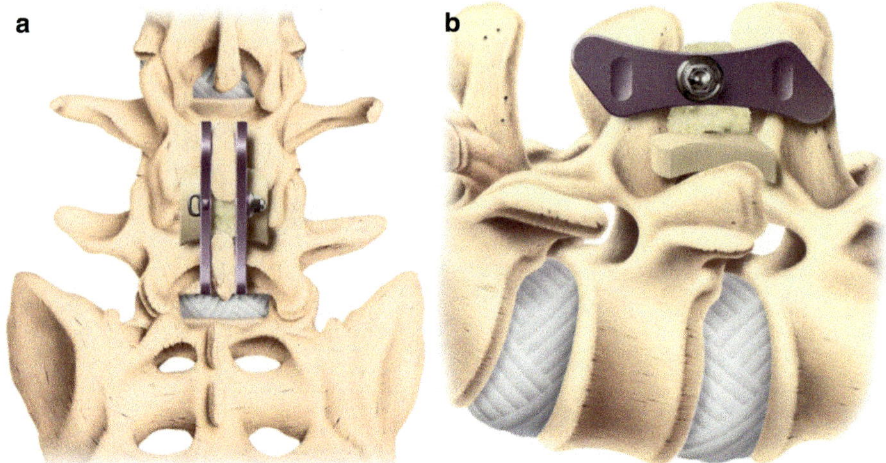

Fig. 7.9 Posterior (**a**) and lateral view (**b**) of the final ILIF construct consisting of ExtenSure® H2™ interlaminar spacer, biologic graft material, and Affix® (NuVasive, Inc.) spinous process plate

corresponding plate can be attached to the inserter and positioned on the lateral aspects of the spinous processes. Once the plates are in position, they are compressed at the plate crossbar in the interspinous region to engage the teeth of the plate into the spinous process. Further compression may be applied directly over the spinous processes to contour the plate to the spinous process anatomy and further secure the teeth of the plate into the spinous processes. Using forceps or similar instrument, biologic materials are applied to the construct between the dorsal aspect of the allograft, spinous processes, and spinous process plates. Once biologic material(s) has been applied, retractor can be removed (Fig. 7.9a, b). The wound is closed in a standard fashion.

Patients are encouraged to limit back movement during the rehabilitation period to allow proper bone growth and fusion to occur. Participation in regular low-impact, limited range of motion, cardiovascular exercise (such as walking) may increase blood flow and nutrient delivery to the surgical site to encourage healing.

In summary, ILIF is a minimally disruptive approach to the lumbar spine to perform a distraction laminoplasty followed by interspinous grafting and interspinous fixation. The limited midline exposure avoids trauma to lateral musculature compared to wider exposures used in conventional decompressive or PLF procedures. As patients with LSS often have multiple simultaneous degenerative conditions, one drawback to ILIF is that it alone is not designed to access the intervertebral disc. In patients with discogenic pathology or in patients with hypermobile or normal disc height patients, this may increase the risk of long-term failure of the construct, as with all PLF constructs, where the intervertebral disc remains unaddressed and where continued motion is probable [9, 10, 32, 35, 36, 42]. In these and any other related indications requiring anterior column stability, ILIF can be supplemented with a specialized TLIF procedure through the same midline incision.

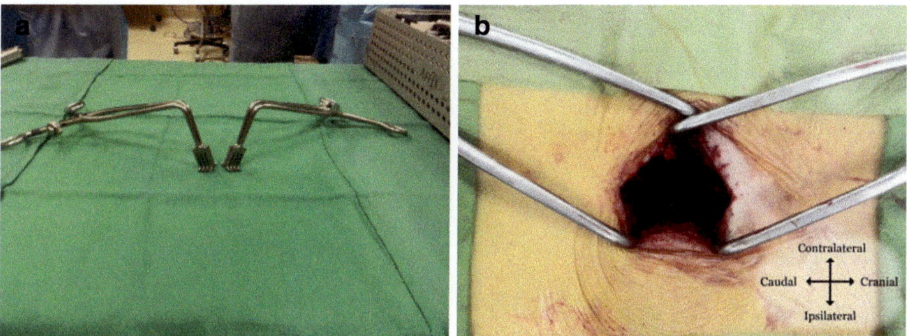

Fig. 7.10 Photographs showing the retractors that can be used to exposure the site for incisional exposure for ILIF (**a**), with preferential unilateral exposure to facilitate the TLIF (ipsilateral) (**b**)

ILIF with Supplemental TLIF

As previously mentioned, some evidence has shown that non-pedicle screw and rod fixation for PLF may have an increased likelihood of long-term construct failure without interbody supplementation, especially when posterior to a highly mobile or less degenerative intervertebral disc [42, 43]. As such, a technique for supplementation of ILIF with a specialized TLIF technique has been developed to better treat both tight foraminal narrowing requiring facetectomy and the presence of instability (degenerative or iatrogenic) requiring interbody fusion. In cases of tight foraminal stenosis, distraction afforded by the ILIF procedure as well as the largely central decompression may not be sufficient alone to provide adequate foraminal decompression. In these cases a more robust decompression is warranted, though this compromises stability following facetectomy and requires supplementation to maintain segmental stability during healing [25].

The approach and initial technique for the TLIF-supplemented ILIF begin the same as for the standard ILIF technique, though the lead author (AT) places the patient in the prone position on a Jackson table, rather than a Wilson frame, to facilitate both compression on the interlaminar graft and segmental lordosis following release of interspinous distraction. The same less invasive (3–5 cm) posterior midline incision located at the junction of the spinous processes of the indicated level is used for the combined approach, following a distraction laminoplasty procedure for a standard central decompression. In the interbody fusion supplementation technique, two self-contained retractors can be overlapped to provide exposure for the ILIF procedure and also preferentially expose one side for the TLIF approach, to minimize contralateral morbidity by maintaining as small an incision as possible (Fig. 7.10a, b). These retractors should be placed in combination with the spinous process distractors to allow for the distraction laminoplasty exposure to be maintained during the TLIF procedure (Fig. 7.11a, b).

To begin, it should be stated that the approach for ILIF differs from a standard TLIF approach, so additional confirmation of the level being treated should be

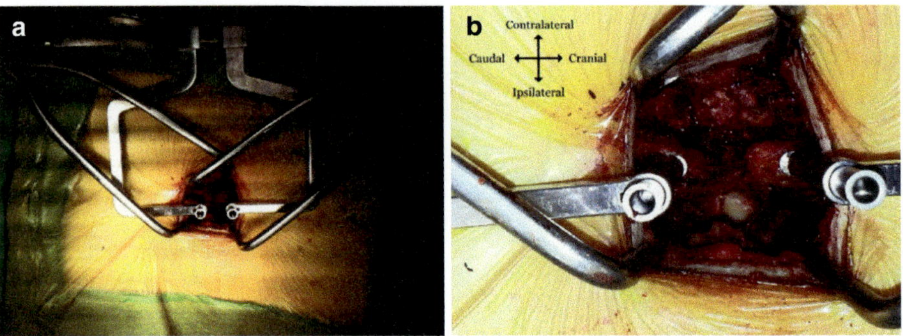

Fig. 7.11 Intraoperative photographs showing surgical setup (**a**) and simultaneous incisional and interspinous distraction for ILIF and TLIF (**b**)

made. In ILIF, interspinous targeting is used to determine the index level and the incision point. A standard TLIF uses a pedicle- or facet-based approach trajectory, and thus, when performing a TLIF through an ILIF exposure, the appropriate facets should be identified on lateral fluoroscopy and marked with a K-wire. For instance, in an L4–5 TLIF through an ILIF exposure, the L5 facet would be marked for access (Fig. 7.12). The start of this technique begins with a partial contralateral facetectomy (approximately 10–15 %, never more than 50 %) of the medial facet aspect to allow for access to the contralateral foramen for decompression without destabilizing the segment [25]. The extent of decompression (out to the medial portions of the facets) can be used in standard ILIF to both adequately decompress the segment and maintain the integrity of the posterior elements, especially in axial rotation. A standard TLIF approach is then used on the ipsilateral side, with facetectomy facilitated by a high-speed burr to resect from the pars through to the lamina, taking the inferior articular facet which allows for access to and visualization of the nerve root (Figs. 7.13a, b). The traversing and existing nerve roots are then isolated retracted medially using a cottonoid and/or wide Penfield elevator for protection during access to the disc space (Fig. 7.14). TLIF annulotomy, discectomy, and endplate preparation are performed in the standard fashion. For the placement of bone graft material and the intervertebral spacer, the primary author (AT) packs the front of the extravasated disc space (posterior to the anterior longitudinal ligament [ALL]) with corticocancellous chips followed by an interdigitating layer of allograft cellular bone matrix (Osteocel® Plus, NuVasive, Inc.). Posterior to this graft material, a curved (banana) TLIF cage is placed in the anterior 1/3 of the disc space with the convexity facing posterior. Posterior to the first cage, a second layer of allograft cellular bone matrix is placed followed by a second curved TLIF cage with its concavity matching the convexity of the first TLIF cage. This graft material–cage–graft material–cage complex should occupy roughly the anterior two-thirds of the disc space, leaving the posterior third free of graft material of intervertebral spacer, to facilitate and maintain a sufficiently decompressed canal and nerve roots during healing (Figs. 7.15 and 7.16).

Fig. 7.12 Lateral intraoperative fluororadiography depicting L5 facet localization in identifying and confirming level during the TLIF approach in the combined ILIF and TLIF procedure. A standard ILIF procedure uses the index level's interspinous space as an approach landmark, and standard TLIF uses a facet-targeting approach, so by identifying the inferior articular facet (L5 for an L4–5 case), the disc space will be identified by a slight cranial trajectory following facetectomy

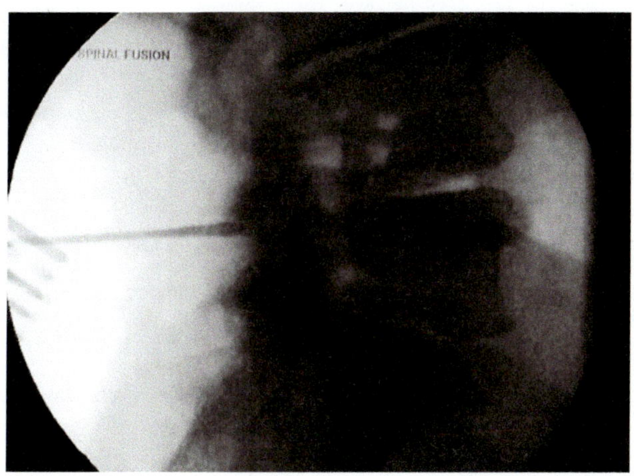

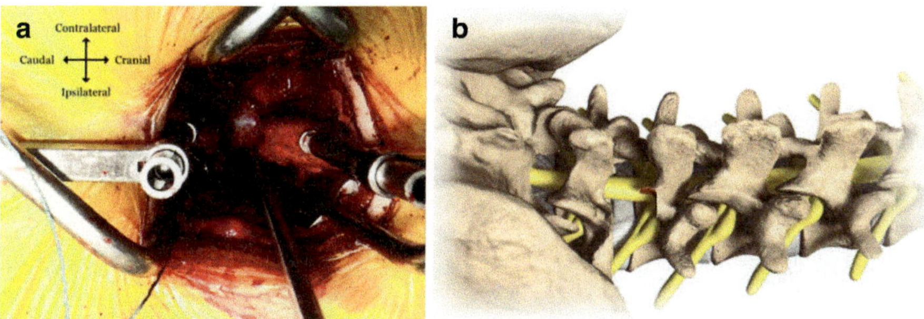

Fig. 7.13 Intraoperative photograph (**a**) and oblique posterior illustration (**b**) showing facetectomy prior to TLIF in the combined ILIF and TLIF procedure

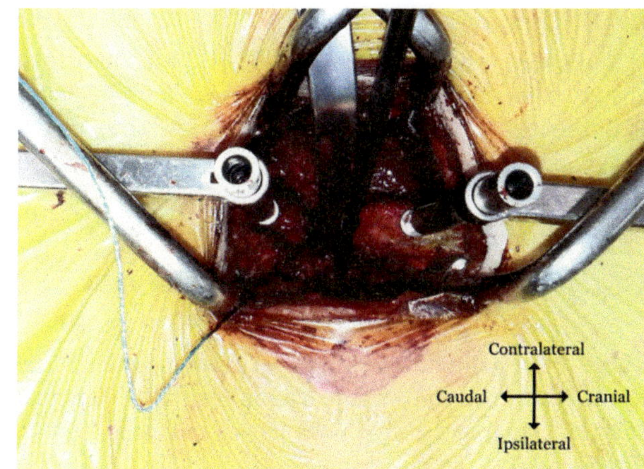

Fig. 7.14 Posterior intraoperative photograph illustrating nerve root retraction prior to annulotomy and discectomy in TLIF through an ILIF exposure

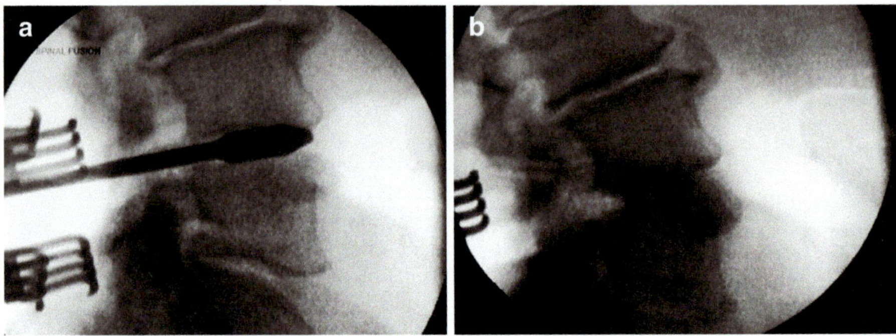

Fig. 7.15 Lateral intraoperative fluororadiography showing TLIF implant trialing (**a**) and the anterior column post-TLIF (**b**)

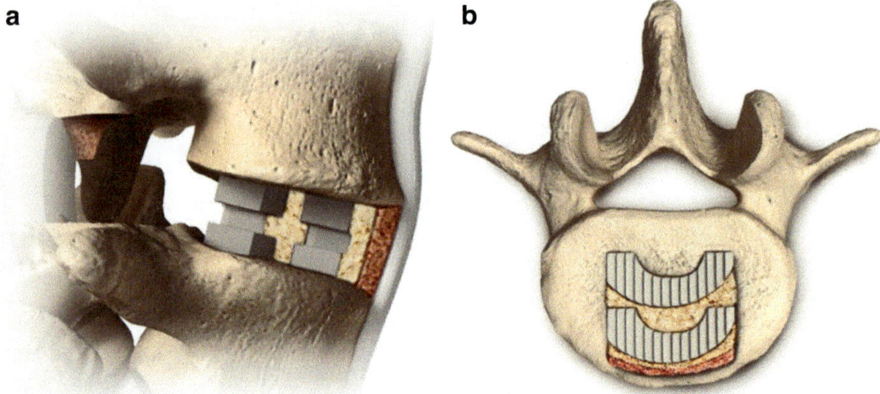

Fig. 7.16 Lateral (**a**) and axial (**b**) illustrations showing TLIF cage and biologic material placement in the specialized TLIF approach to supplement ILIF

Following completion of the TLIF procedure, placement of the interspinous spacer, posterior graft material, and interspinous plate is performed to finalize the ILIF procedure. Closure of the surgical site is then performed in the standard fashion (Figs. 7.17, 7.18, and 7.19).

Outcomes Including Literature Review

There are few literature results describing the characteristics of and outcomes following ILIF, as the procedure was only introduced in the past several years. However, several testing and early outcome references do exist, showing encouraging results for future evaluation.

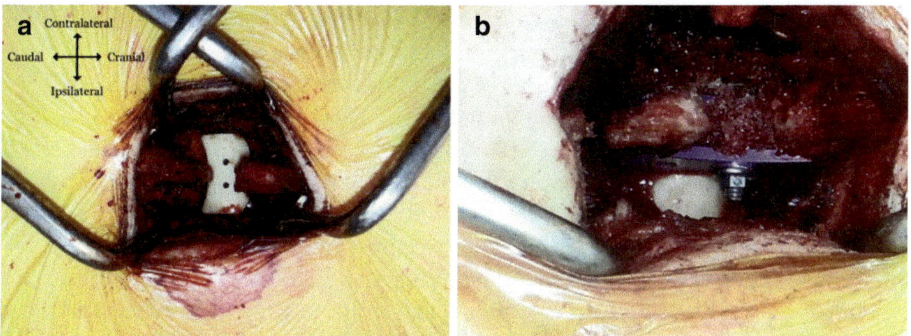

Fig. 7.17 Intraoperative photographs showing placement of the ExtenSure H2 interlaminar graft (**a**) and the final ILIF construct (**b**) following TLIF

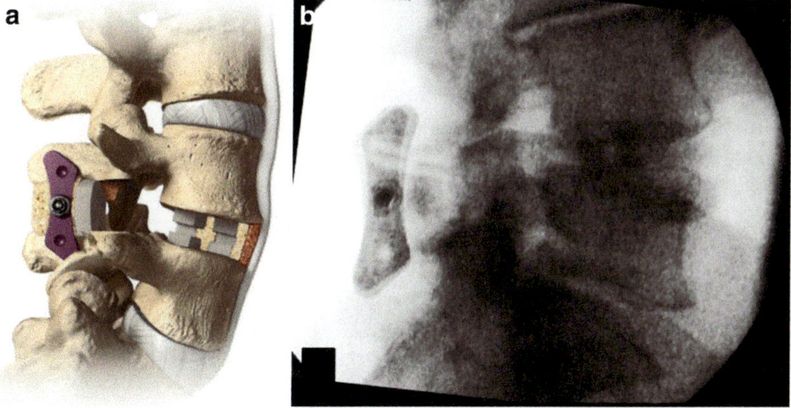

Fig. 7.18 Lateral illustration (**a**) and fluororadiograph (**b**) showing the final ILIF construct supplemental with TLIF. Note that the interspinous plate can be placed in either vertical orientation

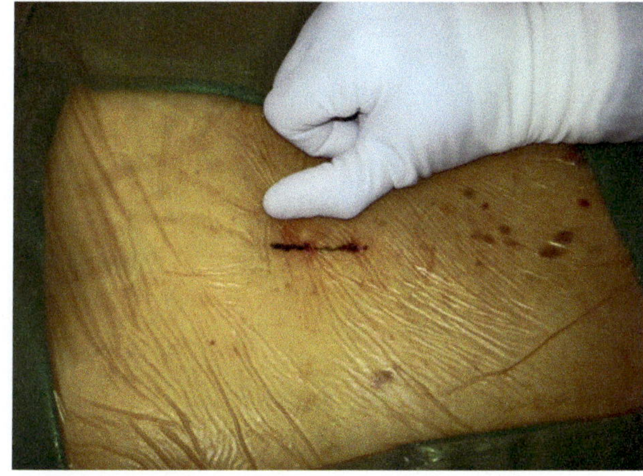

Fig. 7.19 Intraoperative photograph showing the closed incision following a single-level ILIF with supplemental TLIF

A cadaveric study was undertaken by Pradhan et al. [44] to assess the biomechanical characteristics of ILIF (interspinous spacer with spinous process plate) and to compare those results to the results of alternative methods of PLF. In the study, 8 continuous L1–L5 spines underwent nondestructive multidirectional testing across a series of different conditions at L3–4. Test conditions included (1) the intact spine (control), (2) bilateral pedicle screws, (3) bilateral laminotomy, (4) ILIF, (5) partial laminectomy, (6) partial laminectomy plus unilateral pedicle screws, and (7) partial laminectomy plus bilateral pedicle screws. Three cycles of unconstrained, pure-moment flexion and extension, lateral bending, and axial rotation were carried out without compressive load. Data were evaluated from only the third cycle. The most rigid construct, intuitively, was the construct fixation with bilateral pedicle screws without destabilization. ILIF, however, was statistically similar to bilateral pedicle screw fixation with a destabilizing decompression in flexion/extension and axial rotation, though was superior in stiffness to ILIF in lateral bending. In lateral bending, ILIF was found to not differ statistically from unilateral pedicle screw fixation following laminectomy.

Several examples of clinical outcomes following ILIF have been reported or presented. In a retrospective, multicenter review, Bae [45] evaluated pain (visual analog score [VAS]), disability (Oswestry disability index [ODI]), and radiographic outcomes from a series of 52 patients who underwent single-level ILIF. Average operative time and length of hospital stay were 68.5 min and 1.7 days, respectively. Estimated blood loss was <100 mL 93.7 % of patients treated. Two wound complications occurred and three surgical-site reoperations were performed. Reoperations included two rhizotomies and 1 additional decompression for recurrent stenosis. Eighty percent of the patient reached the threshold for minimum clinically important difference (MCID) on VAS and ODI [33].

In a second study of a different patient series, Bae [46] reported interim 12-month clinical and radiographic results from an ongoing multicenter prospective study of ILIF. Evaluations included pain (VAS), disability (ODI), Zurich claudication scores (ZCQ), patient satisfaction, segmental and global lordosis measures, and fusion assessment. Of the 66 patients enrolled 21 were available for 12-month follow-up. Average operative time and length of stay were 71 min and 1.8 days, respectively. Estimated blood loss, similar to the previous study, was <100 mL in 86 % of patients. ODI improved, on average, 31 %, while ZCQ improved 23 %. VAS improved at least 20 mm in 90 % (19/21) of patients. 82 % (17/21) of patients were satisfied with their outcome. On average, global and segmental lordosis changed less than 2° from preoperative, and 71 % of patients exhibited radiographic evidence of interspinous bridging bone. Two instances of asymptomatic spinous process fractures were observed. No revision surgeries were performed.

A recent study by Berjano et al. [47] reported results of ILIF supplemented with interbody fusion as a small subset of a larger series of interbody fusions carried out using extreme lateral interbody fusion (XLIF®, NuVasive, Inc.). In the series, the authors treated 10 % (10/97) patients with ILIF following XLIF, though results were reported only as a whole, not by fixation types as subgroups. Regardless, in the series, low back pain, leg pain, and ODI improved 61, 64, and 55 % (28 point mean absolute ODI improvement), respectively. Clinical success was achieved in 92 % of patients. The authors noted two instances of implant subsidence, both in stand-alone interbody procedures, without any instances of subsidence in patients with supplemental internal fixation (including ILIF).

Complications of Treatment

For the ILIF procedure, standard surgical risks for PLF are a concern, though many are theoretically mitigated through the less invasive incision. The most common concerns for PLF and decompressive surgery, including in ILIF, are dural tears and any resultant sequelae and wound complications. Complications unique to the ILIF procedure, as evidenced in the literature [45], include spinous process fractures. However, all reported spinous process fractures in the literature were asymptomatic.

Conclusions/Personal View

ILIF in the treatment of many classifications of LSS appears to be a viable option based on testing, early literature results, and the outcomes of related techniques for decompression and PLF. The minimally invasive nature of the procedure is advantageous in that it is associated with low operative time and blood loss compared to conventional approaches, with less morbidity and hastened postoperative recovery. Flexibility in being able to deliver a supplemental TLIF through the same exposure provides a mechanism to better address a wider range of lumbar conditions while maintaining the benefits of ILIF alone.

References

1. Deyo RA, Gray DT, Kreuter W, Mirza S, Martin BI. United States trends in lumbar fusion surgery for degenerative conditions. Spine. 2005;30:1441–5.
2. Deyo RA, Mirza SK, Martin BI, Kreuter W, Goodman DC, Jarvik JG. Trends, major medical complications, and charges associated with surgery for lumbar spinal stenosis in older adults. JAMA. 2010;303:1259–65.
3. Bae HW, Rajaee SS, Kanim LE. Nationwide trends in the surgical management of lumbar spinal stenosis. Spine (Phila Pa 1976). 2013;38(11):916–26.
4. Fischgrund JS. The argument for instrumented decompressive posterolateral fusion for patients with degenerative spondylolisthesis and spinal stenosis. Spine (Phila Pa 1976). 2004;29:173–4.
5. Herkowitz HN, Kurz LT. Degenerative lumbar spondylolisthesis with spinal stenosis. A prospective study comparing decompression with decompression and intertransverse process arthrodesis. J Bone Joint Surg Am. 1991;73:802–8.
6. Kovacs FM, Urrutia G, Alarcon JD. Surgery versus conservative treatment for symptomatic lumbar spinal stenosis: a systematic review of randomized controlled trials. Spine. 2011;36:E1335–51.

7. Mardjetko SM, Connolly PJ, Shott S. Degenerative lumbar spondylolisthesis. A meta-analysis of literature 1970–1993. Spine (Phila Pa 1976). 1994;19:2256S–65.
8. Simotas AC, Dorey FJ, Hansraj KK, Cammisa Jr F. Nonoperative treatment for lumbar spinal stenosis. Clinical and outcome results and a 3-year survivorship analysis. Spine. 2000;25: 197–203.
9. Postacchini F. Surgical management of lumbar spinal stenosis. Spine. 1999;24:1043–7.
10. Sengupta DK, Herkowitz HN. Lumbar spinal stenosis. Treatment strategies and indications for surgery. Orthop Clin North Am. 2003;34:281–95.
11. Yone K, Sakou T, Kawauchi Y, Yamaguchi M, Yanase M. Indication of fusion for lumbar spinal stenosis in elderly patients and its significance. Spine (Phila Pa 1976). 1996;21:242–8.
12. Deyo RA. Treatment of lumbar spinal stenosis: a balancing act. Spine J. 2010;10:625–7.
13. Karikari IO, Grossi PM, Nimjee SM, et al. Minimally invasive lumbar interbody fusion in patients older than 70 years of age: analysis of peri- and postoperative complications. Neurosurgery. 2011;68:897–902.
14. Rodgers WB, Cox CS, Gerber EJ. Early complications of extreme lateral interbody fusion in the obese. J Spinal Disord Tech. 2010;23:393–7.
15. Rodgers WB, Gerber EJ, Rodgers JA. Lumbar fusion in octogenarians: the promise of minimally invasive surgery. Spine. 2010;35:S355.
16. Okubadejo GO, Buchowski JM. The textbook of spinal surgery. 3rd ed. Philadelphia: Lippincott Williams & Wilkins; 2011. p. 394–401.
17. Porter RW. Spinal stenosis and neurogenic claudication. Spine. 1996;21:2046–52.
18. Guigui P, Barre E, Benoist M, Deburge A. Radiologic and computed tomography image evaluation of bone regrowth after wide surgical decompression for lumbar stenosis. Spine. 1999;24: 281–8.
19. Johnsson KE, Rosen I, Uden A. The natural course of lumbar spinal stenosis. Clin Orthop Relat Res. 1992;279:82–6.
20. Tomkins-Lane CC, Battié MC. Validity and reproducibility of self-report measures of walking capacity in lumbar spinal stenosis. Spine. 2010;35:2097.
21. Posner I, White III AA, Edwards WT, Hayes WC. A biomechanical analysis of the clinical stability of the lumbar and lumbosacral spine. Spine (Phila Pa 1976). 1982;7:374–89.
22. Manchikanti L, Cash KA, McManus CD, Pampati V, Abdi S. Preliminary results of a randomized, equivalence trial of fluoroscopic caudal epidural injections in managing chronic low back pain: part 4 – spinal stenosis. Pain Physician. 2008;11:833–48.
23. Weinstein JN, Tosteson TD, Lurie JD, et al. Surgical versus nonsurgical therapy for lumbar spinal stenosis. N Engl J Med. 2008;358:794–810.
24. Chen E, Tong KB, Laouri M. Surgical treatment patterns among Medicare beneficiaries newly diagnosed with lumbar spinal stenosis. Spine J. 2010;10:588–94.
25. O'Leary PF, McCance SE. Distraction laminoplasty for decompression of lumbar spinal stenosis. Clin Orthop Relat Res. 2001;384:26–34.
26. Fritsch EW, Heisel J, Rupp S. The failed back surgery syndrome: reasons, intraoperative findings, and long-term results: a report of 182 operative treatments. Spine. 1996;21:626–33.
27. Long DM. Failed back surgery syndrome. Neurosurg Clin N Am. 1991;2:899.
28. Postacchini F, Cinotti G. Bone regrowth after surgical decompression for lumbar spinal stenosis. J Bone Joint Surg Br. 1992;74:862–9.
29. Martin G. Recurrent disc prolapse as a cause of recurrent pain after laminectomy for lumbar disc lesions. N Z Med J. 1980;91:206–8.
30. Deschuyffeleer S, Leijssen P, Bellemans J. Unilateral laminotomy with bilateral decompression for lumbar spinal stenosis: short-term risks in elderly individuals. Acta Orthop Belg. 2012;78:672–7.
31. Kaymaz M, Borcek AO, Emmez H, Durdag E, Pasaoglu A. Effectiveness of single posterior decompressive laminectomy in symptomatic lumbar spinal stenosis: a retrospective study. Turk Neurosurg. 2012;22:430–4.
32. Knaub MA, Won DS, McGuire R, Herkowitz HN. Lumbar spinal stenosis: indications for arthrodesis and spinal instrumentation. Instr Course Lect. 2005;54:313–9.

33. Glassman SD, Carreon LY, Djurasovic M, et al. Lumbar fusion outcomes stratified by specific diagnostic indication. Spine J. 2009;9:13–21.
34. Fischgrund JS, Mackay M, Herkowitz HN, Brower R, Montgomery DM, Kurz LT. 1997 Volvo Award winner in clinical studies. Degenerative lumbar spondylolisthesis with spinal stenosis: a prospective, randomized study comparing decompressive laminectomy and arthrodesis with and without spinal instrumentation. Spine (Phila Pa 1976). 1997;22(24):2807–12.
35. Boden SD. The use of radiographic imaging studies in the evaluation of patients who have degenerative disorders of the lumbar spine. J Bone Joint Surg Am. 1996;78:114–24.
36. Boden SD, Wiesel SW. Lumbar spine imaging: role in clinical decision making. J Am Acad Orthop Surg. 1996;4:238–48.
37. Rihn JA, Patel R, Makda J, et al. Complications associated with single-level transforaminal lumbar interbody fusion. Spine J. 2009;9:623–9.
38. Bowers C, Amini A, Dailey AT, Schmidt MH. Dynamic interspinous process stabilization: review of complications associated with the X-stop device. Neurosurg Focus. 2010;28:E8.
39. Albee FH. The classic. Transplantation of a portion of the tibia into the spine for Pott's disease. A preliminary report. Jama, 57: 885, 1911. Clin Orthop Relat Res. 1972;87:5–8.
40. Hibbs RA. An operation for progressive spinal deformities: a preliminary report of three cases from the service of the orthopaedic hospital. 1911. Clin Orthop Relat Res. 2007;460:17–20.
41. Howorth MB. Evolution of spinal fusion. Ann Surg. 1943;117:278–89.
42. Heggeness MH, Esses SI. Translaminar facet joint screw fixation for lumbar and lumbosacral fusion. A clinical and biomechanical study. Spine (Phila Pa 1976). 1991;16:S266–9.
43. Boden SD, Riew KD, Yamaguchi K, Branch TP, Schellinger D, Wiesel SW. Orientation of the lumbar facet joints: association with degenerative disc disease. J Bone Joint Surg Am. 1996;78:403–11.
44. Pradhan BB, Turner AW, Zatushevsky MA, Cornwall GB, Rajaee SS, Bae HW. Biomechanical analysis in a human cadaveric model of spinous process fixation with an interlaminar allograft spacer for lumbar spinal stenosis: laboratory investigation. J Neurosurg Spine. 2012;16:585–93.
45. Bae HW. A multi-center review of single-level interlaminar lumbar instrumented fusion (ILIF): early clinical and radiographic outcomes. Society For Minimally Invasive Spine Surgery (SMISS): 2012 annual meeting; Miami Beach, Sept 2012.
46. Bae HW. 12-month clinical and radiographic results from an ongoing prospective, multicenter evaluation of interlaminar lumbar instrumented fusion (ILIF). Society For Minimally Invasive Spine Surgery (SMISS): 2012 annual meeting, Miami Beach, Sept 2012.
47. Berjano P, Balsano M, Buric J, Petruzzi M, Lamartina C. Direct lateral access lumbar and thoracolumbar fusion: preliminary results. Eur Spine J. 2012;21 Suppl 1:S37–42.

Chapter 8
Minimal Invasive Posterior Dynamic Stabilization: A New Treatment Option for Disc Degeneration (Yoda)

Gianluca Maestretti, Lorin Michael Benneker, Riccardo Ciarpaglini, and Etienne Monnard

Introduction

Background

Disorders related to intervertebral disc (IVD) degeneration are widespread causes of morbidity and severe life quality deterioration. In particular, IVD degeneration is a major cause of neck and low back pain (LBP), affecting a large percentage of the population at some point in their lives [1]. The lifetime prevalence of LBP is 70–80 %, and approximately 18 % of the population is suffering from LBP at any time leading to enormous costs due to treatment and work absenteeism [2]. With regard to treatment modalities, there is still an ongoing debate among spine specialists, which patients should be selected for surgical treatment and which operative intervention is superior. Various nonsurgical treatment regimens have shown satisfactory results, especially in short term, but in severe chronic LBP and patients with advanced disc degeneration and segmental instability, studies have shown that fusion is more efficient in reducing pain and disability [3, 4]. Although with modern implants high fusion rates can be achieved [5], one must consider that besides the high costs, approximately every fifth patient requires reoperations in the long term,

G. Maestretti, M.D. (⌧) • R. Ciarpaglini, MD
Department of Orthopaedic Surgery,
Hospital Cantonal Fribourg, Fribourg, Switzerland
e-mail: maestrettig@hopcantfr.ch

L.M. Benneker, MD
Department of Orthopaedic Surgery,
Inselspital Bern, Bern, Switzerland

E. Monnard, MD
Department of Radiology,
Hospital Cantonal Fribourg, Fribourg, Switzerland

P.P.M. Menchetti (ed.), *Minimally Invasive Surgery of the Lumbar Spine*,
DOI 10.1007/978-1-4471-5280-4_8, © Springer-Verlag London 2014

often due to adjacent level disease that develops as a consequence of altered biomechanical stresses and is seen in radiographs of every third patient after fusion [5–8]. Disc arthroplasty and dynamic stabilization techniques have evolved as a result of this frequent complication with the hope that this technology can prevent degeneration of adjacent segments, but up to date the benefit of these newer procedures could not be demonstrated [9, 10]. Although these treatment options are effective in short term, they are associated with high costs and long-term problems and are reserved for advanced degenerated segments only; therefore it would be beneficial to start treatment at an earlier stage of the disc degeneration cascade, prior to the loss of mechanical function and visible segmental instability. These early stages are within the scope of "biological" therapies where regeneration of degenerative changes should be achieved by application of growth factor, gene, or cell therapies. Despite intensive research and promising early results in vitro or in animal models, such regenerative therapies are far from clinical application and might be restricted to very early stages of disc degeneration [11–15]. In the short term there is, besides physical therapy, no adequate treatment option for patients with discogenic low back pain at early stages of disc degeneration that would prevent further deterioration of the disease. This is the background for the YODA concept presented in this chapter, where a minimal invasive technique is investigated with the intention to mechanically stabilize the segments and prevent further degradation resulting from micromotion.

Etiology of Disc Degeneration

The etiology of IVDD is multifactorial, and degenerative changes can be observed to some extent in a majority of adult IVDs [16, 17]. It has been suggested that IVD degeneration may mimic age-related changes but occurs at an accelerated rate [18, 19]. Apart from environmental and biomechanical reasons, genetic predisposition plays a major role in the development of IVD and explains over 70 % of variance in IVDD; these genes at risk are associated with various structures and functions of healthy IVDs as macromolecules (collagens, aggrecans), enzymatic activity, cell senescence, and more [20, 21]. However, the most relevant factor in IVD biology and early degeneration is the limited nutrition as the human IVD is the largest avascular structure in the human as the blood vessels in the cartilaginous endplate obliterate in childhood [22]. Metabolite transport therefore has to occur through small openings in the vertebral endplate (marrow contact channels) via diffusion for smaller molecules and fluid flow coupled for larger molecules [22, 23]. This transport route becomes even more impaired with aging and degeneration where calcifications of the marrow contact channels are observed [24, 25]. This hostile environment with limited metabolite transport and low oxygen tension limits density, viability, and activity of disc cells and explains the reduced capability of the IVD for regeneration and recovery from mechanical injury [22, 26]. In fact, probably as a repairing reaction to destruction and failure of disc matrix, an increase in cell proliferation has been observed in disc degeneration [27]. On the other hand, there is increased cell senescence in degenerated discs [9, 28]. It has been suggested that replicate senescence may naturally occur during aging, while stress-induced premature senescence may be the result of exposure to reactive oxygen species, mechanical load, or inflammatory mediators, contributing to degeneration [29, 30]. Apart from the cell density, viability, and activity, phenotypic changes during aging and degeneration have been extensively studied. As a result of altered phenotype, IVD cells exhibit multiple functional changes, including compromised capability of synthesizing correct matrix components, enhanced catabolic activity, altered synthesis of growth factors and their receptors, and increased levels of inflammatory mediators [29]. Age-related changes in the concentration of matrix macromolecules have recently been documented comprehensively [31]. These changes often result in an insufficiency to maintain a highly hydrated matrix in the NP, which in turn severely affects the mechanical integrity of the IVD. The IVD mechanical function of distributing axial loads and absorbing shock, while providing flexibility, strongly relies on the hydrodynamic capabilities of the NP. Reduced disc pressure in dehydrated, degenerated discs leads to eccentric loading patterns of the endplates, and reduced disc height transfers the load to the posterior elements of the segment, which can initiate annular lesions, herniations, and ultimately facet joint arthrosis [32]. The segment presents an abnormal motion pattern, defined as segmental instability, which is one of the most common causes for LBP [33].

Imaging of Early Lumbar Intervertebral Disc Degeneration

The assessment of advanced lumbar intervertebral disc degeneration is possible with multiple radiologic modalities such as conventional radiography, CT scan, and discography. Thanks to the progress of the magnetic resonance imaging (MRI), this is nowadays the best diagnostic tool to describe and assess not only the advanced lumbar intervertebral disc degeneration (IVDD) but also the first signs of the intervertebral disc degeneration. Conventional clinical MR imaging emphasizes the signal intensity and morphologic changes of intervertebral discs in T2-weighted imaging [34]. Pfirrmann et al. therefore suggested to use a semiquantitative score for the grading of IVDD [35]. Four morphological parameters are evaluated for the Pfirrmann's score: the structure of the disc in T2, the distinction of the nucleus pulposus and annulus, the signal intensity, and the height of the intervertebral disc. Due to its simplicity Pfirrmann's score is frequently used, however, this score shows a lack of correlation between histology and biochemistry or with the clinic [36, 37]. Standard T2-weighted MRI scores are of limited value discriminating early degenerative changes when correlated to biochemical alterations [38]. This is the reason why the use of other sequences to quantitatively evaluate the early degenerative changes on the matrix content of intervertebral discs has recently been suggested. Since the intervertebral disc is the largest avascular structure in the body, its nutrition largely depends on the diffusion of fluid either from the vertebral bodies or through the annulus fibrosus. Reduction in apparent diffusion coefficient (ADC) has been associated with reduction in nutrient supply in IVDD [39]. A strong correlation between the ADC and a T2 signal/CSF signal ratio has been demonstrated [40]. However, a recent study proved that the diffusion-weighted imaging is less sensitive to detect early morphologic changes in intervertebral disc compared with the T2-weighted imaging [41]. The most significant change that occurs in an early degenerative disc is the loss of proteoglycans [42]. T1rho imaging has the advantage of showing the interaction between water molecules and their macromolecular environment and early biochemical changes in the intervertebral disc [42, 43]. Modern, quantitative MRI techniques as T2 mapping or T1rho imaging have the advantage of showing the interaction between water molecules and their macromolecular environment and early biochemical changes in the intervertebral disc [44–46] (Fig. 8.4). The T1rho sequence was significantly associated with clinical symptoms. It was also more sensitive in order to detect early degenerative changes in the disc in low Pfirrmann score. Furthermore, the signal intensity was weaker in the Pfirrmann grade 2 than in Pfirrmann grade 1. T1rho and T2 were strongly correlated and more sensitive in order to detect the early degenerative changes in the intervertebral disc [36]. The T1rho-weighted sequence has demonstrated a wide range in signal intensity in Pfirrmann's score 1 and 2, and therefore it was suggested to create a quantitative scale in early degenerated discs [47]. It is also important to mention that the T1rho sequence has been proved to reflect the swelling pressure in the disc and therefore its mechanical function [48]. T2 mapping sequences also allow to quantitatively measure water content and are also sensitive for fiber orientation of structures like the annulus fibrosus [45, 46]. Especially on axial images early changes at the nucleus-annulus interface can be observed, as they represent the mucinous infiltration and invagination of the inner annulus fibrosus fibers which is according to Thompsons macroscopic grading one of the first signs for degeneration [49].

Recently the feasibility of using MR spectroscopy has been examined in cadaveric and bovine spine. A correlation between biochemical reduction in glycosaminoglycan content and N-acetyl/Lac + Lip and N-acetyl/Chol ratios was demonstrated [50]. The feasibility and the clinical application of MR spectroscopy for the demonstration of early IVDD have never been demonstrated. In conclusion, MRI is the gold standard to detect early degenerative changes in the lumbar spine. Currently the Pfirrmann's score is the most used classification scheme; in the near future quantitative and more sensitive sequences as T2 mapping or T1rho imaging are likely to be used in clinical practice. The DWI-weighted sequence has been shown to be less sensitive.

Rational of Interspinous Implants

Discogenic low back pain and spinal stenosis due to hypertrophy of the ligamentum flavum, protrusion of the annulus, and hypertrophic arthrosis of the intervertebral articulations are well-known pathologies in our society. At the beginning of the degenerative process, before alteration of disc height, an increase in range of motion with segmental laxity was demonstrated by Ebara et al. [51] and Mimura et al. [52]. The cascades of disc degeneration begin with loss of disc height and overcharging of the facet joint leading to an intermediate stage of abnormal segment motion in the middle staging before structural lumbar changing appears. This late stage characterized by severe disc degeneration, decrease of disc height and reduced intervertebral mobility, is followed later by structural degenerative deformity and stenosis. The interspinous spacers are implants which are introduced between the spinous processes of the lumbar spine to achieve a segmental distraction. The posterior element tension banding restores the loss of stability missed in the early stage of disc degeneration. This indirect tension, if the implant is correctly positioned, has a positive effect with retention of the posterior annulus and realignment of facet joint without changing the physiological spine balance. The interspinous implants can be classified in two groups depending on the function concept: flexion/extension stabilizer and extension stabilizer. The flexion/extension stabilizer devices have an anchorage in the spinous processes. An example is the DIAM invented by J. Taylor [53]. It is a silicone "bumper" wrapped into a polyester sheath connected to artificial ligaments, positioned in the interspinous space and fixed with the ligament around the superior and inferior spinous processes. The Wallis invented by J. Sénégas [54] is a similar implant with the same fixation system, but the "bumper" is realized in plastic. The surgical technique of the described implants is similar. The SLL (supraspinous lumbar ligament) needs to be detached and the interspinous ligament resected. The difference between these implants is the final stiffness created by the axial load of the "bumper." The DIAM is a less rigid implant than the Wallis. This rigidity has to be considered in the choice of the implant and in the patient selection. These implants have a limited long-term function and efficacy with a tendency of a spontaneous segment fusion. After a long experience with different type of implants, we felt the strong request to develop the YODA (created by SpineArt with the collaboration of G. Maestretti and P. Mangion) a new implant with the capacity to maintain a long-term segment motion and to stabilize the disc.

Implant Description and Surgical Principle

The YODA (Fig. 8.1) posterior dynamic device is realized in Phynox and is designed with a central spring and inferior and superior holding elements, fitting securely between the spinous processes. The interspinous central body is used as a "stand-alone" device. YODA device exists in two sizes (small and large) and is introduced unilaterally preserving the supraspinous ligament. This supple and dynamic implant is intended to unload the disc and maintain mobility and height between two spinous processes allowing flexibility of the implant to accommodate the natural flexion and extension movements of the spine. The elasticity of the implant is the main difference comparing it to other implants in the market that are placed in the interspinous space. The elasticity of the YODA implant is the key feature, which is

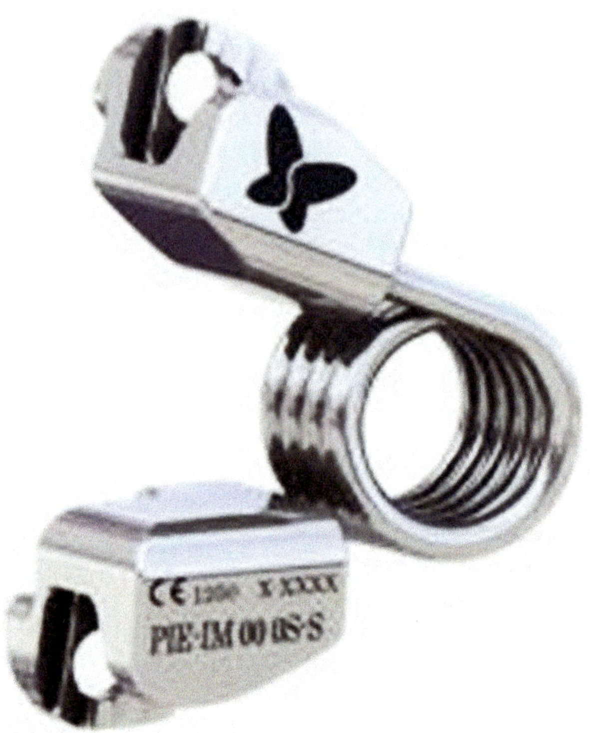

Fig. 8.1 Particular of YODA implant design

designed to rebalance and stabilize the spinal segment. A biomechanical study (Kiami cadaveric test with 3D stereotypic measurement) showed that the YODA is an implant which modifies the kinematics of a lumbar segment where the disc has been injured. The insertion of the YODA significantly reduced the deformation of the interspinous space in the lumbar spines tested, showing a stabilizing effect of the implant regarding the segment. The change in the flexion angulations shows that the YODA has a restabilizing function, putting the segment under tension, relieving the intervertebral disc. The stabilizing effect was quantified in flexion with a 7° reduced flexion and increased 4° extension in comparison with a non-instrumented segment. Furthermore, the tests showed an opening of the foramen by an average of 11 %. This is not a simple spacer; it is designed to put the treated segment back under tension by opening the foramen. The YODA is flexible and dynamic and does not behave as an inert rigid interspinous wedge. It combines a posterior "end-stop" effect, due to its obligatory interspinous filling, with a mechanical return in extension and ligament tensioning in flexion. Another advantage of the YODA implant is its minimal invasive fitting technique which retains part of the interspinous ligaments and above all, the entire supraspinous ligament. These ligaments are pre-stressed and put under tension after fitting the implant by opening the interspinous space. If the more anterior ligaments (anterior and posterior longitudinal ligaments and the ligamentum flavum) are unharmed, they will also be stretched to a lesser degree, because they are farer from the center of the YODA implant. This distraction of the interspinous space, as shown by the reopening of the foramina, occurs within a vertebral unit where the ligaments are all preserved and leads to strain the supraspinous and interspinous ligaments.

Advantages

Technical Advantages

- Minimally unilateral open posterior approach
- Less invasive surgical technique with only consecutive interspinous distraction preserving the muscle
- No detaching or damage of supraspinous lumbar ligament
- Due to the shape and composition in Phynox, the YODA is more elastic than other products in titanium with decrease spinous process stress fracture and future osteolysis
- Two size choices to better fit the interspinous process space
- Simple and compact set instruments to decrease the overall cost

Clinical Advantages

- Restore the missed stability by distracting the posterior elements and posterior annulus relieving low back pain due to degenerative instability
- Indirect disc stabilization with reduced and controlled flexion
- Indirect increase foramen size with reducing root impingement
- Maintain the movement in flexion and extension
- Lateral clamp stabilization to reduce implant migration
- Adapted for multilevel utilization
- Simple surgical technique with reduction of operative time
- Negligible blood loss
- Full reversible procedure with preservation of intact anatomical structures after implant removal

Disadvantages

- No rotational stabilization
- Simple surgical technique with risk of wrong utilization and enlarged indication
- Possible wrong size choice or incorrect implant positioning with risk of secondary displacement

Indications

- Young-middle age patients with history of back pain (>6 months), presenting a disc degeneration with maintained segment mobility
- Disc degeneration grade III and IV following the MRI Pfirrmann classification [35] with ± Modic I change [55]
- In association with the surgical treatment of a voluminous discal hernia or in recurrent discal hernia
- Central, lateral, and foraminal lumbar spinal stenosis with leg, buttock, or groin pain, which can be relieved during flexion due to a large bulging disc
- Topping off pathology adjacent to fusion

Contraindications

- General contraindication for a surgical treatment
- Infection and tumors
- Fractures
- Conus/cauda syndrome
- Severe structural spinal stenosis lacking a dynamic component
- Degenerative spondylolisthesis at index level of grade >I according to Meyerding
- Spondylolisis
- Scoliotic deformity at index level
- Not mobile or hypomobile segment
- DDD with fixed retrolisthesis
- Spinous process and Baastrup/or lamina dysplasia
- Grade V Pfirmann disc degeneration [35]
- Grade IV Weishaupt facet degeneration [56]
- Nonspecific discogenic low back pain
- Severe osteoporosis
- Morbid obesity (BMI >40)
- Psychological disorders
- Pregnancy

Surgical Technique

Preoperative Planning

The patient's selection is the key of surgery success. The history of patient pain, the plain flexo-extension films, and MRI investigations must be correlated with clinical examination. To confirm the discogenic pain, a discography with double test is

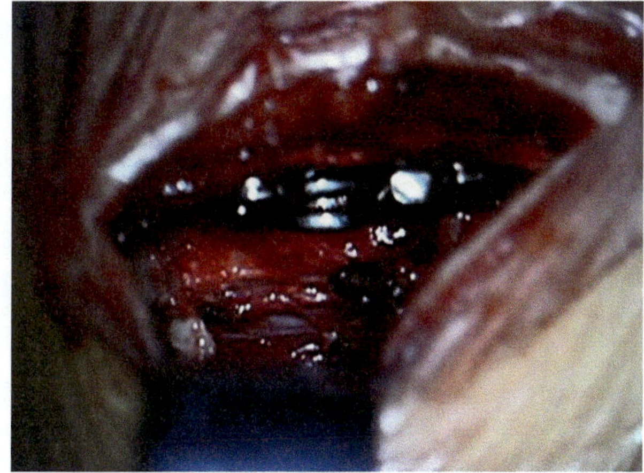

Fig. 8.2 Microscopic intraoperative view of minimal invasive unilateral posterior approach. The image shows the integrity of the supraspinous ligament after YODA implantation

performed. In addition facet joint and sacroiliac joint infiltrations are utilized to find the pain origin. For the soft stenosis, a functional MRI with myelographic sequences or a conventional myelography with CT scan is preformed to assess the clinical indication.

Anesthesia

The procedure is performed with the patient in general or in spinal anesthesia depending on the indications and on the patient. An antibiotic prophylaxis in single shoot is administered at the induction.

Patient Positioning

The patient is placed in prone position on a radiolucent table. An increased flexion of the spine is useful to optimize the implant placement and does not increase the risk a postoperative segmental lumbar kyphosis because, against other products, the implant is flexible.

Surgical Steps

Minimally Invasive Posterior Approach

Mini open approaches centered at the interspinous and associated approach for disc herniation decompression are utilized (Fig. 8.2).

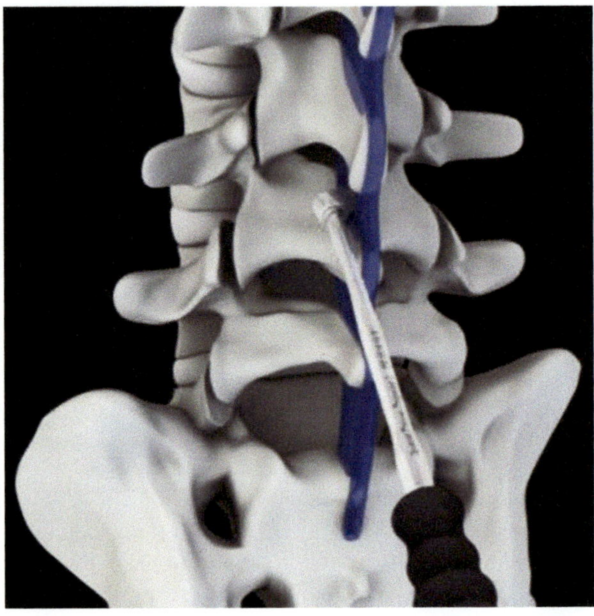

Fig. 8.3 Tridimensional drawing of inferior spinous process preparation using the dedicated instrument to detach the muscular insertion

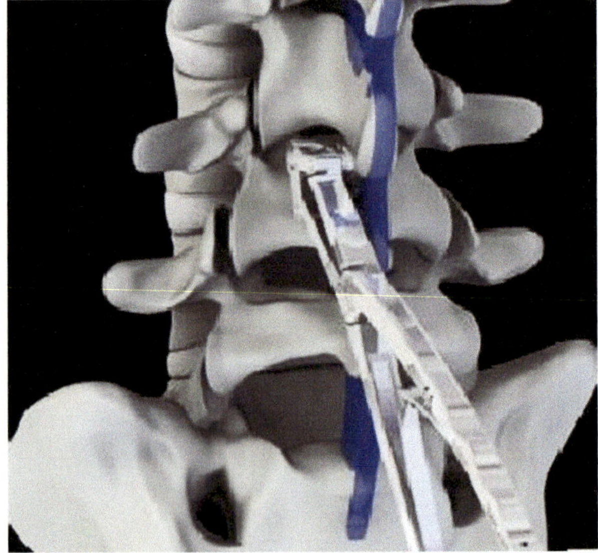

Fig. 8.4 Drawing of the insertion of the YODA implant in the interspinous space

1. Interspinous process preparation (Fig. 8.3)
   This consists in different two instruments inserted directly in the interspinous space for the spinous process preparation.
2. Implant size selection
   With a special footprint insertion instruments, the size of implant is decided.
3. Implant insertion (Fig. 8.4)
   After implant placement on the implant holder, it is inserted between the spinous processes and released.

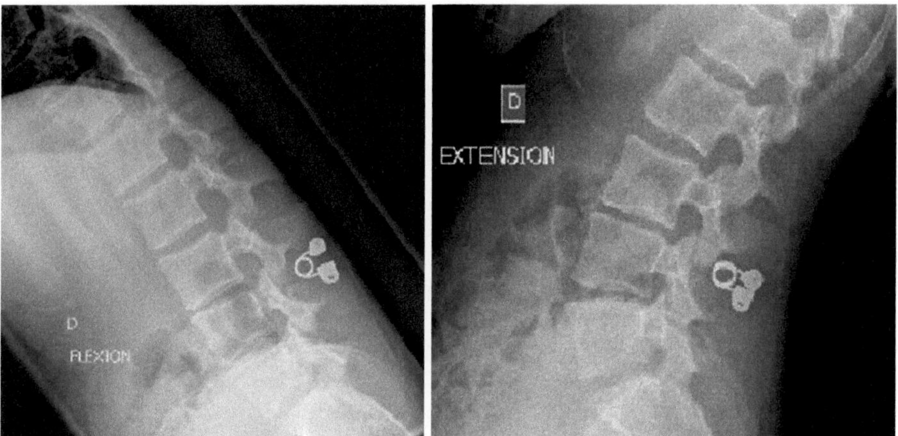

Fig. 8.5 Postoperative flexo-extension X-rays of a case of L3–L4 YODA implantation

Postoperative Care

Free mobilization is allowed since first postoperative day with extreme flexo-extension and heavy (weight-lifting) limitations. Physiotherapy for spine rebalancing is necessary in the first postoperative months in patients with discogenic pain. X-rays are performed at the first mobilization and in the follow-up at 6 weeks and 3, 12, and 24 months to assess the long-term result in association at the clinical score (Fig. 8.5). The sport activity can be early restarted after few weeks depending on the axial loading stress. A book publication from Calvosa and Dubois [57] presents the rehabilitation program in detail after dynamic stabilization with Dynesys. The main of the therapy are similar and finally are adapted for all dynamic stabilization systems including YODA.

Results and Discussion

Over 150 cases of YODA have been performed all over the world, and in these cases the postoperative evaluation demonstrates promising clinical results. So far 28 patients have been treated in our institution since the end of 2009. From February 2010, 20 patients (11 men and 9 females) with mean age of 44 years (19–77) were enrolled in a prospective study. In 17 patients we treated one level, in 2 patients two levels, and in 1 patient three levels were treated. The treated levels were especially L3–L4 and L4–L5. The indication was in 18 patients a back pain history (>6 months) associated to radiological disc degeneration (>Pfirrmann IV) and a deficitary disc herniation or a dynamic stenosis due to a large bulging disc. Two patients presented chronic discogenic pain and radiological evidence of a two levels discopathy. Patients presenting disc herniation underwent to a microscopic disc decompression at the same time. The average of our patients presented, for the different indications, a leg and back VAS higher than 6 with pathological Oswestry rate. At 1-year preliminary data analysis, the leg and back VAS and Oswestry were improved.

The preliminary clinical and radiological analysis shows promising good short-term results. In patients with pure discogenic pain, results seemed to be better than expected but necessitate a postoperative rehabilitation program to restore the spinal balance. These patients presented persistent muscular tension pain due to the preexisting history of back pain. Only after 3 months with physiotherapeutic treatment, a clinical benefit was observed.

Conclusions

The YODA is not indicated to treat degenerative stenosis in the aging spine, because of the difference in the design compared to other interspinous implants. In our opinion if the rare cases of dynamic stenosis are excluded, the indication should be reserved for patients with large herniated disc with low back pain. Quite different is the concept for patients suffering from discogenic chronic low back pain. The less invasiveness, the early mobilization, and the short rehabilitation time offer a concrete temporary alternative for the patient suffering from low back pain. These reversible solutions do not compromise any future treatments. The mini invasive open approach offers the possibility to treat patients with multilevel lumbar disc pathology. The difficulty in this special treatment remains the patient selection. The results after 1 year in this demanding category of patients demonstrate a positive clinical outcome similar to other more invasive surgical techniques (fusion, total disc replacement). The efficacy of the implant to protect the adjacent segment against accelerated disc degeneration needs years of follow-up to establish whether this theoretical advantage is actually achieved. G. Dubois, J. Sénégas, and J. Taylor observed in some patients at the follow-up MRI a certain capacity of the degenerated black disc to rehydrate after dynamic stabilization. N. Specchia presented cases with histological disc amelioration after Dynesys implantation. These observations are very promising for the future and may be a prospective treatment for young patients suffering from chronic discogenic low back pain. The new biological cellular stem cell or fibroblast research can be one of the more promising future disc treatments. For those eventual possibilities, it is important to maintain the natural patient scaffold (disc) with the interspinous spacers. At the moment with a too short follow-up, it is impossible to answer if the YODA is a really good solution to avoid future disc degeneration at the target level or if it has the same capacity like other interspinous implants to give a sufficient posterior disc stabilization and to provide disc rehydration.

References

1. Freemont AJ, Watkins A, Le Maitre C, et al. Current understanding of cellular and molecular events in intervertebral disc degeneration: implications for therapy. J Pathol. 2002;196(4):374–9.
2. Andersson GB. Epidemiological features of chronic low-back pain. Lancet. 1999;354(9178): 581–5.
3. Mannion AF, Muntener M, Taimela S, et al. A randomized clinical trial of three active therapies for chronic low back pain. Spine. 1999;24(23):2435–48.

4. Fritzell P, Hagg O, Wessberg P, et al. 2001 Volvo Award Winner in Clinical Studies: Lumbar fusion versus nonsurgical treatment for chronic low back pain: a multicenter randomized controlled trial from the Swedish Lumbar Spine Study Group. Spine. 2001;26(23):2521–32.
5. Fritzell P, Hagg O, Wessberg P, et al. Chronic low back pain and fusion: a comparison of three surgical techniques: a prospective multicenter randomized study from the Swedish lumbar spine study group. Spine. 2002;27(11):1131–41.
6. Martin BI, Mirza SK, Comstock BA, et al. Reoperation rates following lumbar spine surgery and the influence of spinal fusion procedures. Spine. 2007;32(3):382–7.
7. Etebar S, Cahill DW. Risk factors for adjacent-segment failure following lumbar fixation with rigid instrumentation for degenerative instability. J Neurosurg. 1999;90(2 Suppl):163–9.
8. Kumar MN, Jacquot F, Hall H. Long-term follow-up of functional outcomes and radiographic changes at adjacent levels following lumbar spine fusion for degenerative disc disease. Eur Spine J. 2001;10(4):309–13.
9. Grob D, Benini A, Junge A, et al. Clinical experience with the dynesys semirigid fixation system for the lumbar spine: surgical and patient-oriented outcome in 50 cases after an average of 2 years. Spine. 2005;30(3):324–31.
10. van den Eerenbeemt KD, Ostelo RW, van Royen BJ, Peul WC, van Tulder MW. Total disc replacement surgery for symptomatic degenerative lumbar disc disease: a systematic review of the literature. Eur Spine J. 2010;19(8):1262–80. Review.
11. Masuda K. Biological repair of the degenerated intervertebral disc by the injection of growth factors. Eur Spine J. 2008;17 Suppl 4:441–51.
12. Nishida K, Suzuki T, Kakutani K, et al. Gene therapy approach for disc degeneration and associated spinal disorders. Eur Spine J. 2008;17 Suppl 4:459–66.
13. Sakai D. Future perspectives of cell-based therapy for intervertebral disc disease. Eur Spine J. 2008;17 Suppl 4:452–8.
14. Hohaus C, Ganey TM, Minkus Y, et al. Cell transplantation in lumbar spine disc degeneration disease. Eur Spine J. 2008;17 Suppl 4:492–503.
15. Alini M, Roughley PJ, Antoniou J, Stoll T, Aebi M. A biological approach to treating disc degeneration: not for today, but maybe for tomorrow. Eur Spine J. 2002;11 Suppl 2:S215–20. Review.
16. Jensen MC, Brant-Zawadzki MN, Obuchowski N, Modic MT, Malkasian D, Ross JS. Magnetic resonance imaging of the lumbar spine in people without back pain [see comments]. N Engl J Med. 1994;331:69–73.
17. Boden SD, Davis DO, Dina TS, Patronas NJ, Wiesel SW. Abnormal magnetic-resonance scans of the lumbar spine in asymptomatic subjects. A prospective investigation. J Bone Joint Surg Am. 1990;72(3):403–8.
18. Adams MA, Roughley PJ. What is intervertebral disc degeneration, and what causes it? Spine. 2006;31(18):2151–61.
19. Le Maitre CL, Freemont AJ, Hoyland JA. Accelerated cellular senescence in degenerate intervertebral discs: a possible role in the pathogenesis of intervertebral disc degeneration. Arthritis Res Ther. 2007;9(3):R45.
20. Battié MC, Videman T. Lumbar disc degeneration: epidemiology and genetics. J Bone Joint Surg Am. 2006;88 Suppl 2:3–9. Review. PubMed PMID: 16595435.
21. Chan D, Song Y, Sham P, Cheung KM. Genetics of disc degeneration. Eur Spine J. 2006;15 Suppl 3:S317–25. Review.
22. Urban JP, Smith S, Fairbank JC. Nutrition of the intervertebral disc. Spine. 2004;29(23):2700–9.
23. Ferguson SJ, Ito K, Nolte LP. Fluid flow and convective transport of solutes within the intervertebral disc. J Biomech. 2004;37:213–21.
24. Bernick S, Cailliet R. Vertebral end-plate changes with aging of human vertebrae. Spine. 1982;7(2):97–102.
25. Benneker LM, Heini PF, Alini M, Anderson SE, Ito K. 2004 Young Investigator Award Winner: vertebral endplate marrow contact channel occlusions and intervertebral disc degeneration. Spine (Phila Pa 1976). 2005;30(2):167–73.

26. Horner HA, Urban JP. 2001 Volvo Award Winner in Basic Science Studies: Effect of nutrient supply on the viability of cells from the nucleus pulposus of the intervertebral disc. Spine. 2001;26(23):2543–9.

27. Sakai D, Mochida J, Yamamoto Y, et al. Transplantation of mesenchymal stem cells embedded in Atelocollagen gel to the intervertebral disc: a potential therapeutic model for disc degeneration. Biomaterials. 2003;24(20):3531–41.

28. Roberts S, Evans EH, Kletsas D, et al. Senescence in human intervertebral discs. Eur Spine J. 2006;15 Suppl 3:S312–6.

29. Zhao CQ, Wang LM, Jiang LS, et al. The cell biology of intervertebral disc aging and degeneration. Ageing Res Rev. 2007;6(3):247–61.

30. Kim KW, Chung HN, Ha KY, et al. Senescence mechanisms of nucleus pulposus chondrocytes in human intervertebral discs. Spine J. 2009;9(8):658–66.

31. Singh K, Masuda K, Thonar EJ, et al. Age-related changes in the extracellular matrix of nucleus pulposus and annulus fibrosus of human intervertebral disc. Spine (Phila Pa 1976). 2009;34(1):10–6.

32. McNally DS, Shackleford IM, Goodship AE, et al. In vivo stress measurement can predict pain on discography. Spine. 1996;21(22):2580–7.

33. Kirkaldy-Willis WH, Farfan HF. Instability of the lumbar spine. Clin Orthop Relat Res. 1982;165:110–23.

34. Modic MT, Ross JS. Lumbar degenerative disk disease. Radiology. 2007;245:43–61.

35. Pfirmann CWA, Metzordf A, Zanetti M, et al. Magnetic resonance classification of lumbar intervertebral disc degeneration. Spine. 2001;26:4873–8.

36. Blumenkrantz G, zuo J, Li X, et al. In vivo 3.0 Tesla magnetic resonance T1rho and T2 relaxation mapping in subjects with intervertebral disc degeneration and clinical symptoms. Magn Reson Med. 2010;63:1193–200.

37. Buirski G, Silberstein M. They symptomatic lumbar disc in patients with low-back pain. Magnetic resonance imaging appearances in both a symptomatic and control population. Spine. 1993;18:1808–11.

38. Benneker LM, Heini PF, Anderson SE, Alini M, Ito K. Correlation of radiographic and MRI parameters to morphological and biochemical assessment of intervertebral disc degeneration. Eur Spine J. 2005;14(1):27–35.

39. Nguyen-minh C, Riley 3rd L, Ho KC, et al. Effect of degeneration of the intervertebral disk on the process of diffusion. AJNR Am J Neuroradiol. 1997;18:435–42.

40. Niinimäki J, Korkiakoski A, Ojala O, et al. Association between visual degeneration of intervertebral discs and the apparent diffusion coefficient. Magn Reson Imaging. 2009;27:641–7.

41. Niu G, Yang J, Wang R, Dang S, Wu EX, Guo Y. MR Imaging assessment of lumbar intervertebral disk degeneration and age-related changes: apparent diffusion coefficient versus T2 quantification. AJNR Am J Neuroradiol. 2011;32:1617–23.

42. Raj PP. Intervertebral disc: anatomy-physiology-pathophysiology-treatment. Pain Pract. 2008;8:18–44.

43. Antoniou J, Pike GB, Steffen T, Baramki H, Poole AR, Aebi M, Alini M. Quantitative magnetic resonance imaging in the assessment of degenerative disc disease. Magn Reson Med. 1998;40(6): 900–7.

44. Johannessen W, Auerbach JD, Wheaton AJ, Kurji A, Borkhatur A, Reddy R, Elliott DM. Assessment of human disc degeneration and proteoglycan content using T1-rho weighted magnetic resonance imaging. Spine. 2006;31:1253–7.

45. Watanabe A, Benneker LM, Boesch C, Watanabe T, Obata T, Anderson SE. Classification of intervertebral disk degeneration with axial T2 mapping. AJR Am J Roentgenol. 2007;189(4):936–42.

46. Hoppe S, Quirbach S, Mamisch TC, Krause FG, Werlen S, Benneker LM. Axial T2* mapping in intervertebral discs: a new technique for assessment of intervertebral disc degeneration. Eur Radiol. 2012;22(9):2013–9.

47. Zobel BB, Vadalà G, Vescovo RD, Battisti S, Martina FM, Stellato L, Leoncini E, Borthakur A, Denaro V. T1rho magnetic resonance imaging quantification of early lumbar intervertebral disc degeneration in healthy young adults. Spine (Phila Pa 1976). 2012;37(14):1224–30. PAP.

48. Nguyen AM, Johannessen W, Yoder JH, et al. Noninvasive quantification of human nucleus pulposus pressure with use of T1rho-weighted magnetic resonance imaging. J Bone Joint Surg Am. 2008;90:796–802.
49. Thompson JP, Pearce RH, Schechter MT, Adams ME, Tsang IK, Bishop PB. Preliminary evaluation of a scheme for grading the gross morphology of the human intervertebral disc. Spine (Phila Pa 1976). 1990;15(5):411–5.
50. Zoo J, Saadat E, Romeno A, Look K, Li X, Link TM, Kunhanewicz J, Majumdan S. Assessment of intervertebral disc degeneration with magnetic resonance single-voxel spectroscopy. Magn Reson Med. 2009;62:1140–6.
51. Ebara S, Harada T, Hosono N, et al. Intraoperative measurement of lumbar spinal instability. Spine. 1992;17:44–50.
52. Mimura M, Panjabi M, Oxland TR, et al. Disc degeneration affects the multidirectional flexibility of the lumbar spine. Spine. 1994;19:1371–80.
53. Taylor J, Ritland S. Technical and anatomical consideration for the placement of a posterior interspinous stabilizer. In: Mayer HM, editor. Chapter 50: Minimally invasive spine surgery. 2nd ed. Berlin/Heidelberg: Springer; 2006.
54. Sénégas J. Mechanical supplementation by non rigid fixation in degenerative intervertebral lumbar segment: the Wallis system. Eur Spine J. 2002;11 suppl 2:164–9.
55. Modic M, Pavlicek W, Weinstein M, et al. Magnetic resonance imaging of intervertebral disc disease. Radiology. 1984;152:103–11.
56. Weishaupt D, Zanetti M, Boos N, Hodler J. MR imaging in osteoarthritis of the lumbar facet joints. Skeletal Radiol. 1999;28:215–9.
57. Calvosa G, Dubois G. Rehabilitation in the dynamic stabilization of the lumbosacral spine, vol. 7. Heidelberg: Springer cap; 2008. p. 21–5.

Chapter 9
Percutaneous Pedicle Screws in the Lumbar Spine

Nicola Di Lorenzo and Francesco Cacciola

Introduction

Spinal fixation with transpedicular screw instrumentation has come a long way in the last four decades. Ever since the first description of transpedicular screws with posterior plates in 1970 by Roy-Camille, who reported on his experience with the technique since 1963, a substantial amount of research has gone into improvement of the hardware and refinement of operative technique and indications [1].

Nowadays, a vast gamut of sophisticated screw-rod systems enable the spinal surgeon to perform not only in situ fusions but also three-dimensional remodeling and fusion of the spine in case of deformity.

What has remained the same, however, for the majority of spinal surgeons, is the initial phase of the fixation procedure, and that is the exposure of the posterior aspect of the vertebral column. Meticulous dissection of the posterior elements, in order to identify the landmarks for entry into the pedicle, is crucial for a safe positioning of pedicle screws. This requires mobilization of the important bulk of paravertebral muscles represented mainly by multifidus and erector spinae.

The dissection of these muscles is even more extensive in the lower lumbar and lumbosacral levels due to the need to obtain a lateral to medial converging screw trajectory requiring generous lateral mobilization of the muscles [2–9].

With increasing diffusion of more extensive spinal operations and thus the need for more extensive muscle dissections in the last decades, during the course of the 90s, the spinal scientific community started to increasingly investigate whether the extent of dissection would have any consequences on trunk muscle performance and be potentially related to a major incidence of postoperative back pain [10, 11].

N. Di Lorenzo, MD (✉)
Department of Neurosurgery, Florence University, Florence, Italy
e-mail: dilorenzo@unifi.it

F. Cacciola, MD
Department of Neurosurgery, Siena University, Siena, Italy

P.P.M. Menchetti (ed.), *Minimally Invasive Surgery of the Lumbar Spine*,
DOI 10.1007/978-1-4471-5280-4_9, © Springer-Verlag London 2014

Particular attention had been paid to the multifidus muscles that represent the deepest muscle group in the lumbar region [12] and consist of multiple bands arising from each vertebral lamina and inserting from two to five segments below the level of origin [13]. The principal action of the multifidus muscle is rotation in the sagittal plane having therefore the strongest influence in stiffening the lumbar functional unit. From these anatomic and functional studies of the multifidus muscle, it seemed clear that damage to the muscle could result in back muscle dysfunction after surgery and negative repercussions on segmental stability and the evolution of back pain.

Various groups had therefore conducted studies that used mainly magnetic resonance imaging (MRI) and investigation of clinical parameters in order to establish whether there was any correlation between muscle dissection and retraction and the change of these parameters.

The general conclusion of all of these studies was that postoperative signal changes on MRI, a reduced functional capacity and increased low back pain all correlated positively with the duration and thus also the extent of paraspinal muscle retraction during surgery [10].

As a consequence, in order to reduce muscle mobilization and damage, less invasive screw and rod insertion techniques have been studied and developed throughout the years.

In 1995, Mathews and Long described a percutaneous lumbar fixation technique with connecting plates inserted suprafascially [14]. In 2000 Lowery and Kulkarny described a similar technique in which rods were used, but the position of the rods would still be suprafascial and thus distant from the actual segment that needs to be stabilized with an obvious biomechanical disadvantage [15].

In 2001 Foley et al. described their experience with percutaneous pedicle screws (PPS) and a rod insertion device that relying on geometrical constraint would permit the introduction of a rod in a standard submuscular position through a separate stab incision. With this technique the final construct and thus the biomechanical result would be entirely similar to what can be achieved with a construct placed with a standard open technique [16].

Nowadays almost all producers of spinal instrumentation offer also a set for percutaneous insertion of pedicle screws and rods with slight differences in the technical layout.

In this chapter we describe the technique of PPS instrumentation.

After an overview on the indications for PPS in the lumbar spine and some concrete examples of the most recent studies, considerations on radiation exposure as pertaining to spinal surgery will be made before the description of the operative technique.

Indications

Indications for the use of PPS in the lumbar spine are continuously growing [17–19]. This comes as no surprise when we consider that the end product, as mentioned earlier, is similar to what is possible with an open technique, without, however, the same burden for the patient. Small tubular retractors can additionally be used through the same incision required for screw placement in order to reach the transverse processes and/or the disc space for decortication and fusion (Fig. 9.10a, b).

Thus, minimally invasive surgery (MIS) techniques have the potential to replace the standard open technique in virtually all conditions where instrumented fusion is necessary, leaving the open technique to those cases where extensive decompression is required or in case of complex deformities that require release osteotomies and remodeling.

Overall superiority of MIS techniques with respect to traditional open procedures has not yet been demonstrated in high quality studies, but various studies have shown a reduction of blood loss, postoperative analgesics, infection, and length of hospital stay in patients operated on with a percutaneous technique as compared to the open technique [20, 21].

In a recent study on neurologically intact thoracolumbar burst fractures treated with PPS, Wen-Fei et al. treated 36 adult patients, who had single thoracolumbar AO type A3 fractures and a load-sharing score of 6 or less, with short-segment PPS fixation [22]. The operation consisted in implanting a construct of bilateral pedicle screws in the two adjacent vertebra above and below the fracture, which were then connected with bilateral rods.

The authors report an average operative time of 78 min and an average intraoperative blood loss of 75 mL. Average hospital stay was 5 days.

This compared very favorably with a similar series by Verlaan et al. of open surgeries with short-segmental pedicle screw fixation [23]. In that study operation time and intraoperative blood loss averaged 153 min and 828 mL, respectively.

Furthermore, in terms of realignment and maintenance of correction, the average sagittal Cobb angle and vertebral body height were comparable between the PPS and the open surgery study.

In the PPS study the average preoperative kyphotic angle changed from 18.7° to 3.6° immediately after surgery. At the final follow-up, the kyphotic angle was 7.6° with an average loss of kyphotic correction of 4°.

The average preoperative percentage of vertebral height (VBH) loss was 42.2 %, and the percentage was reduced to 8.3 % immediately after surgery. At the final follow-up, the percentage of VBH loss averaged 10.2 %.

Adogwa et al. carried out a retrospective cohort comparison between MIS- and open-transforaminal lumbar interbody fusion (TLIF) [24]. In that study 15 patients underwent MIS-TLIF and another 15 patients open-TLIF for grade I degenerative spondylolisthesis associated with back and leg pain. The primary aim of this study was to determine whether the MIS technique with PPS resulted in reduced postoperative narcotic use, quicker return to work, or improved 2-year outcomes.

The MIS group had been operated with discectomy and insertion of an interbody graft and PPS as in the technical description following in this chapter. No autologous bone graft had been placed posterolaterally between the transverse processes. The open group had been operated by a standard open technique for screw insertion, placement of an interbody graft, and posterolateral grafting with autologous bone.

No mention is made as to the nature of the interbody graft material in both MIS and open cases.

MIS-TLIF versus open-TLIF cohorts were similar at baseline. Median length of hospitalization after surgery was significantly less for MIS-TLIF versus open-TLIF with an average of 3 versus 5.5 days. MIS-TLIF versus open-TLIF patients showed similar 2-year improvement in visual analog score (VAS) for back pain, VAS for leg pain, Oswestry disability index (ODI), and European Quality of Life (EuroQol) 5D scores.

Median length of postoperative narcotic use was 2 weeks in the MIS group versus 4 weeks in the open group. Time to return to work was 8.5 weeks in the MIS group versus 17.1 weeks in the open group. All of the differences were statistically significant.

As far as long-term follow-up is concerned, Rouben et al. published on a series of 169 consecutive patients treated with MIS-TLIF and an average follow-up of 49 months (range 36–60 months) [25]. Patients were treated with 1or 2-level MIS-TLIF and evaluated based on clinical outcomes, reoperation rates, and fusion status. Forty-five patients required 2-level fusions, whereas 124 patients required 1-level fusions. The operation consisted in placement of PPS and placement of an interbody graft augmented with autologous bone and rhBMP-2 (Medtronic Spinal and Biologics, Memphis, TN). Average surgery time was 183 min (range, 90–390). Surgical blood loss averaged 171 cc (range, 50–750). Patients with 2-level fusions (218 cc) had a little greater blood loss than 1-level fusion patients (154 cc). Ninety-one percent of all patients (154/169) were discharged in 24 h or less hours after surgery. The longest hospital patient stay was 3 days. In terms of disability and pain improvement, ODI and VAS on a 100-point scale improved both from around 70 to around 30, with the improvement being maintained or only slightly lost over the entire follow-up period. All improvements were statistically significant.

The series reported above are by far not exhaustive in terms of representation of what is being published in the literature on the topic but are representative for the techniques adopted and the respective outcomes. The advantages over open procedures are certainly tangible when adopted in well-selected cases [26].

Fusion rates could represent a concern when one considers the limited exposures and therefore the lack of posterolateral fusion with the usual decortication of the posterolateral elements and application of bone graft, but several studies have shown how in the treatment of thoracolumbar fractures, the addition of bone fusion to the instrumentation does not seem to offer advantages versus instrumentation alone, resulting, on the contrary, in a better tolerance of the operation due to reduced operative times and less blood loss.

Wang et al., in 2006, performed a prospective randomized study wherein they sought to answer the question whether fusion is necessary for surgically treated burst fractures of the thoracolumbar spine [27]. In their series of 59 patients randomly assigned to a fusion and nonfusion group, they found no statistically significant difference in loss of kyphotic angle and residual back pain at follow-up, but a statistically significant difference in blood loss and operative time. They concluded that the short-term results of short-segmental fixation without fusion for surgically treated burst fractures of the thoracolumbar spine were satisfactory. The advantages of instrumentation without fusion are the elimination of donor site complications, saving more motion segments, and reducing blood loss and operative time.

Dai et al. in 2009 published a study on 73 patients randomly assigned to a fusion versus nonfusion group in short-segment instrumentation for the treatment of Denis type B thoracolumbar burst fractures [28]. Their minimum follow-up in that series was 5 years. No significant difference in radiographic or clinical outcomes was noted between the patients managed with the two techniques. Both operative time and blood loss were significantly less in the nonfusion group compared with the fusion group ($p < 0.05$). Twenty-five of the 37 patients in the fusion group still had some degree of donor-site pain at the time of the latest examination.

They concluded that posterolateral bone grafting is not necessary when a Denis type B thoracolumbar burst fracture associated with a load-sharing score of ≤ 6 is treated with short-segment pedicle screw fixation.

Jindal et al. in 2012 conducted another randomized fusion versus nonfusion study on 50 patients treated with short-segment fusion for thoracolumbar burst fractures [29]. They came to the same conclusions as the previous authors. According to their findings, there were no clinical or radiological differences in outcome between the groups (all outcomes $p > 0.05$). They conclude that the results of their study suggest that adjunctive fusion is unnecessary when managing patients with a burst fracture of the thoracolumbar spine with short-segment pedicle screw fixation.

Considerations on Radiation Exposure

Every fluoroscopically assisted percutaneous technique raises the issue of radiation exposure. Some basic knowledge about the amount of radiation involved in a procedure and which measures to adopt to keep radiation levels low is important.

Modern fluoroscopy systems have the capability of operation in a number of dynamic imaging modes: normal fluoroscopy, high-dose fluoroscopy, and conventional and digital cine fluoroscopy.

These different imaging modes have different dose characteristics, which can make dosimetry a difficult task and we recommend each operator to become familiar with their specific system and modes.

Rampersaud et al. have determined radiation levels for open pedicle screw insertion in a cadaver model. Hand dose of the operating surgeon, just to cite one of the measurements, was quantified as 58 millirem (mrem) per minute of fluoroscopy time. Considering the individual fluoroscopy time needed for a certain case and with a recommended annual hand exposure limit of 50.000 mrem, one can get a rough idea of how many cases can be done over a certain amount of time without exceeding the recommendations. Another useful piece of information in this study is the fact that radiation to the surgeon is more than 20 times as high when standing next to the beam source as opposed to standing on the opposite side, next to the image intensifier end, with the radiation thus having traversed the patient [30].

Mehlman and Di Pasquale published another interesting study in which they investigated the amount of radiation exposure in relation to the distance from the C-arm. They concluded that individuals working 24 in. (70 cm) or less from a fluoroscopic beam receive significant amounts of radiation, whereas those working 36 in. (91.4 cm) or greater from the beam receive an extremely low amount of radiation [31].

Operative Technique

Operating Room Setup

The main requirements for a successful percutaneous procedure are an appropriately radiolucent table and a C-arm fluoroscopy unit. When positioning the patient care must be taken to make sure that the C-arm can freely swing between the antero-posterior (AP) and lateral (LL) projection.

The C-arm should be positioned in an AP projection with the radiation source underneath the table in order to take advantage of the dose reduction as mediated by the patient's body. The LL position is then obtained by simply rotating the radiation source up- and sidewards making sure to have it covered on the side by a previously placed large drape (Figs. 9.1a, b and 9.2). Thus only the image intensifier end needs to be covered with a sterile plastic cap. Surgeon and scrub nurse should, if possible, always stand on the side of the image intensifier end.

Before draping the patient it is useful to get both an AP and LL image of the levels that need to be instrumented and to make sure that there are no obstacles between the C-arm positions as frequent changes are required quite often, at least in the initial learning phase. Furthermore one has to make sure to not have any radiodense objects like electrocardiogram (ECG) electrodes, cautery wires, or towel clips along the path of the x-rays and that could lead to an obscuration of the relevant surgical landmarks.

Once position and setup is completed and checked, the patient is draped in a standard fashion.

Pedicle Screw Trajectory Determination

The operation is started with the C-arm in the AP position. The vertebra that needs to be instrumented should be represented in a way that the superior endplate is perfectly parallel to the x-rays thus appearing as a horizontal line. Next, the pedicles are identified, and a Jamshidi needle is placed on the skin with the tip lateral to the lateral border of the pedicle by about 2 cm (Fig. 9.3). The needle is then inserted through a stab incision, and once bone contact is reached, the tip should lie just lateral to or on the lateral border of the pedicle. The needle is now carefully impacted into the pedicle

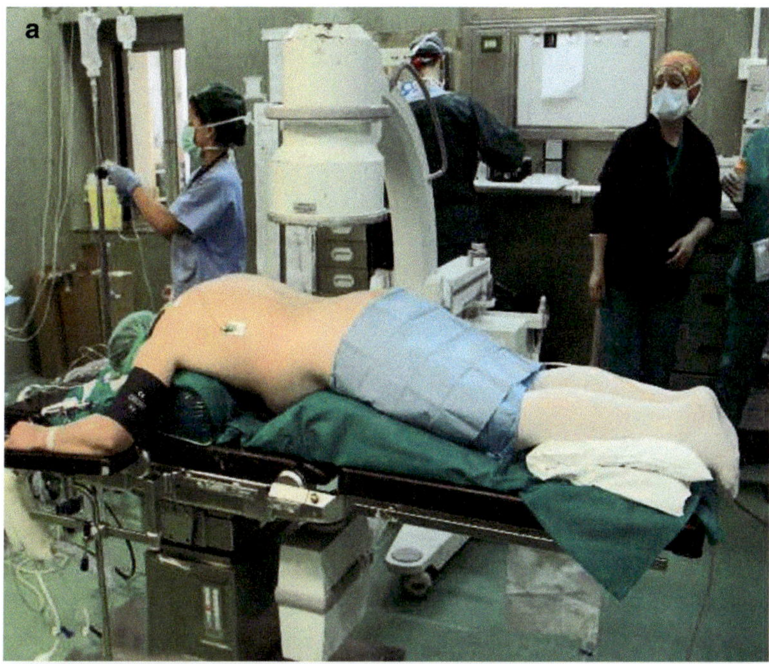

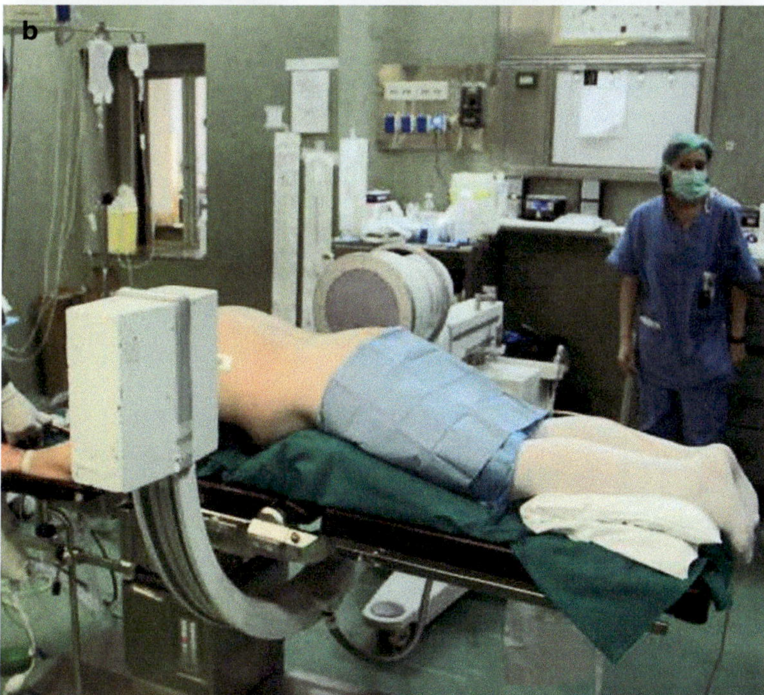

Fig. 9.1 (**a, b**) Operating table setup for a lower lumbar percutaneous pedicle screw fixation. (**a**) Anteroposterior position of the C-arm with the source emission part under the table. (**b**) By simply swinging the C-arm the lateral projection is obtained

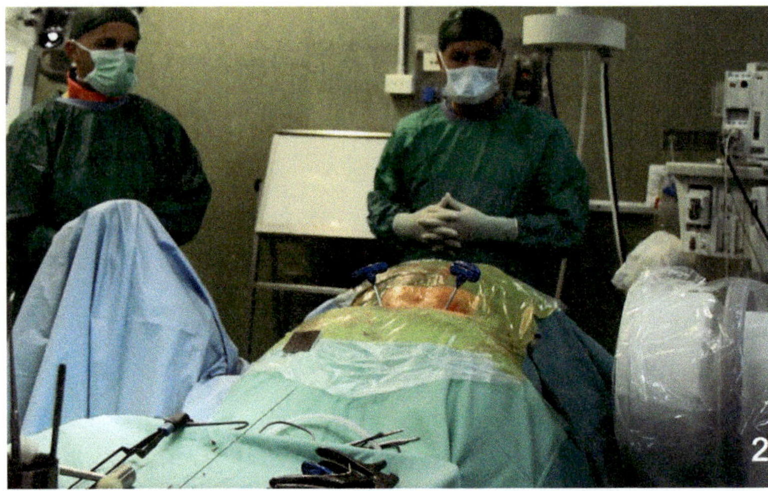

Fig. 9.2 Intraoperative picture with two Jamshidi needles inserted and the C-arm in the lateral projection. Note the intensifier end covered with a transparent sterile cap while the beam source is under the large drape fitted to the patient's side

Fig. 9.3 Fluoroscopic image in AP projection with previously positioned bilateral S1 screws. The next step is making the trajectories for the L5 screws. Note how the upper endplate of L5 appears as a single line. The *black arrow* indicates the medial and inferior margins of the L5 pedicle. The *white arrow* indicates the tip of the Jamshidi needle on the skin of the patient

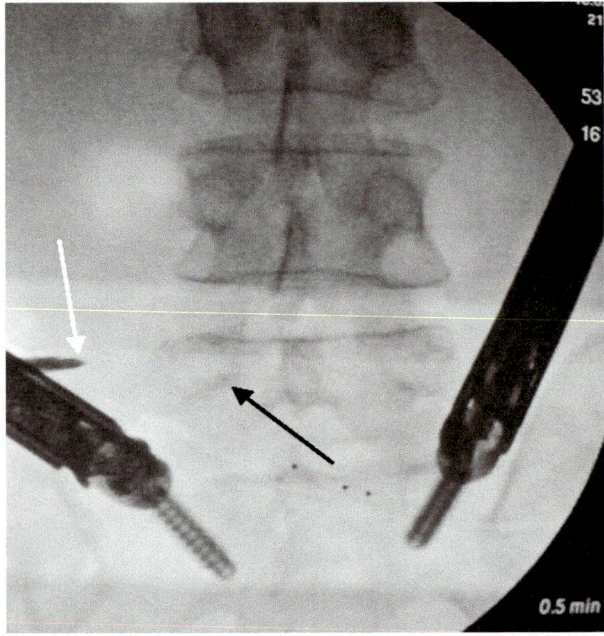

with a mallet and following the medially convergent trajectory. Frequent image controls are needed at this stage as the tip of the needle should never go beyond the medial edge of the pedicle in the AP view (Fig. 9.4). Once the medial edge is reached, the C-arm should be swung to the LL view. If the LL view shows the needle to be inside

Fig. 9.4 Same case as in Fig. 9.3. The Jamshidi needle has now been impacted into the pedicle, and the tip is resting at the medial margin of the L5 pedicle (*white arrow*). Once this point is reached, a lateral fluoroscopic image is needed to verify whether the tip of the needle is already inside the vertebral body

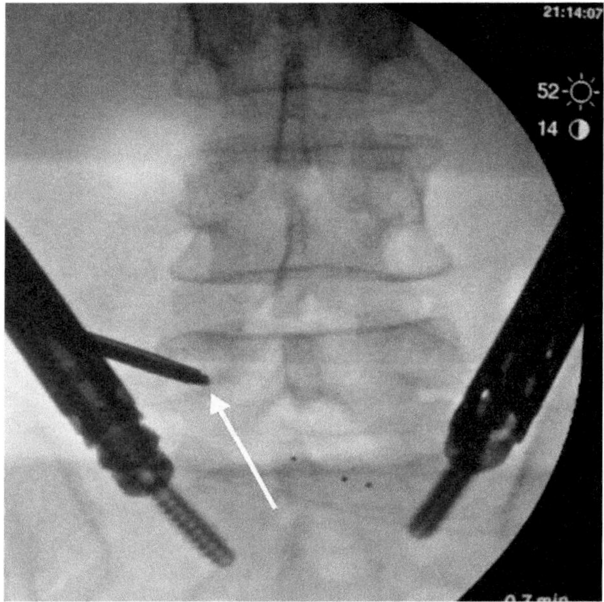

Fig. 9.5 Lateral fluoroscopic image projection. Two Jamshidi needles have been inserted into both L5 pedicles. Note that the tip of both is lying within the vertebral body (*black line* delineates the posterior wall). As long as the needles do not invade the medial pedicle wall on AP projections (see Fig. 9.4) and are within the vertebral body on the lateral projection, there is no risk of pedicle breach or invasion of the spinal canal

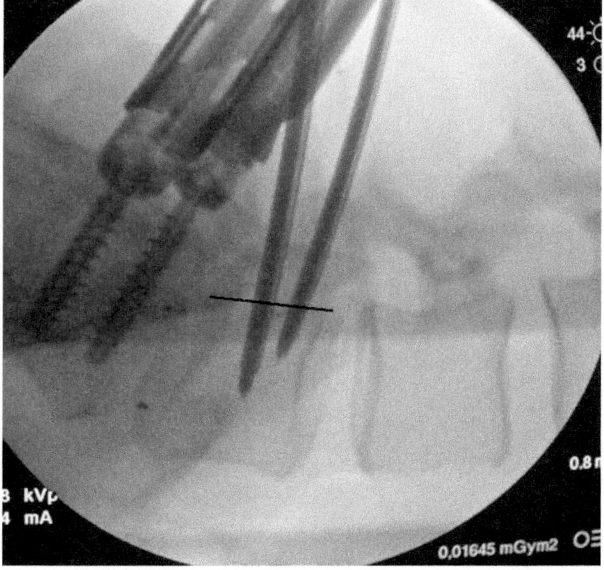

the vertebral body, there is no risk of pedicle violation, and the needle can be further impacted ready for the next step which is placement of the K-wire (Fig. 9.5). If on the LL view, however, the tip of the needle is still inside the pedicle, the trajectory is too converging and further impaction would cause medial pedicle wall breach. The C-arm needs thus to be put back into AP and the trajectory needs to be corrected.

Fig. 9.6 (**a**) Intraoperative picture showing bilateral inserted Jamshidi needles with insertion of a K-wire in one of them. (**b**) Lateral fluoroscopic image showing two K-wires in L5 after the Jamshidi cannulae have been withdrawn. The *black arrow* points at the K-wire in position, the *white arrow* shows the tapping device inserted over the other K-wire

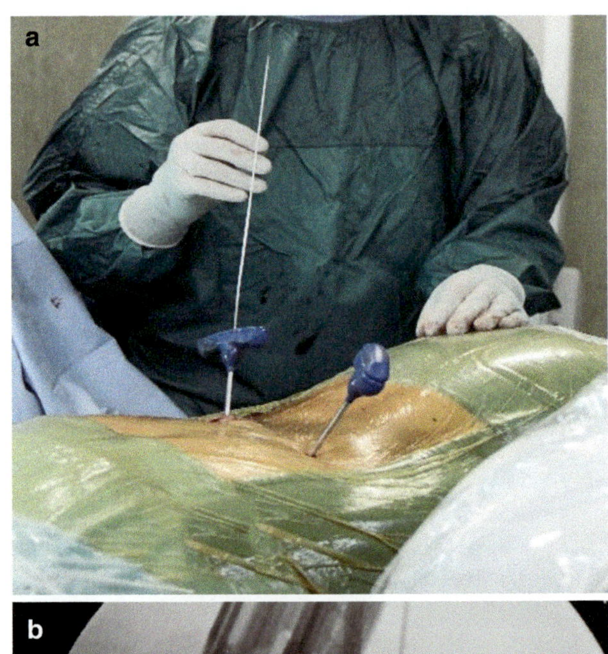

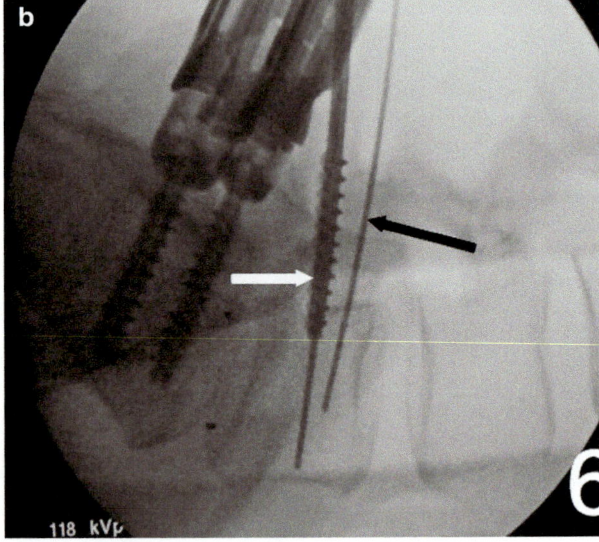

Once the Jamshidi needle is in the vertebral body as seen on the LL view, K-wires can be inserted through the needles and advanced until the tip rests well inside the vertebral body. The needles are now withdrawn making sure that the K-wires do not move (Fig. 9.6a, b). The next step consists in inserting serial

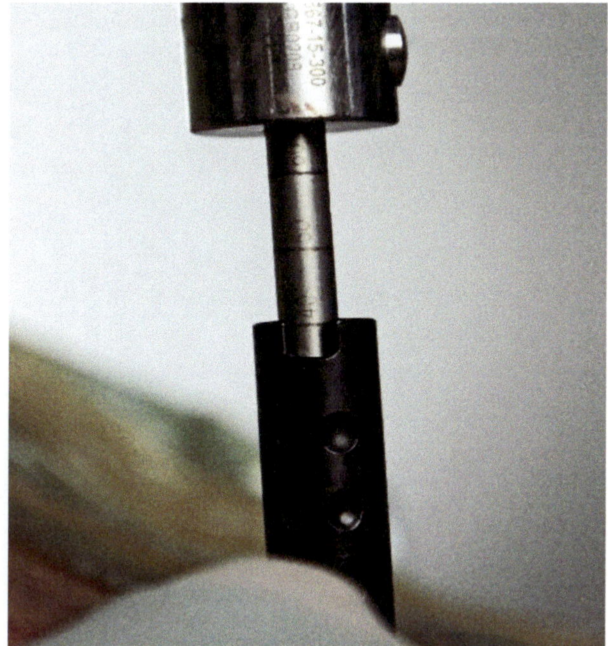

Fig. 9.7 Intraoperative picture showing a close-up of the tapping device inserted into the dilator cannula. The latter is docked against bone at the screw entry site. With the tap thus being inserted up to the desired length, the length of the screw can be identified from the marking on the tap in relation to the upper border of the cannula (Viper 2 system, DePuy, Johnson & Johnson)

dilators over the K-wire so as to split and dilate the muscles. The dilator will now rest at the height of the screw entry point and the K-wire within the vertebral body.

Tapping of the Pedicle Screw Trajectory

At this stage the screw trajectory needs to be tapped and screw length determined.

Tapping is usually done with a diameter that is one millimeter smaller than the desired screw diameter to permit for increased insertional torque which appears to correlate with pullout strength.

Under lateral control the tap is thus inserted over the K-wire, and the tip is brought to lie at the desired depth at which the tip of the screw should be. Most systems have depth markings on the taps, which when read against the upper margin of the dilator indicate the depth of insertion of the tap and thus the screw length needed (Figs. 9.6b and 9.7). The inserted tap length is read on the dilator cannula and subsequently a screw of appropriate length and diameter inserted. The screws are mounted on cannulae that will remain attached to the screw once disengaged from the screwdriver.

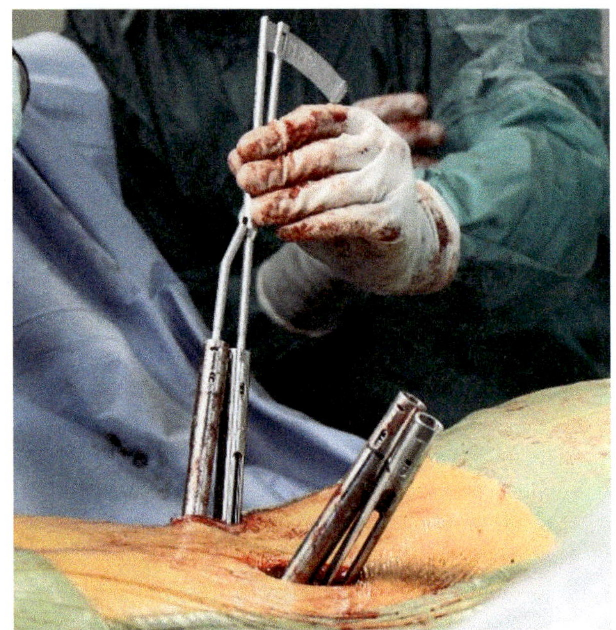

Fig. 9.8 Intraoperative picture showing four screws inserted with their respective cannulae. A caliper is inserted in the two adjacent screws to determine rod length

Insertion of the Rods and Final Tightening

Once all the pedicle screws are inserted, the respective cannulae that hold them will be standing out of the incisions and will guide both the insertion of the rods as well as the compression-distraction maneuvers and final tightening. The first step is determination of rod length. As the screws' heads are not accessible, the determination of the distance between two adjacent tulips is generally determined with the insertion of a caliper that indicates the distance at the level of the screw heads (Fig. 9.8).

Subsequently the appropriate length rod is chosen and inserted either through the same incision as the one used for the screws or through a separate stab incision. The respective procedures vary according to the systems. The various systems will have specific tools to permit for compression-distraction and final tightening of the screw nuts. Finally, once everything is tightened, the screw cannulae are removed and a final fluoroscopic image is taken in both projections (Fig. 9.9a, b).

The images used so far for the description of the operative technique belong to a case of L5–S1 recurrent disc herniation on the left with an important amount of low back pain. The patient was treated with a minimally invasive TLIF and PPS. As can be seen in Fig. 9.10a, the discectomy and subsequent oblique

Fig. 9.9 (**a**, **b**) Fluoroscopic images of the same patient in Fig. 9.8. (**a**) Anteroposterior image showing final construct of L5–S1 instrumentation with transforaminal interbody fusion (TLIF). (**b**) Note the radiodense markers in the polyether ether ketone (PEEK) interbody cage inserted obliquely (*white arrows*)

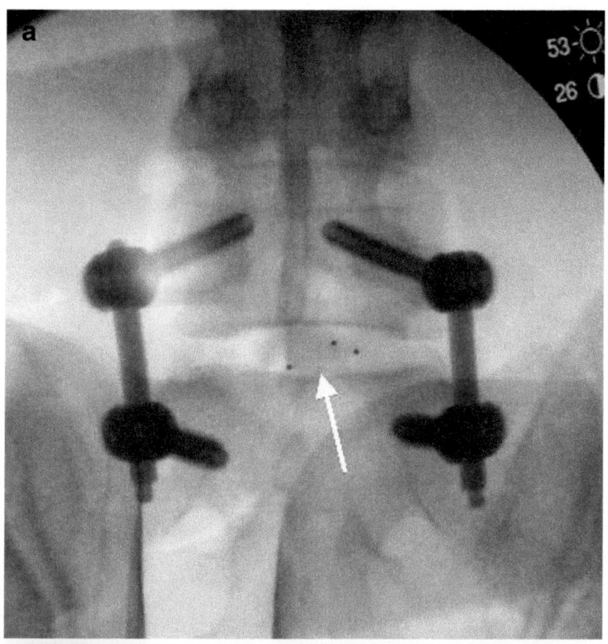

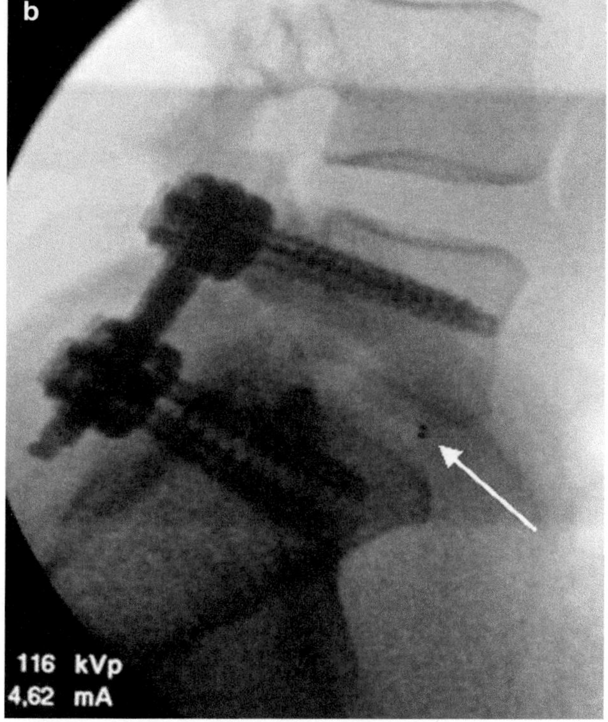

Fig. 9.10 (**a**, **b**)
Intraoperative image (Same
patient as in previous
pictures). (**a**) Tubular
retractor (Pipeline, DePuy,
Johnson & Johnson) in
position for transforaminal
discectomy, decompression,
and interbody cage insertion.
(**b**) Postoperative picture of
patient showing the two
bilateral small incisions for
the L5–S1 fixation and TLIF
procedures

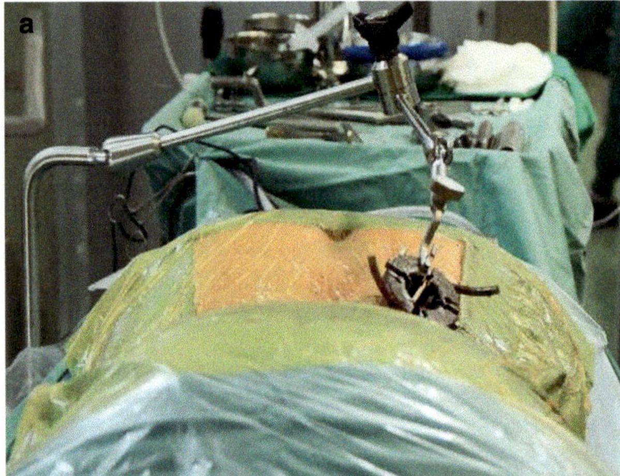

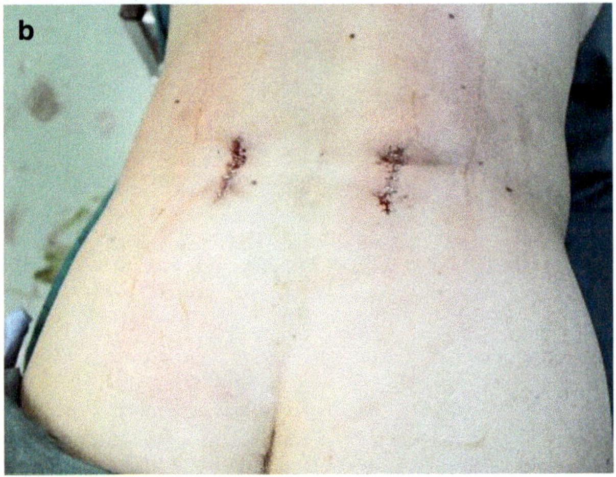

insertion of a straight PEEK cage was performed through a tubular retractor
through a small paramedian incision on the left. This same incision was then
used to insert the PPS on the same side and another incision made on the contralateral side for the PPS on the right. In Fig. 9.10b the size and location of the
incisions can be appreciated. No median incisions were made, and no muscle
stripping, or scar dissection, as this patient had undergone a previous discectomy, was needed.

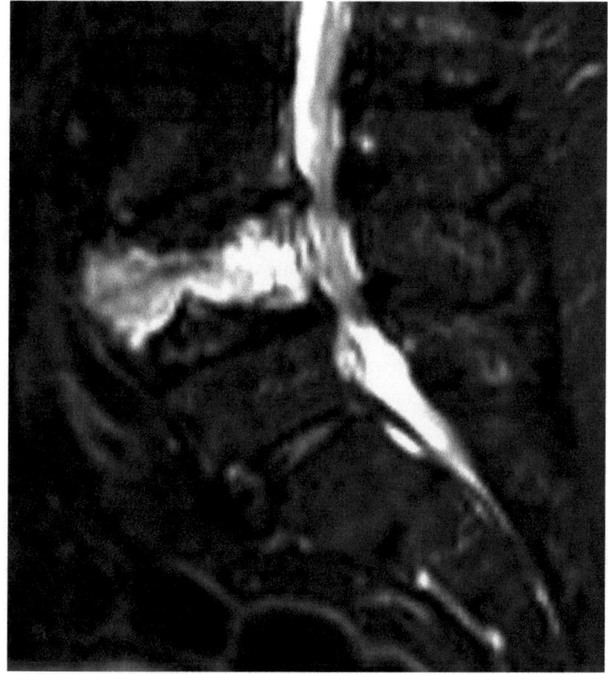

Fig. 9.11 MRI STIR sequence showing how the entire body of L4 is replaced by a hyperintense mass lesion

Case Examples

Following is the description of three further cases to illustrate the modality and indications for use of lumbar PPS in different settings.

Case 1

This 72-year-old patient came to our observation after having performed imaging studies of the lumbar spine for non-remitting low back pain with increasing intensity over the previous 3 months. An MRI scan of the spine revealed a lesion replacing almost the entire body of L4, hypointense on T1WI and intensely hyperintense on T2WI and STIR sequences (Fig. 9.11).

A CT scan to further investigate the bony anatomy of the lesion revealed a significant destruction of the bone with impeding risk of vertebral collapse (Fig. 9.12). The case was reviewed with our neuroradiologists, and a differential diagnosis of aggressive angioma versus metastatic lesion was made. Tumoral workup revealed no primary tumor, and with the working diagnosis of aggressive angioma we discussed with the patient a treatment plan of preoperative angiography with potential embolization and subsequently an anterolateral retroperitoneal approach with placement of an expandable intervertebral cage in L4.

Due to the extensive bony destruction, we felt that any percutaneous augmentative procedure like vertebroplasty or kyphoplasty would neither be safe in terms of cement migration nor sufficient for structural support.

His general conditions were determined by overweight, type II diabetes, and chronic obstructive pulmonary disease (COPD), which together with the other data made an American Association of Anesthetists (ASA) score of 3.

After discussion of the risks with the patient, he was then scheduled for the proposed surgery. Preoperative angiography revealed modest vascularization, and intraoperative histology revealed a chordoma. The tumor was removed partially and an expandable cage fitted between L3 and L5 to keep the surgery as short as possible given the general conditions of the patient. It took the patient over 1 week to recover from the anterior surgery, and at that point posterior fixation was needed.

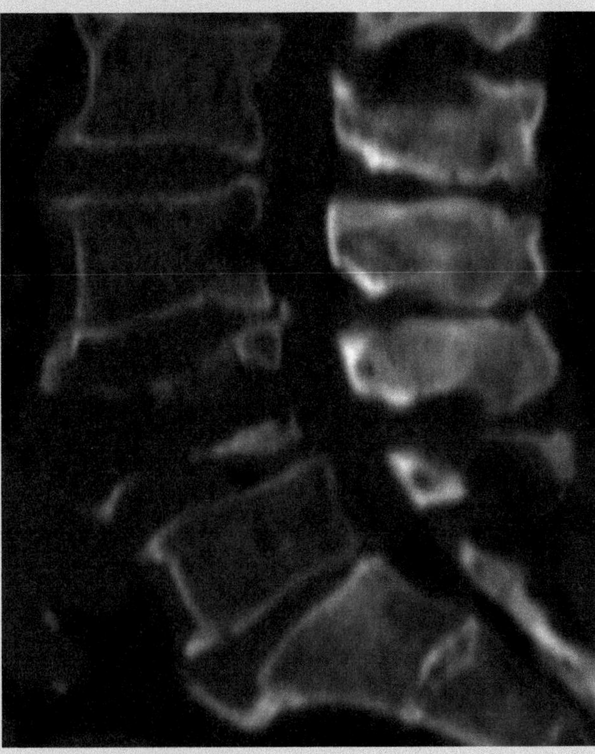

Fig. 9.12 CT scan with bony window of the same patient. The entire bony anatomy has been subverted in L4. Note in particular the absence of a posterior wall

Given the conditions of the patient and the need for a procedure that would be least invasive, percutaneous pedicle screw fixation appeared to be the only option.

Thus he underwent L3–L5 fixation in a procedure that lasted less than 1 h and with neglectable blood loss (Fig. 9.13). Postoperative course was very favorable and the patient mobilized standing on postoperative day 2.

Postoperative x-rays revealed good position of the implants. This is maintained at two and a half years follow-up with a control CT scan that revealed no progression of the disease. The patient mobilizes autonomously and is able to do his routinary daily activities with minimum pain.

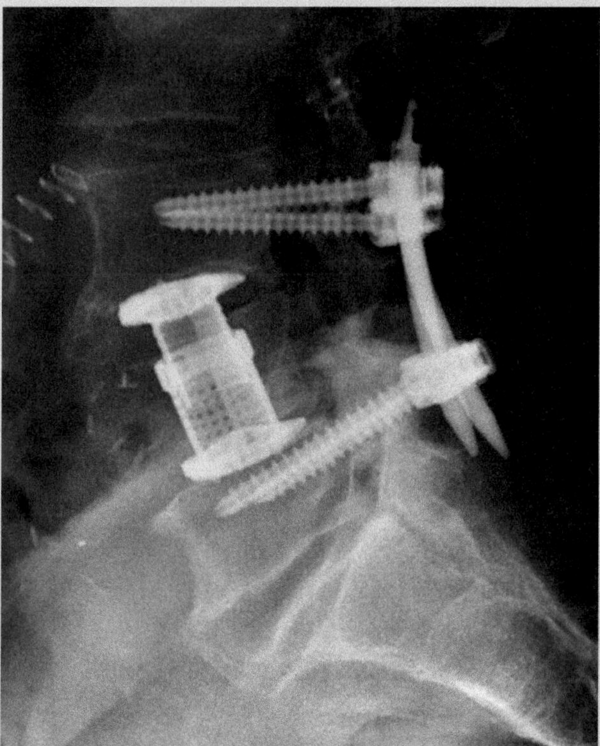

Fig. 9.13 Postoperative radiograph showing the expandable titanium cage in L4 inserted in the first step surgery via an anterolateral retroperitoneal approach (Synex, Synthes). In the second surgery L3 and L5 pedicle screws were inserted percutaneously (Sextant, Medtronic)

Case 2

This 56-year-old self-employed male was involved in a motorcycle accident that resulted in a three-column fracture of L4. It was essentially a burst fracture, but given two coronal fracture lines through the bases of the pedicles, there was instability of the posterior column as well with diastasis of the zygapophyseal joints bilaterally (Figs. 9.14a, b and 9.15). The patient had no deficit.

We discussed with the patient the option of conservative treatment in a lumbar brace with however a significant risk of future instability due to the bilateral joint rupture.

He discarded any attempt at conservative treatment and sought for an option that permitted quick recovery and return to work.

We therefore performed a percutaneous L4–5 pedicle screw fixation. The operation went well with less than 1 h operative time, neglectable blood loss, and discharge home after autonomous mobilization on the first postoperative day. The patient resumed his working activity after 2 weeks. At almost 3 years follow-up, he does not complain of any problems, and control x-rays show regular position of the implant (Fig. 9.16).

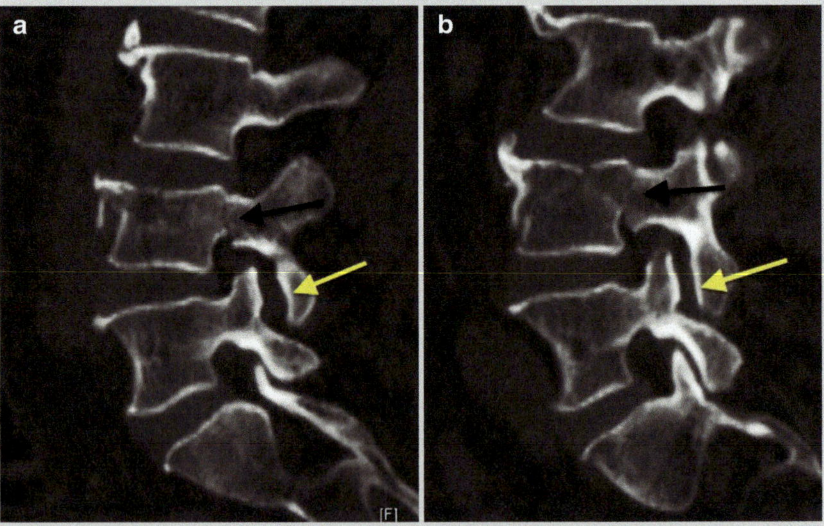

Fig. 9.14 (**a, b**) CT scan sagittal reconstruction in bone window. Figure (**a**) goes through the right joint and figure (**b**) through the left. Note the fracture lines at the base of the pedicles (*black arrows*) and note the diastasis on both sides (*yellow arrows*)

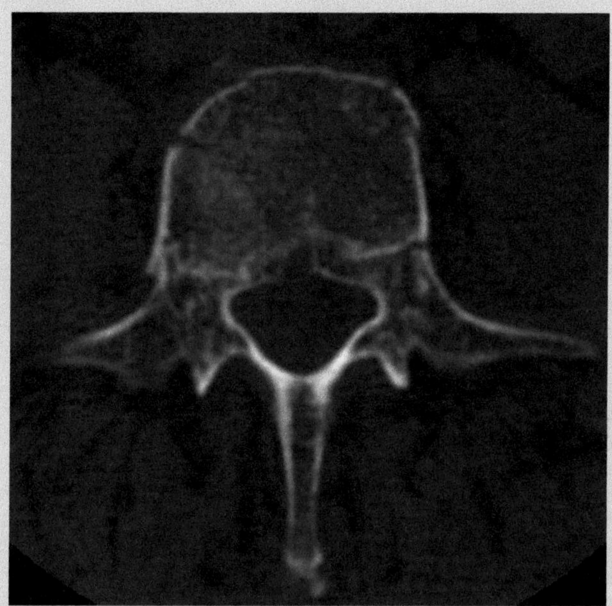

Fig. 9.15 CT scan image axial in bone window. Note the fracture lines at the base of the pedicles

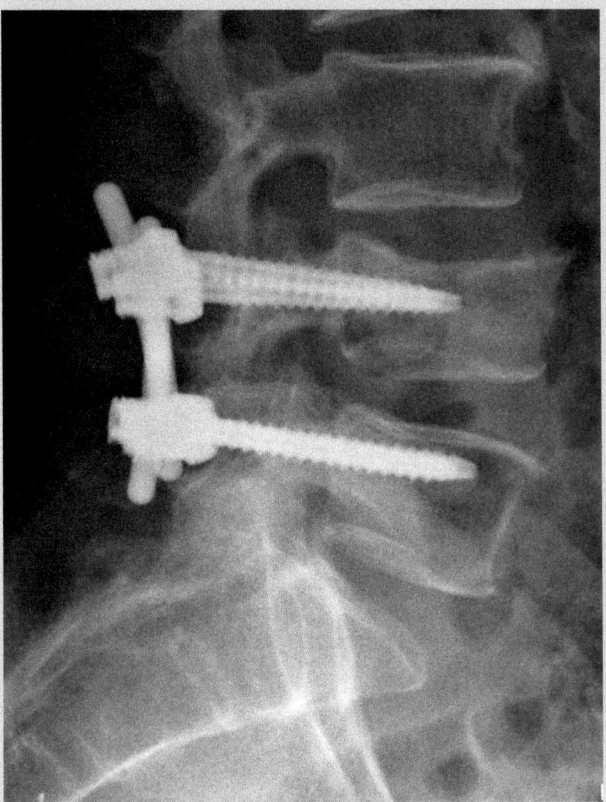

Fig. 9.16 Two-year postoperative radiograph after percutaneous L4–L5 pedicle screw instrumentation (Icon, Blackstone Medical)

Case 3

This 74-year-old lady came to our observation after a minor fall that had resulted in a L3 burst fracture. Being a severe osteoporotic she had already had a L1 fracture a couple of years prior that had healed with no problems but with some kyphosis. Given the poor quality of the bone and the risk of progression with further kyphosis adding to the already existing, as well as the need for early and efficient mobilization, we decided to offer the patient operative much rather than conservative treatment (Fig. 9.17).

She underwent percutaneous kyphoplasty in L3 and percutaneous placement of cement augmented pedicle screws in L2 and L4.

Her postoperative course was characterized by immediate improvement of back pain and mobilization with autonomous walking on the second postoperative day. After 5 days the pain from the intervention was very well controlled with paracetamol, and the patient was discharged home. At the latest control one and a half years postoperative, she is pain free and independent. X-rays show a good position of the implants and good maintenance of lordosis (Fig. 9.18).

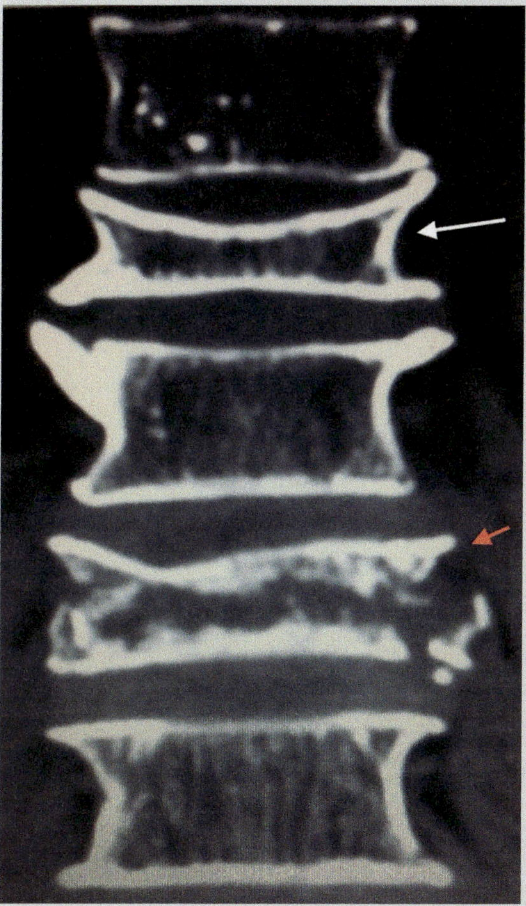

Fig. 9.17 CT scan coronal section showing the L3 burst fracture and the poor bone quality (*red arrow*). Note also the previous fracture in L1 (*white arrow*) which is healed but with a considerable amount of loss of height

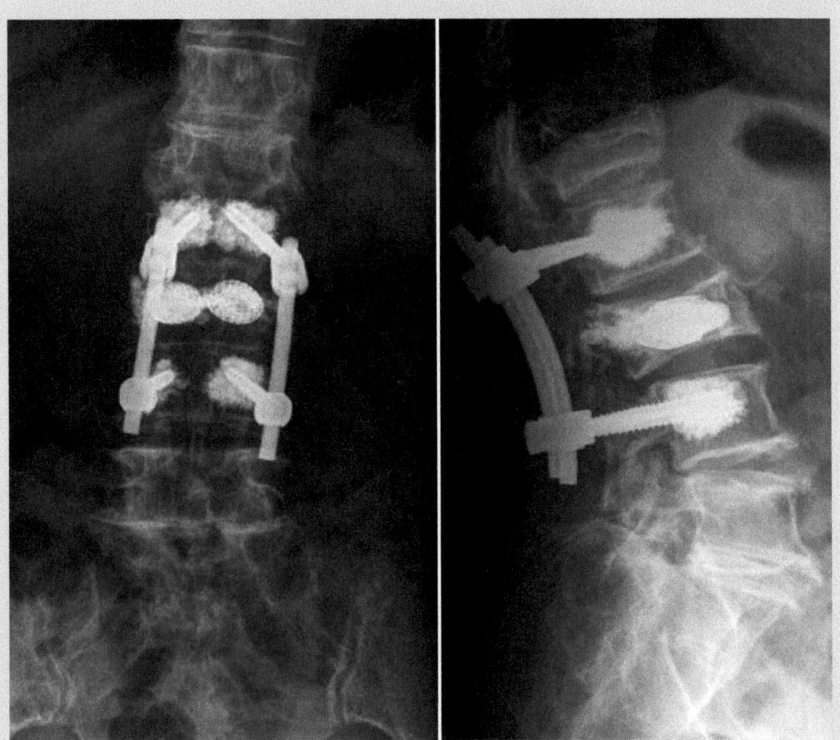

Fig. 9.18 Postoperative radiograph showing the fixation with cement-augmented pedicle screws in L1 and L3 and the kyphoplasty in L2 (Pangea and VBS, Synthes). Note the maintenance of segmental lordosis at the operated level and the kyphosis at the level of the previously fractured L1 vertebra

Accuracy and Safety

Two main factors need to be taken into account when it comes to accuracy and safety of pedicle screws: the rate of misplacement in terms of pedicle breach and in terms of violation of the superior adjacent articulation. As far as the former is concerned, the rate of medial pedicle breaches should ideally be nil or as close to as possible due to the obvious risk of nerve root damage or irritation that goes along with a significant breach. As for superior facet violation, the immediate effects might not be evident but could potentially show in the future under the form of superior adjacent segment degeneration, caused by a zygapophyseal joint that has been rendered insufficient by violation of its integrity from a suboptimal placed pedicle screw.

Accuracy and safety of pedicle screw placement depends both on the level of training of the surgeon and on the technique used.

As described above, the authors use a 2-dimensional (2D) or biplanar fluoroscopy technique without any computer guidance. By strictly observing the radiological landmarks and making sure that the needle is within the vertebral body on the lateral projection once it has reached the medial wall on the AP before advancing it any further, in our personal series of over 70 patients with more than 350 screws placed in both the lumbar and dorsal spine, no instance of clinically evident screw malposition was noted and thus no revision needed. We have, however, not carried out any computed tomography (CT) study to investigate on breach rate and entity.

Kim et al. retrospectively evaluated 488 pedicle screws in 110 consecutive patients and noted an incidence of cortical encroachment of 12.5 % with frank penetration of the medial cortex in the majority of these [32]. However, only 0.4 % of patients had to undergo revision for pain and foot drop, respectively. Knox et al. report on 61 consecutive patients in which seven cortical breaches were noted for a rate of 2.48 %. One of these had to undergo screw revision [33]. These authors also investigated the frequency of superior facet violation which resulted in 11.48 % of the cases.

Patel et al. carried out a cadaver study in which a total of 48 screws were inserted and classified [34]. The placement of 28 screws (58 %) resulted in violation of facet articulation, with 8 of these screws being intra-articular. The largest and most recent series to our knowledge was reported by Smith et al. on 151 consecutive patients with 601 screws placed percutaneously [35]. Radiological misplacement as investigated with CT scan was 6.2 % with over half of these considered significant (>3 mm). Clinical complications in that series occurred in two patients and were transitory without the need for revision surgery.

Biplanar non-navigated fluoroscopy was used in all the series.

Conclusion

Percutaneous pedicle screw placement appears to be a safe and accurate technique with various series in the literature documenting a low rate of complications. The technique compares well to the traditional open technique in which pedicle breach rates have been described as high as 29 %, although the criteria for quantifying and thus identifying a cortical breach are not homogeneous, thus making direct comparison of the series difficult.

Biplanar non-navigated fluoroscopy appears to be reliable, and both the experience of the authors, as well as the cited series in the literature, compare well with reports where 2D and 3D computer-assisted techniques were implemented [36, 37].

The learning curve for safe performance of percutaneous techniques can be quite steep initially and requires the skill of 3D imagination of the operator based on 2D images. As the learning process progresses, radiation exposure to both the patient and the surgeon reduces significantly, and we recommend the acquisition of the initial skills either in cadaver labs or on models. This spares the patients the exposure to excessive radiation, and the nature of the technique lends itself to be acquired close-to-reality on a model or even better a cadaver specimen.

Finally, once in the armamentarium of the spinal surgeon, the placement of percutaneous pedicle screws might expand its application beyond minimally invasive techniques but can also be implemented in open procedures. In cases, for example, where open central decompression is indicated, especially in the L5–S1 segment, initial placement of the screws percutaneously with subsequent midline opening and application of the rods will still significantly reduce muscle dissection, damage, and bleeding and thus reduce the burden of the procedure on the patient.

References

1. Roy-Camille R, Demeulenaere C. Osteosynthese du rachis dorsal, lombaire et lombosacree par plaque metalliques vissees dans les pedicles vertebraux et les apophyses articulaires. Presse Med. 1970;78:1447–8.
2. Roy-Camille R. Current trends in surgery of the spine. Int Orthop. 1989;13(2):81–7.
3. Vaccaro AR, Garfin SR. Internal fixation (pedicle screw fixation) for fusions of the lumbar spine. Spine (Phila Pa 1976). 1995;20(24 Suppl):157S–65.
4. Boos N, Webb JK. Pedicle screw fixation in spinal disorders: a European view. Eur Spine J. 1997;6(1):2–18.
5. Michelsen C, Jackson R, Lowe T, Farcy JP, Deinlein D. A multi-center prospective study of the CD spinal system in patients with degenerative disc disease. J Spinal Disord. 1998;11(6):465–70.
6. Gaines Jr RW. The use of pedicle-screw internal fixation for the operative treatment of spinal disorders. J Bone Joint Surg Am. 2000;82-A(10):1458–76.
7. Dickman CA, Detwiler PW, Porter RW. The role of pedicle screw fixation for lumbar spinal stabilization and fusion. Clin Neurosurg. 2000;47:495–513.
8. Park P, Garton HJ, Gala VC, Hoff JT, McGillicuddy JE. Adjacent segment disease after lumbar or lumbosacral fusion: review of the literature. Spine (Phila Pa 1976). 2004;29(17):1938–1944.
9. Polly Jr DW, Santos ER, Mehbod AA. Surgical treatment for the painful motion segment: matching technology with the indications: posterior lumbar fusion. Spine (Phila Pa 1976). 2005;30(16 Suppl):S44–51.
10. Kawaguchi Y, Matsui H, Tsuji H. Back muscle injury after posterior lumbar spine surgery. Part 1: histologic and histochemical analyses in rats. Spine. 1994;19:2590–7.
11. Kong WZ, Goel VK, Gilbertson LG, Weinstein JN. Effects of muscle dysfunction on lumbar spine mechanics. A finite element study based on a two motion segment model. Spine. 1996;21:2197–206.
12. Bogduk N. A reappraisal of the anatomy of the human lumbar erector spinae. J Anat. 1980;131:525–40.
13. Kalimo H, Rantanen J, Viljianen T, et al. Lumbar muscles: structure and function. Ann Med. 1989;21:353–9.
14. Mathews HH, Long BH. Endoscopy assisted percutaneous anterior interbody fusion with subcutaneous suprafascial internal fixation: evolution, techniques and surgical considerations. Orthop Int Ed. 1995;3:496–500.
15. Lowery GL, Kulkarni SS. Posterior percutaneous spine instrumentation. Eur Spine J. 2000;9 Suppl 1:S126–30.
16. Foley KT, Gupta SK, Justis JR, Sherman MC. Percutaneous pedicle screw fixation of the lumbar spine. Neurosurg Focus. 2001;15:10(4).

17. Hsieh PC, Koski TR, Sciubba DM, et al. Maximizing the potential of minimally invasive spine surgery in complex spinal disorders. Neurosurg Focus. 2008;25(2):E19.
18. Mobbs RJ, Sivabalan P, Li J. Minimally invasive surgery compared to open spinal fusion for the treatment of degenerative lumbar spine pathologies. J Clin Neurosci. 2012;19(6):829–35.
19. Molina CA, Gokaslan ZL, Sciubba DM. A systematic review of the current role of minimally invasive spine surgery in the management of metastatic spine disease. Int J Surg Oncol. 2011;2011:598148.
20. Park Y, Ha JW. Comparison of one-level posterior lumbar interbody fusion performed with a minimally invasive approach or a traditional open approach. Spine (Phila Pa 1976). 2007;32(5):537–43.
21. Adorer O, Parker SL, Bydon A, Cheng J, McGirt MJ. Comparative effectiveness of minimally invasive versus open transforaminal lumbar interbody fusion: 2-year assessment of narcotic use, return to work, disability, and quality of life. J Spinal Disord Tech. 2011;24(8):479–84.
22. Ni W-F, Huang Y-X, Chi Y-L, et al. Percutaneous pedicle screw fixation for neurologic intact thoracolumbar burst fractures. J Spinal Disord Tech. 2010;23:530–7.
23. Verlaan JJ, Diekerhof CH, Buskens E, et al. Surgical treatment of traumatic fractures of the thoracic and lumbar spine. Spine. 2004;29:803–14.
24. Adogwa O, Parker SL, Bydon A, et al. Comparative effectiveness of minimally invasive versus open transforaminal lumbar interbody fusion 2-year assessment of narcotic use return to work, disability, and quality of life. J Spinal Disord Tech. 2011;24:479–84.
25. Rouben D, Casnellie M, Ferguson M, et al. Long-term durability of minimal invasive posterior transforaminal lumbar interbody fusion a clinical and radiographic follow-up. J Spinal Disord Tech. 2011;24:288–96.
26. Payer M. "Minimally invasive" lumbar spine surgery: a critical review. Acta Neurochir (Wien). 2011;153(7):1455–9.
27. Jindal N, Sankhala SS, Bachhal V. The role of fusion in the management of burst fractures of the thoracolumbar spine treated by short segment pedicle screw fixation: a prospective randomised trial. J Bone Joint Surg Br. 2012;94(8):1101–6.
28. Dai LY, Jiang LS, Jiang SD. Posterior short-segment fixation with or without fusion for thoracolumbar burst fractures. A five to seven-year prospective randomized study. J Bone Joint Surg Am. 2009;91(5):1033–41.
29. Wang ST, Ma HL, Liu CL, Yu WK, Chang MC, Chen TH. Is fusion necessary for surgically treated burst fractures of the thoracolumbar and lumbar spine? A prospective, randomized study. Spine (Phila Pa 1976). 2006;31(23):2646–52; discussion 2653.
30. Rampersaud YR, Foley KT, Shen AC, Williams S, Solomito M. Radiation exposure to the spine surgeon during fluoroscopically assisted pedicle screw insertion. Spine (Phila Pa 1976). 2000;25(20):2637–45.
31. Mehlman CT, DiPasquale TG. Radiation exposure to the orthopaedic surgical team during fluoroscopy: "how far away is far enough?". J OrthopTrauma. 1997;11(6):392–8.
32. Kim MC, Chung HT, Cho JL, et al. Factors affecting the accurate placement of percutaneous pedicle screws during minimally invasive transforaminal lumbar interbody fusion. Eur Spine J. 2011;20(10):1635–43.
33. Knox JB, Dai 3rd JM, Orchowski JR. Superior segment facet joint violation and cortical violation after minimally invasive pedicle screw placement. Spine J. 2011;11(3):213–7.
34. Patel RD, Graziano GP, Vanderhave KL, et al. Facet violation with the placement of percutaneous pedicle screws. Spine (Phila Pa 1976). 2011;36(26):E1749–52.
35. Smith ZA, Sugimoto K, Lawton CD, Fessler RG. Incidence of lumbar spine pedicle breach following percutaneous screw fixation: a radiographic evaluation of 601 screws in 151 patients. J Spinal Disord Tech. 2012 Jun 7 [Epub ahead of print].
36. Ravi B, Zaharai A, Rampersaud R. CLinical accuracy of computer-assisted two-dimensional fluoroscopy for the percutaneous placement of lumbosacral pedicle screws. Spine. 2001;36(1):84–91.
37. Villavicencio AT, Burneikiene S, Bulsara KR, et al. Utility of computerized isocentric fluoroscopy for minimally invasive spinal surgical techniques. J Spinal Disord Tech. 2055;18(4):369–75.

Chapter 10
Dynamic Stabilization of the Lumbar Spine: Current Status of Minimally Invasive and Open Treatments

Carlo Doria, Francesco Muresu, and Paolo Tranquilli Leali

Introduction

In recent years, the number of systems for dynamic stabilization of the lumbar spine has grown significantly. These nonfusion systems are designed to maintain or restore the intersegmental motion of the intact spine and have no adverse effects on adjacent segments [1–3]. However, today the gold standard system for the stabilization of the lumbar spine remains internal fixation, although the idea of dynamic fixation has aroused increasing interest in surgery of the lumbar spine.

The fusion systems make use of different technical solutions, ranging from complete replacement of the disk, to keeping the core intact annulus, to maintenance of the disk but keeping under control the whole segment motion. Internal fixators are generally used as an adjunct to fusion, where, in many instances, the disc is replaced by either intervertebral cages, allograft, or autologous bone graft [4–6].

Improvements are needed in the predictability of pain relief, the reduction of treatment-related morbidities, and overall clinical success rates of pain reduction and function [7]. Recent advances in fusion techniques have elevated arthrodesis rates, without an equivalent improvement in relief of pain. Fusion is intended to alleviate pain secondary to abnormal motion or instability. Recent reports, however, have demonstrated relative success with implants that permit movement rather than eliminate it [7].

Abnormal patterns of load transmission are recognized as a principal cause of osteoarthritic changes in other joints. Spinal osteoarthritic changes may be caused by similar forces across the lumbar disc. Dynamic stabilization, or "soft stabilization," systems seek to alter the mechanical loading of the motion segment by

C. Doria, MD (✉)
U.O.C. Orthopedics and Traumatology, San Martino Hospital, ASL 5, Oristano, Italy
e-mail: reemad@tiscali.it

F. Muresu, MD • P.T. Leali, MD
Department of Orthopedics, University of Sassari, Sassari, Italy

P.P.M. Menchetti (ed.), *Minimally Invasive Surgery of the Lumbar Spine*,
DOI 10.1007/978-1-4471-5280-4_10, © Springer-Verlag London 2014

unloading the disc, without the loss of motion required by fusion surgery [7, 8]. Low-back symptoms often implicate abnormal loading rather than motion as the primary source of pain. Many patients complain of postural or positional pain as a prevailing symptom [9]. Radiographs of these patients often fail to demonstrate motion on dynamic studies. Furthermore, many patients with low-back pain fail to improve following a successful lumbar fusion [9]. These observations suggest that low-back pain may have etiologies related to load, and successful treatments may exist beyond fusion.

Pain at a symptomatic motion segment may originate from the vertebral end-plates, the disc anulus, vertebral periosteum, facet joints, and/or surrounding supportive soft tissue structures [10]. As the lumbar spine ages, these structures undergo well-described degenerative changes, such as disc space dehydration and collapse, and corresponding facet arthropathy. The increased stiffness that accompanies these changes may further aggravate global spinal function by diminishing sagittal balance and disrupting coronal and sagittal contour [11–13].

Rationale for Dynamic Stabilization

Dynamic stabilization has several theoretical advantages over fusion. By allowing limited motion, dynamic stabilization may negate the deleterious effects of fusion on adjacent levels and on overall sagittal balance [7, 14]. Fusion has been implicated in accelerated disease of adjacent motion segments and, in the case of surgical posterior distracting procedures, major deformities such as flat back syndrome [7, 15]. Even well-performed fusions impose considerable postural stress on levels above the fusion. Fusions from L4 to S1 place considerable rotatory stress on the sacroiliac joints during sitting [7, 16]. Dynamic systems may allow the motion segment to be altered in an anatomic fashion when subjected to postural changes. Furthermore, solid posterolateral fusions do not stop loading of the disc. Although the pattern of load transmission may be altered, fusion may also prevent the spine from taking up a position where normal loading occurs [7].

Spinal fusion remains the gold standard for surgical management of instability and mechanical low-back pain. However, even in carefully selected patients, successful clinical results can be difficult to achieve. Reasons for failure include pseudarthrosis and adjacent segment disease. Although dynamic stabilization seems promising in some clinical reports, a cautious approach should be taken to any new spinal-implant system. Whereas an implant for fusion only has to provide temporary stabilization until fusion has taken place, a dynamic stabilization system has to provide stability throughout its life. Implant loosening following fusion surgery is common in the presence of pseudarthrosis. With dynamic stabilization, the implant has to stay anchored to the bone despite allowing movement. Any mismatch between the kinematics of the implant system and the motion segment and, in particular, any discrepancy between their instantaneous axis of rotation would result in the implant bearing unexpected load at certain ranges of motion. The need for strict bench testing in the laboratory, therefore, is critical. The few dynamic stabilization systems that have had clinical applications so far have produced some clinical outcomes comparable to that of fusion [17].

In the course of the degenerative process, during which the segment undergoes various anatomic alterations, there are significant changes in both the motion characteristics of, and the load distribution across, the affected (and possibly also neighboring) segments [18–20]. The loading pattern and motion are, to a certain extent, interdependent, and alterations in either (or both) may contribute to the generation of pain [18–20]. The concept of spinal fusion originally arose from the notion that a degenerated motion segment is often "unstable" or shows "movement abnormalities," and that, accordingly, the elimination of motion in the affected segment would prevent it from undertaking the movements associated with the generation of pain. Recent thinking, however, suggests that the prevention of movement may not be the most important factor accounting for the success of fusion [18–20].

Different Strategies for Dynamic Stabilization of the Lumbar Spine

Lumbar dynamic stabilization devices provide dynamic or "soft" stabilization by providing a posterior tension band. This places the motion segment in extension while allowing limited movements in other planes. The dynamic stabilization devices that have been described from time to time and used clinically may be classified into four categories:

1. Ligaments across pedicle screws

   - Graf ligament
   - Dynesys device

2. Interspinous distraction devices

   - Minns silicone distraction device
   - Wallis system
   - X-STOP

3. Interspinous ligament devices

   - Elastic ligament (Bronsard's ligament across the spinous processes)
   - Loop system

4. Semi-rigid metallic devices across the pedicle screws

   - FASS system
   - DSS system

Graf Ligament

The Graf ligament system was one of the first such devices used. It consists of a posterior nonelastic band that serves as a ligament between two pedicle-based screws [7, 21]. The inventor, Henri Graf, thought that abnormal rotatory motion was responsible for pain generation; therefore, the device was primarily designed to control rotatory movement by locking the lumbar facets in the extended position. Limited flexion was allowed within the range of normal movement. By providing posterior tensioning, the system probably unloads the anterior disc and may redistribute the load transmission of the painful disc. Although widely used, the clinical effects of the Graf system have not been rigorously studied. Some analyses, however, have demonstrated clinical success of the Graf ligamentoplasty similar to fusion procedures [6, 7, 22]. In two separate studies, clinical rates of excellent to good outcomes were in the 75 % range at 2-year follow-up [7, 22, 23]. It is recommended by the authors that the device be used in younger patients with adequate lumbar musculature, and in whom facet arthropathy is minimal.

The Graf ligament stabilizes the lumbar segment through the coaptation of the bilateral facet joints, and it is the first posterior dynamic stabilization device to be widely clinically evaluated. The Graf procedure reportedly has the potential to treat flexion instability but cannot correct vertebral slippage or deformity. The most common surgical indication is degenerative lumbar disorder with less than 25 % of vertebral slip, minimal disc space narrowing, and facet arthrosis. In the mid- and long term, Graf ligamentoplasty may reduce the risk of adjacent segment degeneration. Kanayama et al. [17, 24] reported the adjacent-segment morbidity after Graf ligamentoplasty compared to posterolateral lumbar fusion at a minimum of 5-year follow-up in 45 patients.

Although there was no difference in the preoperative adjacent-segment disc condition between the two groups, radiographic evidence of adjacent-segment degeneration at final follow-up was more frequent in the posterolateral-lumbar-fusion group than the Graf group (25 and 6 % at L1–L2, 38 and 6 % at L2–L3, 38 and 18 % at L3–L4, and 43 and 18 % at L5–S1, respectively). One case in the Graf group (6 %) and five cases in the posterolateral-lumbar-fusion group (19 %) required additional surgery for adjacent-segment degeneration. The authors concluded that in well-selected patients, Graf ligamentoplasty lowers the rate of adjacent-segment degeneration [17, 24] (Figs. 10.1 and 10.2).

Dynesys System

The Dynesys system (Zimmer Spine, Warsaw, IN) includes a design that provides both controlled flexion and extension by combining a tension band with a plastic tube, which resides between pedicle screws. In flexion, motion is controlled by tension on the band, while during extension the plastic cylindrical tubes act as a

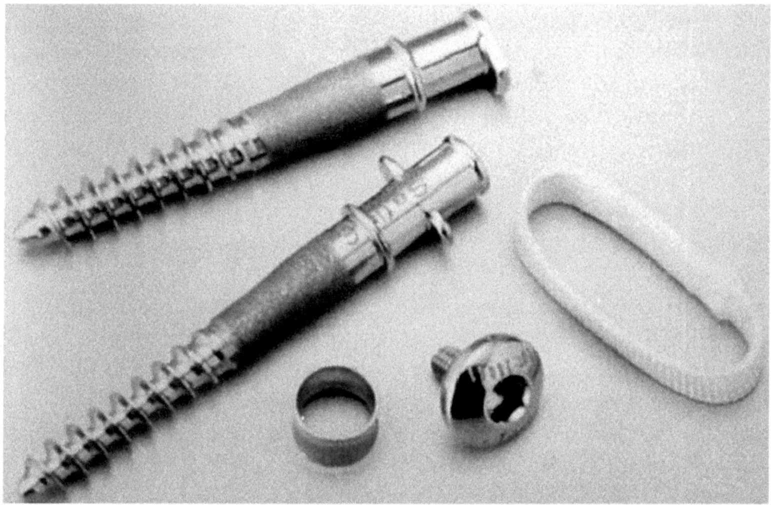

Fig. 10.1 Graf ligamentoplasty: the implant is shown disassembled. The components include a nonelastic band, which is secured around two pedicle screw heads by a metal band

Fig. 10.2 Graf ligamentoplasty: the implant is shown in situ

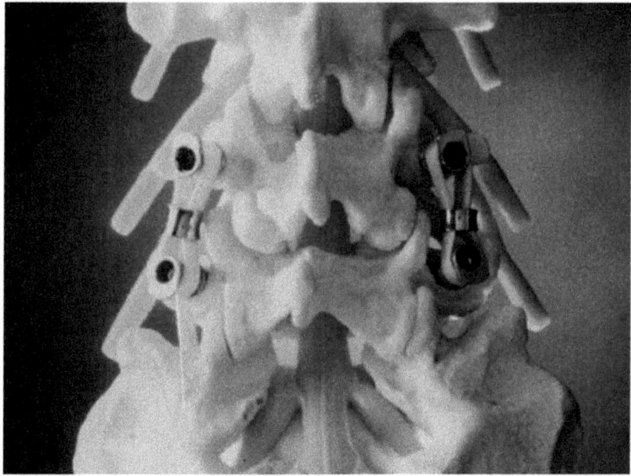

partially compressible spacer, thereby allowing limited extension [7, 25, 26]. Indeed, these plastic cylinders can be partially weight bearing in extension. In order to function properly, application of the Dynesys device must follow careful technical guidelines. Inappropriately long plastic spacers, for example, may cause a focal kyphosis, a scenario that has been associated with poor outcomes [7, 27]. The Dynesys system may have some advantage over pure band-like devices in that it provides some protection against compression of the posterior anulus, a structure known to contribute to painful load bearing.

The dynamic neutralization system for the spine (Dynesys) is a nonfusion pedicle screw stabilization system, which was developed more than 10 years ago [18, 27]. In view of the arguments presented above, and the suggestion that prevention of all movement within fused segments may not only be detrimental to sagittal balance and overall function, but may also elicit accelerated degenerative changes in neighboring segments, "soft stabilization" was developed. Although the system has now been in clinical use for almost a decade, there are few studies in the literature that report on patient-oriented outcome after Dynesys implantation [18, 27].

Dynesys was developed based upon all the current knowledge of and experience with conventional rigid pedicle systems. It establishes a mobile load transfer and controls motion of the segment in all planes, while inducing stability. Thus, the bilateral implant system controls motion in all planes. Stability with controller segmental motion is established, achieving a more physiological condition as compared with the sole decompression of an unstable segment or as compared with fusion of such a segment. In connection with decompressive procedures, the system re-establishes stability and avoids iatrogenic instability. Schnake et al. [17, 28] evaluated whether elastic stabilization with the Dynesys system provides enough stability to prevent instability after decompression for spinal stenosis with degenerative spondylolisthesis. Twenty-six patients with lumbar spinal stenosis and degenerative spondylolisthesis underwent interlaminar decompression and dynamic stabilization with the Dynesys system. Minimum follow-up was 2 years. Mean leg pain decreased significantly ($P<0.01$), and mean walking distance improved significantly to more than 1,000 m ($P<0.01$). There were five patients (21 %) who still had some claudication. A total of 21 patients (87.5 %) were satisfied and indicated that they would undergo the same procedure again. Radiographically, no significant progression of spondylolisthesis could be detected. The implant failure rate was 17 %, and none of the implant failures was clinically symptomatic. In elderly patients with spinal stenosis with degenerative spondylolisthesis, dynamic stabilization with the Dynesys system in addition to decompression leads to similar clinical results as seen in established protocols using decompression and fusion with pedicle screws. Dynesys also maintains enough stability to prevent further progression of spondylolisthesis or instability [17, 28].

Dynamic stabilization may prevent further degeneration of the lumbar spine. Putzier et al. [17, 29] evaluated the addition of dynamic stabilization to lumbar discectomy procedures in an attempt to investigate the effect of dynamic stabilization on segmental degeneration after discectomy. Eighty-four patients with initial-stage disc degeneration (Modic 1) underwent discectomy for symptomatic disc herniation and 35 had the addition of Dynesys stabilization. At mean 34-months follow-up, a significant increase in Oswestry Disability Scores and Visual Analog Scale results was observed only in the nonstabilized group. No progression of disc degeneration was noted in the Dynesys group at follow-up, whereas radiographic signs of accelerated degeneration were noted only in the discectomy group. The authors concluded that dynamic stabilization is useful to prevent progression of initial disc degeneration in segments after lumbar discectomy [17, 29] (Figs. 10.3, 10.4, and 10.5).

Fig. 10.3 Dynesys with the pedicle
screws connected by the synthetic
flexible cords, and spacers

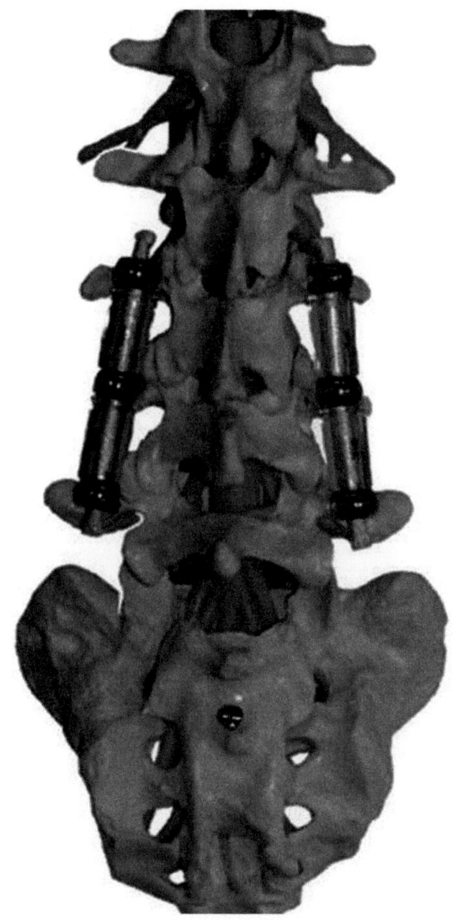

X-STOP Device

Another alternative system to lumbar fusion is the X-STOP interspinous process
distraction device. The X-STOP (Fig. 10.6) implant is a rigid titanium-alloy device
that is placed between the spinous processes to reduce the canal and foraminal
narrowing that occurs in extension. The X-STOP device is designed to distract the
posterior elements of the stenotic lumbar segment and place it in flexion to treat
neurogenic claudication. Anderson et al. [30] reported the results of X-STOP for
the treatment of neurogenic claudication in patients with degenerative spondylolisthesis. Forty-two patients underwent X-STOP surgery and 33 patients were
treated nonoperatively. Two-year follow-up data were obtained in 70 of the 75
patients. There was statistically significant improvement in the SF-36 scores of the
X-STOP device-treated patients but not in those of the nonoperative controls.
Overall clinical success occurred in 63 % of the X-STOP-treated patients and only
13 % of the controls. Spondylolisthesis and segmental kyphosis were unaltered.
The authors concluded that the X-STOP device was more effective than

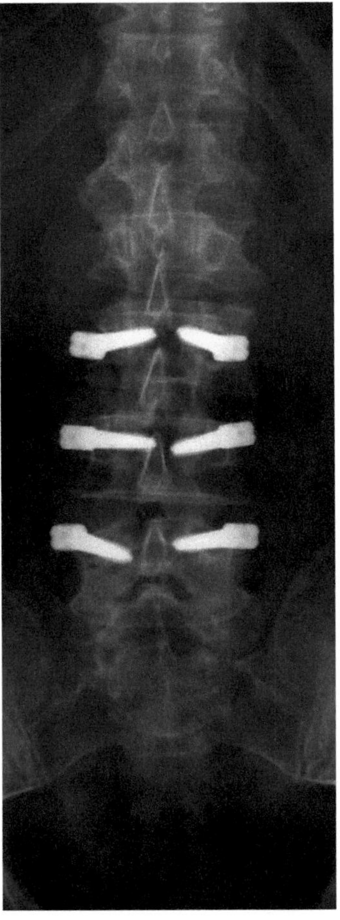

Fig. 10.4 Radiograph AP with Dynesys of the lumbar spine

nonoperative management of neurogenic claudication secondary to degenerative lumbar spondylolisthesis [30].

Spinal fusion has been accepted as the definitive surgical treatment of symptomatic lumbar degenerative disk disease and/or instability. The rationale for spinal arthrodesis as a treatment modality for low-back pain centers on the assumption that abnormal intervertebral motion causes pain and that immobilization of adjacent vertebral bodies will lead to a reduction in mechanical back pain. Unfortunately, the potential benefits and the results of arthrodesis can often be compromised by symptomatic adjacent segment degeneration and/or pseudarthrosis [31–37] (Fig. 10.7).

AccuFlex

The AccuFlex rod (Globus Medical, Inc., Audubon, PA) is designed with helical cuts within its substance to minimize rigidity. This more flexible rod is currently FDA approved as an adjunct for single-level fusions. In a 1-year prospective,

Fig. 10.5 L-L X-ray view of Dynesys

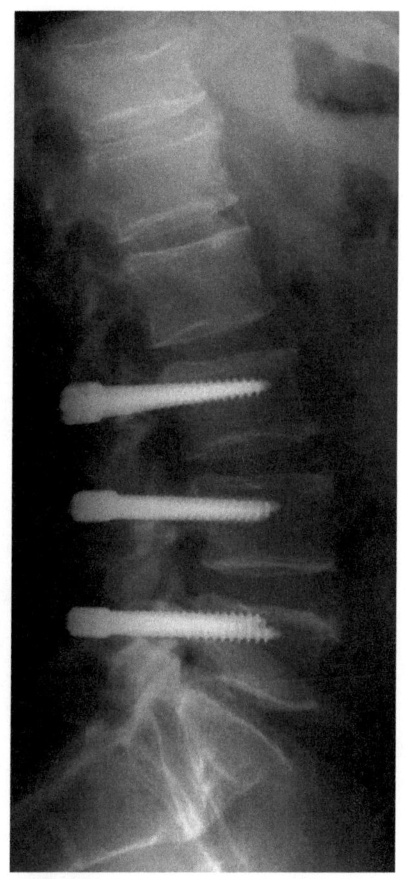

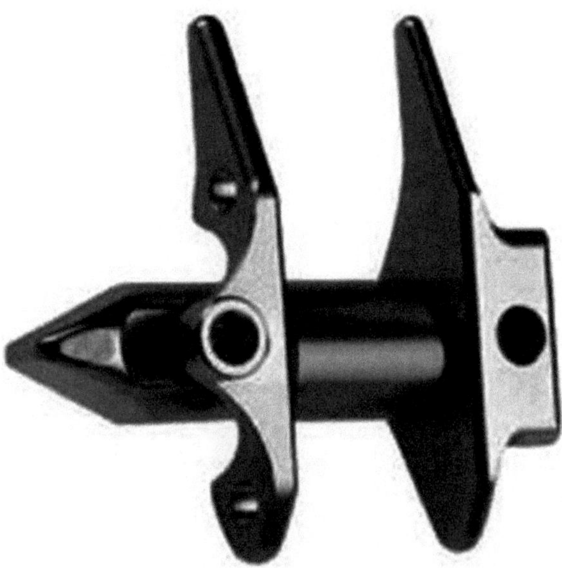

Fig. 10.6 X-STOP device

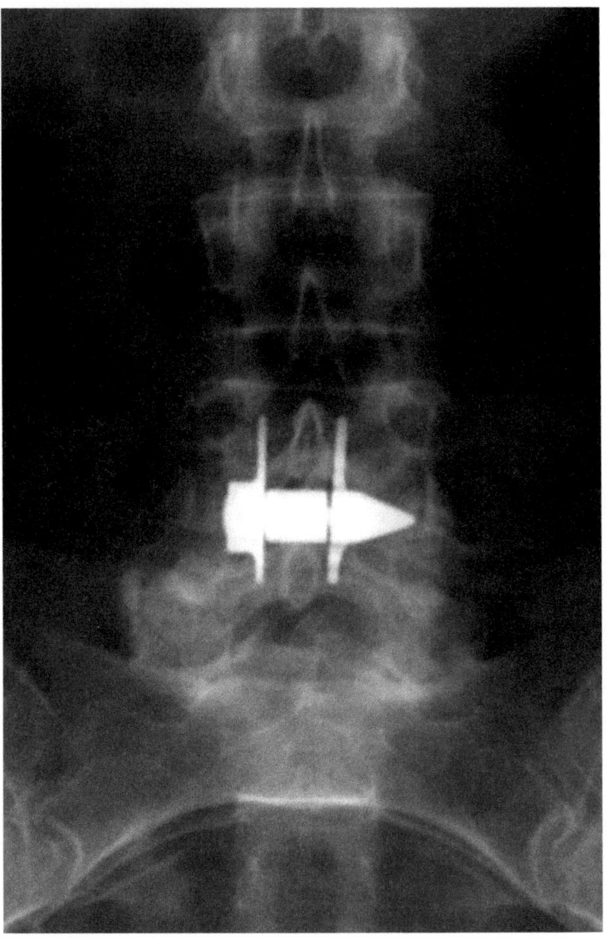

Fig. 10.7 Radiograph AP with X-STOP device of the lumbar spine

randomized study of 170 patients treated with the AccuFlex rod system (Fig. 10.8), comparable fusion rates and clinical outcomes were reported between interbody fusion using the traditional rigid instrumentation versus the flexible rods [38].

Isobar TTL

One of the first introduced semi-rigid rods is the Isobar TTL system (Scient'x USA, Maitland, FL). This implant has been used in Europe for over 10 years and was granted FDA clearance for use as an adjunct to spinal fusion in 1999. Perrin and Cristini reported a retrospective study with a mean follow-up of 8.27 years using the Isobar TTL system (Fig. 10.9) in 22 patients with lumbar spondylolisthesis.

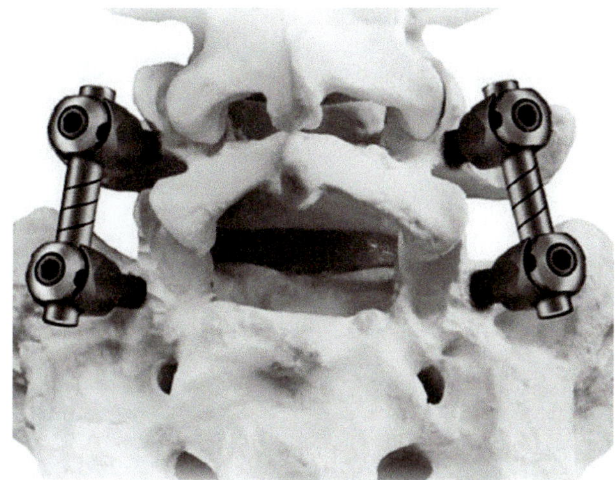

Fig. 10.8 AccuFlex rod device on a spine model

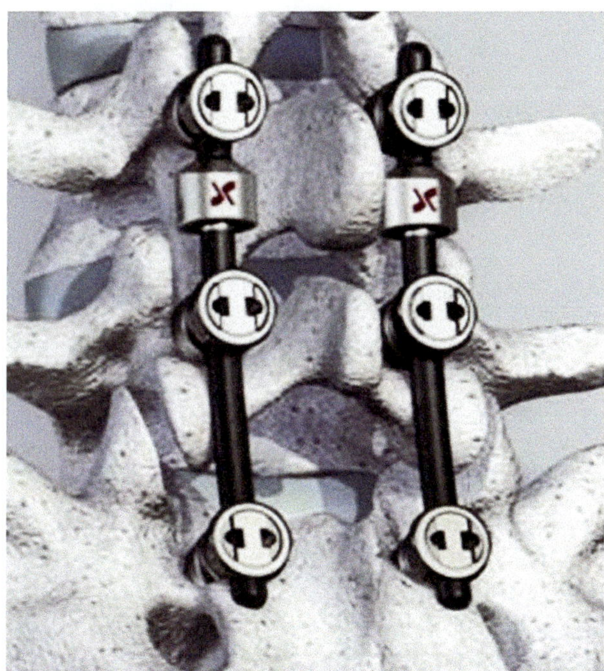

Fig. 10.9 Isobar TLL device

The upper levels were treated with a PEEK cage followed by a two-level posterior fixation with the Isobar TTL system. All patients went on to fusion at the rigidly fixed level, with no device failure or revision surgery required. Long-term clinical outcomes were excellent, with 68.2 % of patients reporting mild leg pain, 72 % no or mild back pain, and 91 % of patients very satisfied with the procedure. The adjacent level also appeared to be protected using this type of rod [15, 31].

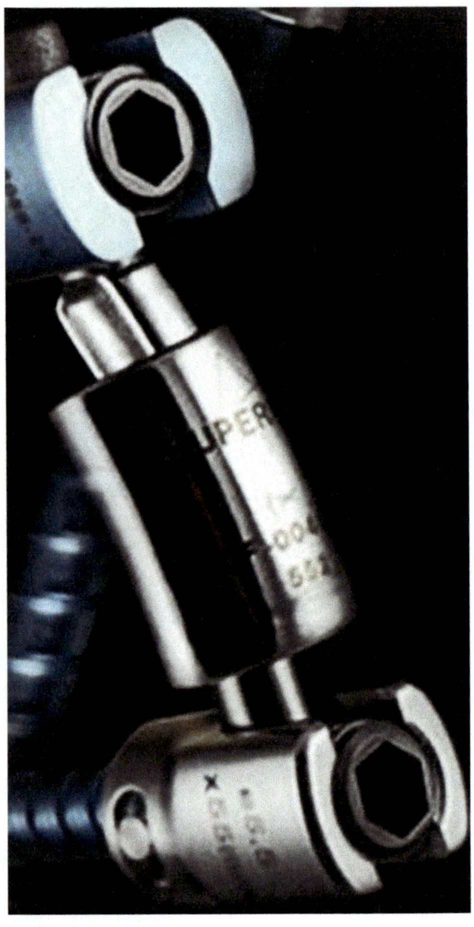

Fig. 10.10 The Truedyne PDS device is a pedicle screw-based adjustable posterior dynamic stabilizer, in which 5 mm of flexion and 3 mm of extension and rotation can be set separately

Truedyne PDS

The Truedyne PDS (Disc Motion Technologies, Boca Raton, FL) is a pedicle screw-based adjustable posterior dynamic stabilizer, in which 5 mm of flexion and 3 mm of extension and rotation can be set separately (Fig. 10.10). It is designed to move in an arc that elongates in flexion, ensuring normal angular segmental motion, and because of its closed design, it is also stable to shear forces. This system is designed to allow synchronous motion resulting in less strain on the disc above. The dynamic pedicle screw still allows motion between the head and shaft of the screw after being locked down. This minimizes screw loosening and also allows the screw to be used for multilevel nonfusion constructs in degenerative scoliosis. This system is currently in preclinical testing [31, 39].

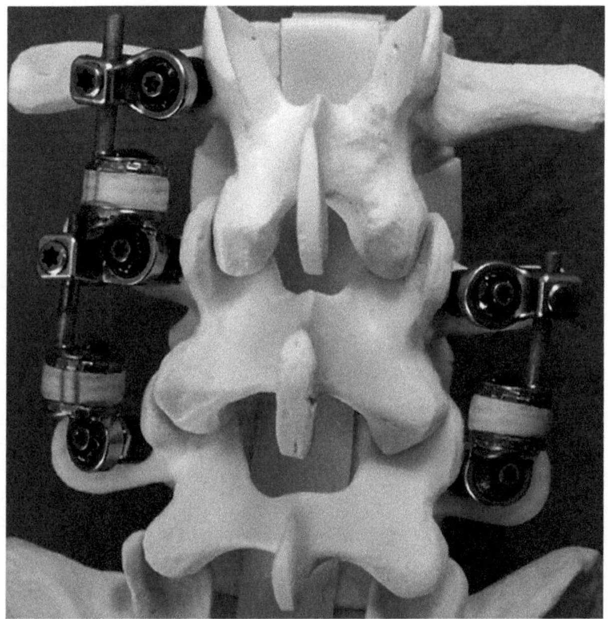

Fig. 10.11 NZ device implanted on a spine model

Stabilimax NZ

The range at which there is minimal resistance to motion by the disc during normal spine motion is referred to as the neutral zone (NZ). The NZ is believed to increase with disc degeneration or injury, resulting in more "instability" and pain. The Stabilimax NZ (Applied Spine Technologies (AST) Inc., New Haven, CT) device (Fig. 10.11) was created to reduce the impact of the NZ on mechanical back pain. The Stabilimax NZ system uses a rod with dual concentric springs to maintain the spinal segment in a neutral position during spinal motion, serving as a sort of internal splint. The Stabilimax NZ is currently undergoing randomized clinical trials for dynamic fusion applications in the United States [31, 40].

Cosmic Posterior Dynamic System

The Cosmic posterior dynamic system (Ulrich GmbH & Co. KG, Ulm, Germany) uses hinged pedicle heads to allow for segmental motion. We have analyzed a study in the literature, carried out by Van Strempel et al., which examined patients with chronic lumbar degenerative disease treated with this system. The results were quite comparable with those obtained in patients treated with spinal fusion. Thus, this system could be an alternative to traditional therapy with arthrodesis. However, long-term follow-up studies are needed to assess its impact on adjacent level degeneration [41].

Fig. 10.12 The BioFlex
System, a pedicle screw-
based system using a Nitinol
rod shaped with loops,
intended to confer stability

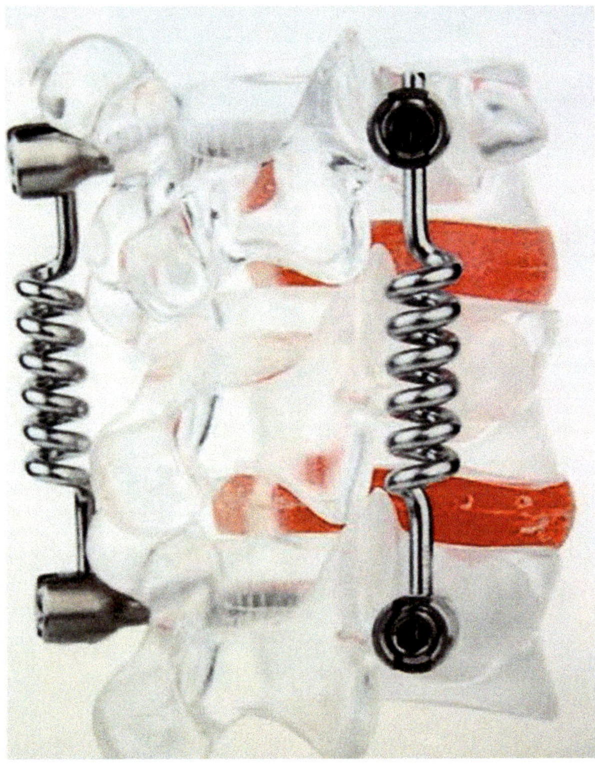

BioFlex Spring Rod Pedicle Screw System

The BioFlex System is a flexible rod system that has been used to preserve motion
at the area of implantation. It is a pedicle screw-based system that uses a Nitinol rod
shaped with one or two loops intended to confer stability in flexion, extension, and
lateral bending (Fig. 10.12). Nitinol is an alloy of nickel and titanium that belongs
to a class of materials called shape memory alloys. Ni and Ti are the chemical sym-
bols for nickel and titanium, and the "nol" of Nitinol stands for the Naval Ordnance
Laboratory, where the material was discovered. Nitinol implants have the following
characteristics: high elasticity, high tensile force, flexibility (below 10 °C) but rigidity (above 30 °C), and biological compatibility [42].

CD Horizon Agile

The CD Horizon® Agile™ (Medtronic Sofamor Danek, Inc. Memphis, TN)
dynamic stabilization device was intended to provide posterior dynamic stabilization through a floating cable design that allows for an axial compressive load
while retaining constant stiffness. This system was designed to provide more
movement than other dynamic stabilization systems. However, because of successive failures it has been withdrawn from the market. The implants were found to

break due to shear-related failure of the cable component, which was more likely to occur with advanced instability.

NFlex

The NFlex controlled stabilization system (Synthes Spine Inc., West Chester, PA) consists of polyaxial titanium alloy pedicle screws that are fixed to a semi-rigid polycarbonate urethane sleeved rod (Figs. 10.13 and 10.14). The integrated

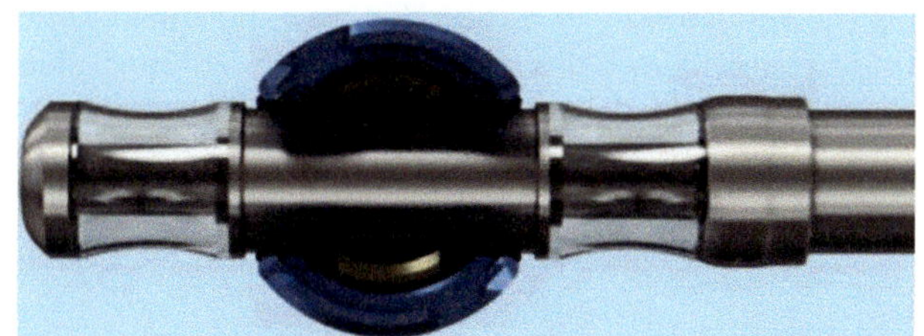

Fig. 10.13 An illustration depicting the motion of the NFlex device

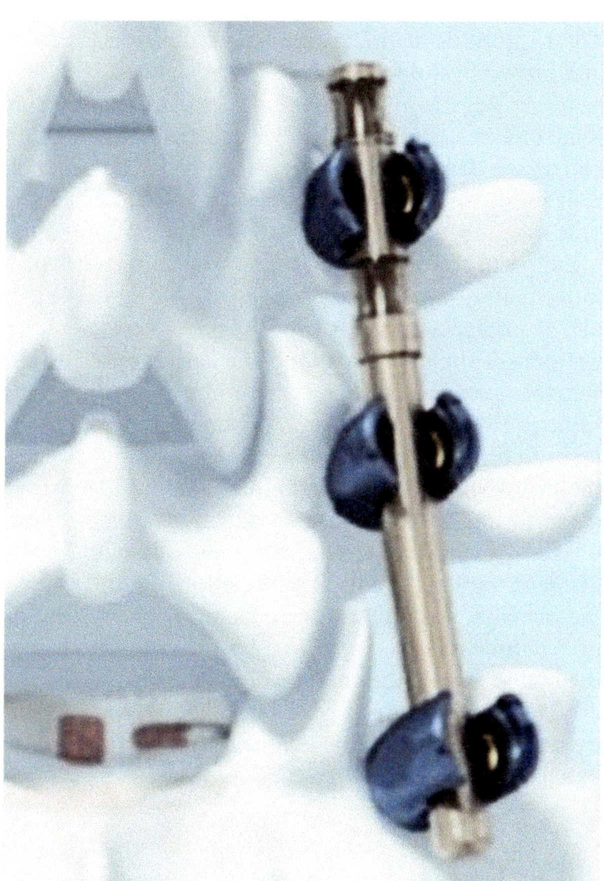

Fig. 10.14 The NFlex controlled stabilization system on a mock-up spine

polycarbonate urethane (PCU) spacer is surrounded by a central titanium ring, to which a pedicle screw is locked. The controlled pistoning of this spacer along the axis of the central titanium core provides a shock absorber effect, reducing the overall rigidity of the construct [31]. The rods are low profile, may be used in single- or multi-level applications, and require a relatively short distance between screws of only 9 mm. The rod may be attached to pedicle screws in the standard fashion, with one pedicle screw attached to the titanium ring of the sleeve and one or more pedicle screws attached to the solid portion of the titanium rod [31, 43, 44]. Biomechanical study of this device demonstrated that, in all loading modes, the NFlex device provided a decompressed lumbar segment with sufficient stability but significantly less rigidity than a similar segment stabilized with a solid rod, suggesting the applicability of this implant as a dynamic fixation device in clinical practice [43]. The system is a viable method of retaining stable motion at the implanted levels and appears comparable to other presently available methods used to preserve segmental motion.

Discussion

The hypothesis behind dynamic stabilization is that control of abnormal motions and more physiological load transmission will relieve pain and prevent adjacent segment degeneration. A remote expectation is that, once normal motion and load transmission is achieved, the damaged disc may repair itself, unless of course the degeneration is too advanced. The pertinent questions in dynamic stabilization, therefore, are (a) how much control of motion is desirable, and (b) how much load should be shared by the system, to unload the damaged disc. The question in the long term is how to prevent implant failure, in view of constant movement of the stabilized segment. A pseudarthrosis often leads to fatigue failure of implants used for rigid fixation, because the rigidity of the implant does not permit them to accommodate any motion originated at the pseudarthrosis. Flexible stabilization may accommodate this movement and may avoid a fatigue failure. However, a closer look at the kinematics of the dynamic stabilization leads to further consideration before its fatigue life may be determined. Normally, the disc is loaded both during flexion and extension. The average disc pressure rises during flexion and also during extension, and is lowest during the early phase of extension. Let us consider a dynamic stabilization system that shares 30 % of the load during flexion, allowing only 70 % of the load to pass through the damaged disc. During extension, if the system forces the instantaneous axis of rotation (IAR) to be shifted posterior to the disc, the disc will be increasingly distracted toward the end of extension. This will be evident by a progressive lowering of the disc pressure toward the end of extension, which indicates that the dynamic stabilization system becomes an increasingly load-bearing structure in extension.

Conclusion

While soft stabilization appears to be promising, a cautious approach should be taken to any new implant system. This implant for fusion only has to serve a temporary stabilization until fusion has taken place; on the other hand, a soft stabilization system has to provide stability throughout its life. After soft stabilization, the implant must stay anchored to the bone and still allow movement. The flexibility of the implant system should be able to protect it from loosening at the anchor point into the bone; the soft stabilization system is intended to load share with the disc and the facet joint only partially and unloads the motion segment. Dynamic stabilization systems have theoretical advantages over rigid spinal implants. They may allow similar or improved patient outcomes compared with fusions in patients in whom disc load characteristics represent a modifiable solution over the sagittal plane of the vertebral endplates. Some design features must be addressed, as well as placement of the devices with preservation of the surrounding spinal structures. Ultimately, a well-designed system would need to prove its clinical effectiveness in a well-designed prospective randomized clinical trial. The few posterior dynamic stabilization systems that have had clinical applications so far have produced outcomes somewhat comparable with fusion. No severe adverse events caused by these implants have been reported. Long-term follow-up data and well-controlled, prospective randomized studies do not exist, but are essential to prove the safety, efficacy, appropriateness, and economic viability of these methods.

References

1. Link HD. History, design and biomechanics of the LINK SB Charite artificial disc. Eur Spine J. 2002;11 Suppl 2:S98–105.
2. Mayer HM, Wiechert K, Korge A, et al. Minimally invasive total disc replacement: surgical technique and preliminary clinical results. Eur Spine J. 2002;11 Suppl 2:S124–30.
3. Ray CD. The PDN, prosthetic disc-nucleus device. Eur Spine J. 2002;11 Suppl 2:S137–42.
4. Stoll TM, Dubois G, Schwarzenbach O. The dynamic neutralization system for the spine: a multi-center study of a novel non-fusion system. Eur Spine J. 2002;11 Suppl 2:S170–8.
5. Freudiger S, Dubois G, Lorrain M. Dynamic neutralisation of the lumbar spine confirmed on a new lumbar spine simulator in vitro. Arch Orthop Trauma Surg. 1999;119:127–32.
6. Grevitt MP, Gardner AD, Spilsbury J, et al. The Graf stabilisation system: early results in 50 patients. Eur Spine J. 1995;4:169–75; discussion 35.
7. Russ P. Nockels dynamic stabilization in the surgical management of painful lumbar spinal disorders. Spine. 2005;30(16S):S68–72.
8. Troum OM, Crues 3rd JV. The young adult with hip pain: diagnosis and medical treatment, circa 2004. Clin Orthop. 2004;418:9–17.
9. Smith D, McMurray N, Disler P. Early intervention for acute back injury: can we finally develop an evidence-based approach? Clin Rehabil. 2002;16:1–11.
10. Gibson JN, Grant IC, Waddell G. The Cochrane review of surgery for lumbar disc prolapse and degenerative lumbar spondylosis. Spine. 1999;24:1820–32.
11. Bogduk N. The innervation of the lumbar spine. Spine. 1983;8:286–93.

12. Fujiwara A, Lim TH, An HS, et al. The effect of disc degeneration and facet joint osteoarthritis on the segmental flexibility of the lumbar spine. Spine. 2000;25:3036–44.
13. Fujiwara A, Tamai K, An HS, et al. The relationship between disc degeneration, facet joint osteoarthritis, and stability of the degenerative lumbar spine. J Spinal Disord. 2000;13: 444–50.
14. Korovessis P, Papazisis Z, Koureas G, et al. Rigid, semirigid versus dynamic instrumentation for degenerative lumbar spinal stenosis: a correlative radiological and clinical analysis of short-term results. Spine. 2004;29:735–42.
15. Okuda S, Iwasaki M, Miyauchi A, et al. Risk factors for adjacent segment degeneration after PLIF. Spine. 2004;29:1535–40.
16. Lazennec JY, Ramare S, Arafati N, et al. Sagittal alignment in lumbosacral fusion: relations between radiological parameters and pain. Eur Spine J. 2000;9:47–55.
17. Robert W. Molinari dynamic stabilization of the lumbar spine. Curr Opin Orthop. 2007;18:215–20.
18. Grob D, Benini A, Junge A, Mannion AF. Clinical experience with the Dynesys semirigid fixation system for the lumbar spine surgical and patient-oriented outcome in 50 cases after an average of 2 years. Spine. 2005;30(3):324–31.
19. Kirkaldy-Willis WH, Farfan H. Instability of the lumbar spine. Clin Orthop. 1982;165: 110–23.
20. Mulholland RC, Sengupta DK. Rationale, principles and experimental evaluation of the concept of soft stabilization. Eur Spine J. 2002;11 Suppl 2:198–201.
21. Graf H. Lumbar instability: surgical treatment without fusion. Rachis. 1992;412:123–37.
22. Brechbuhler D, Markwalder TM, Braun M. Surgical results after soft system stabilization of the lumbar spine in degenerative disc disease–long-term results. Acta Neurochir (Wien). 1998;140:521–5.
23. Markwalder TM, Wenger M. Dynamic stabilization of lumbar motion segments by use of Graf's ligaments: results with an average follow-up of 7.4 years in 39 highly selected, consecutive patients. Acta Neurochir (Wien). 2003;145:209–14.
24. Kanayama M, Hashimoto T, Shigenobu K, et al. Nonfusion surgery for degenerative spondylolisthesis using artificial ligament stabilization: surgical indication and clinical results. Spine. 2005;30:588–92.
25. Rajaratnam SS, Shepperd JAN, Mulholland RC. Dynesis stabilization of the lumbo-sacral spine. Second combined meeting of the BSS BASS BCSS SBSR, Birmingham; 2002
26. Schmoelz W, Huber JF, Nydegger T, et al. Dynamic stabilization of the lumbar spine and its effects on adjacent segments: an in vitro experiment. J Spinal Disord Tech. 2003;16:418–23.
27. Stoll TM, Dubois G, Schwarzenbach O. The dynamic neutralization system for the spine: a multi-center study of a novel non-fusion system. Eur Spine J. 2002;11 Suppl 2:170–8.
28. Schnake KJ, Schaeren S, Jeanneret B. Dynamic stabilization in addition to decompression for lumbar spinal stenosis with degenerative spondylolisthesis. Spine. 2006;31:442–9.
29. Putzier M, Schneider SV, Funk JF, et al. The surgical treatment of the lumbar disc prolapse: nucleotomy with additional transpedicular dynamic stabilization versus nucleotomy alone. Spine. 2005;30:E109–14.
30. Anderson PA, Tribus CB, Kitchel SH. Treatment of neurogenic claudication by interspinous decompression: application of the X STOP device in patients with lumbar degenerative spondylolisthesis. J Neurosurg Spine. 2006;4:463–71.
31. Song JJ, Barrey CY, Ponnappan RK, Bessey JT, Shimer AL, Vaccaro AR. Pedicle screw-based dynamic stabilization of the lumbar spine. PAN Arab J Neurosurg. 2010;14(1):1–141.
32. Barr JS. Ruptured intervertebral disc and sciatic pain. J Bone Joint Surg. 1947;29:429–37.
33. Bono CM, Lee CK. Critical analysis of trends in fusion for degenerative disc disease over the past 20 years: influence of technique on fusion rate and clinical outcome. Spine. 2004;29(4): 455–63; discussion Z5.
34. Coppes MH, Marani E, Thomeer RT, Groen GJ. Innervation of "painful" lumbar discs. Spine. 1997;22(20):2342–9; discussion 2349–50.

35. Fritzell P, Hagg O, Wessberg P, Nordwall A, Swedish Lumbar Spine Study Group. Chronic low back pain and fusion: a comparison of three surgical techniques: a prospective multicenter randomized study from the Swedish Lumbar Spine Study Group. Spine. 2002;27(11): 1131–41.
36. Kirkaldy-Willis WH, Farfan HF. Instability of the lumbar spine. Clin Orthop Relat Res. 1982;165:110–23.
37. Mulholland RC, Sengupta DK. Rationale, principles and experimental evaluation of the concept of soft stabilization. Eur Spine J. 2002;11 Suppl 2:S198–205.
38. Mandigo CE, Sampath P, Kaiser MG. Posterior dynamic stabilization of the lumbar spine: pedicle based stabilization with the AccuFlex rod system. Neurosurg Focus. 2007;22(1):E9.
39. Goel VK, Kiapour A, Faizan A, Krishna M, Friesem T. Finite element study of matched paired posterior disc implant and dynamic stabilizer (360° motion preservation system). SAS J. 2007;1(1):55–61.
40. Yue JJ, Timm JP, Panjabi MM, Jaramillo-de la Torre J. Clinical application of the Panjabi neutral zone hypothesis: the Stabilimax NZ posterior lumbar dynamic stabilization system. Neurosurg Focus. 2007;22(1):E12.
41. Von Strempel A, Moosmann D, Stoss C, Martin A. Stabilisation of the degenerated lumbar spine in the nonfusion technique with cosmic posterior dynamic system. World Spine J. 2006; 1(1):40–7.
42. Kim YS, Zhang HY, Moon BJ, Park KW, Ji KY, Lee WC, et al. Nitinol spring rod dynamic stabilization system and Nitinol memory loops in surgical treatment for lumbar disc disorders: short-term follow up. Neurosurg Focus. 2007;22:E10.
43. Coe JD, Kitchel SH, Meisel HJ, Wingo CH, Lee SE, Jahng T-A. NFlex dynamic stabilization system: two-year clinical outcomes of multi-center study. J Korean Neurosurg Soc. 2012; 51:343–9.
44. Wallach CJ, Teng AL, Wang JC. NFlex. In: Yue JJ, Bertagnoli R, McAfee PC, An HS, editors. Motion preservation surgery of the spine. Philadelphia: Saunders; 2008. p. 505–10.

Chapter 11
Lumbar Nucleus Replacement

Massimo Balsano

Introduction

Lumbar disc arthroplasty is gaining popularity in the spinal surgery community for many reasons, the first being to avoid spinal fusion, which, even with evidence of good and solid clinical outcomes, is a surgical procedure that abolishes the physiological movement of the joints of the spine. Spinal fusion has always been accepted as a "surgical gold standard," but complication rates up to 70 % have been reported, and adjacent segment alterations vary from 31 to 66 % of cases [1, 2].

To overcome these issues, lumbar disc replacement was introduced in the early 1980s for the treatment of degenerative low-back pain [3]. The fundamental goals of artificial disc replacement are to relieve pain in a predictable and successful manner with low morbidity, to restore function and stability to the spine, to restore disc height to open foramina, to decrease stress on the facet joints, and to achieve long-term success.

Artificial disc prosthesis can be divided into two groups: complete disc replacement and nuclear replacement. This classification helps the surgeon to consider that various stages of degeneration of the intervertebral disc give rise to different problems that require different strategies for successful treatment.

Because discogenic back pain can be caused both by a chemical origin and mechanical irritation or instability, and with no definite diagnostic method for the exact pain mechanism, the intradiscal arthroplasty procedure must address both potential pain mechanisms. To eliminate the potential chemical pain, the "diseased" nucleus needs to be removed in the intradiscal arthroplasty procedure. It is well known that removal of the nucleus will cause collapse of the disc height and lead to further instability of the index segment, which in turn can cause mechanical pain. Therefore, an intradiscal arthroplasty device should maintain or restore the disc

M. Balsano, MD
Department of Orthopaedic, Regional Spinal Department,
Santorso Hospital, Via Garziere, 42-36014 Santorso, Vicenza, Italy
e-mail: massimo.balsano@gmail.com

P.P.M. Menchetti (ed.), *Minimally Invasive Surgery of the Lumbar Spine*,
DOI 10.1007/978-1-4471-5280-4_11, © Springer-Verlag London 2014

height and mechanical function of the natural nucleus. Mechanically, in a healthy disc, the nucleus shares the compressive load, with the annulus taking about half of the total load passing through the anterior column [4]. Because of its hydrostatic nature, the nucleus distributes load evenly over the endplates under all physiological loading conditions [5] and presents no restriction to the rotational motion by itself. The resistance to the rotation mainly comes from the annulus and the facet joints.

The need for an artificial intervertebral disc prosthesis is theoretically analogous to that for the hip and knee joint. Degenerative changes affecting a synovial joint can often result in painful inflammation, instability, and abnormal biomechanics. As with the hip and knee joints, pain and inflammation can be reduced or eliminated by removing the offending agent or pain generator, which in this case is the joint. Historically, this has been accomplished by arthrodesis. The abolishment of the movement with a solid fusion restores stability and decreases pain and inflammation. Unfortunately, this leads to an increased stress across the adjacent joints in an attempt to preserve motion and mobility and can lead to an accelerated degeneration of them.

This chapter will provide an overview of the lumbar nuclear replacement using a relatively new device, the NuBac system (Pioneer Surgical Technology, Marquette, MI).

Design Rationale

Different devices have been developed to replace the nucleus. The designs and materials for nucleus replacements vary from different hydrogel or non-hydrogel elastomers, which are either preformed or formed in situ, to non-elastomeric materials such as metal, polymethylmethacrylate (PMMA), and pyrolytic carbon. Most of these devices had complications like subsidence, extrusion, and reactive endplate changes. This could be explained by the fact that most of these devices are either too soft, with risk for extrusion, or use rigid nonarticulating constructs that do not allow for uniform load distribution, resulting in subsidence, extrusion, and end plate changes.

One of the earliest reported experiences with nucleus implants is a stainless steel ball, the Fernström ball. Fernström believed that a ball-formed nucleus device would best restore the articulation of the adjacent vertebrae while preventing anterior or posterior slippage of neighboring vertebrae. Retrospective, nonrandomized, controlled studies showed excellent and good results after short-term [6] and long-term follow-up. After an average follow-up time of 17 years, results for herniated disc patients and discogenic back pain patients were graded excellent and good in 83 and 75 %, respectively [7].

The clinical results obtained with the Fernström ball indicate a nonelastic device that allows motion of the indexed level and is able to relieve discogenic back pain over a long period. Based on the shape of the Fernström ball and its small or nearly pointed contact area, subsidence was to be expected. Results showed that the device was subsiding in 88 % of the patients and that subsidence stopped after 1–3 mm per endplate (Fig. 11.1a, b). It is commonly assumed that subsidence is stopped after reaching a balance between the contact stress of the Fernström ball on the end plates and the strength of the end plates, that is, subsidence increases the contact area of the device, resulting in less contact stress on the end plates.

Newly developed nucleus devices should include the principle of motion-preserving, while preventing subsidence of the device. The NuBac disc arthroplasty is designed to mimic natural kinematics of an intact disc. Free motion is maintained by the two-piece design with an inner ball-and-socket articulation, whereby this motion is constrained by preserving the surrounding annulus and ligaments (Fig. 11.2). To prevent subsidence, the NuBac is developed with a large contact area; for the smallest NuBac implant, the contact area is 2.2 times the contact area of a 12-mm Fernström after 3 mm subsidence. For a medium NuBac implant with a contact area of 191 mm^2, the average contact stress under 400 N is 2.1 MPa. Reported end plate strengths vary from 2.7 MPa [8] to 20 MPa [9], which are larger than the average contact stress for the smallest NuBac device, thus theoretically preventing subsidence of the device.

In total disc replacement, the constraint, or the stability, of the motion segment after an intradiscal or nucleus arthroplasty procedure is largely determined by the surrounding tissues, such as the annulus and ligaments. Because most of these surrounding tissues are preserved in the intradiscal arthroplasty procedure and the annulus is restored to the normal tension stage, the segment mobility and stability after the NuBac implantation will be maintained. It also allows more uniform stress distribution on the endplates under all physiological rotational motions as compared with nonarticulating intradiscal devices (Fig. 11.3a, b).

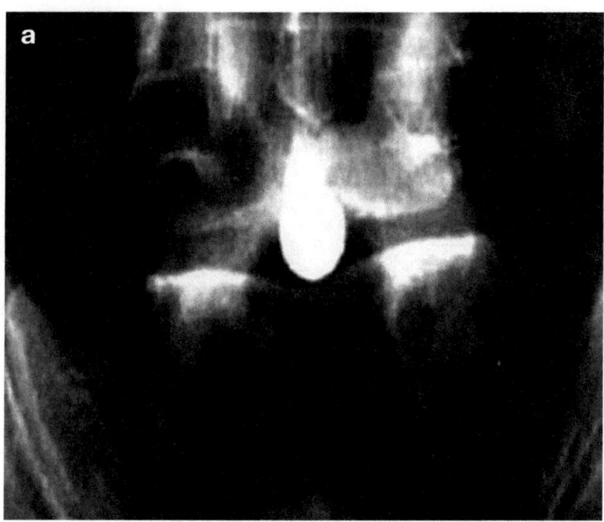

Fig. 11.1 (**a, b**) Fernström ball

Fig. 11.1 (continued)

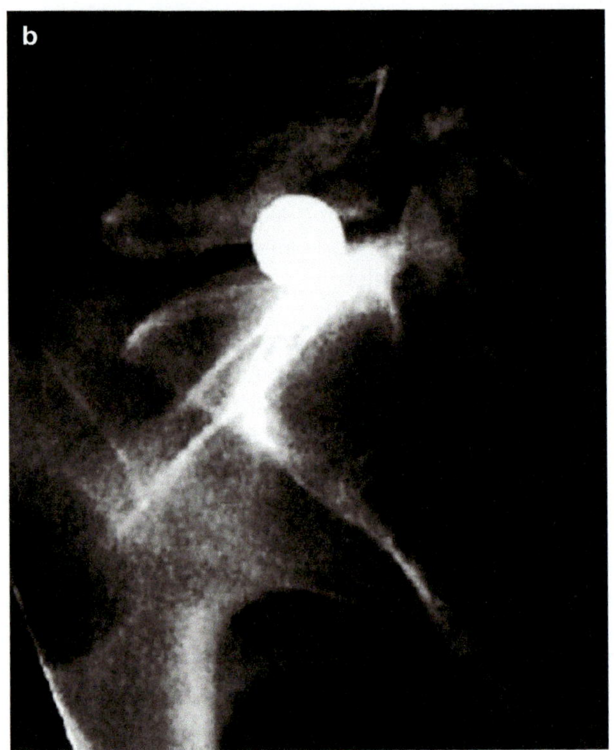

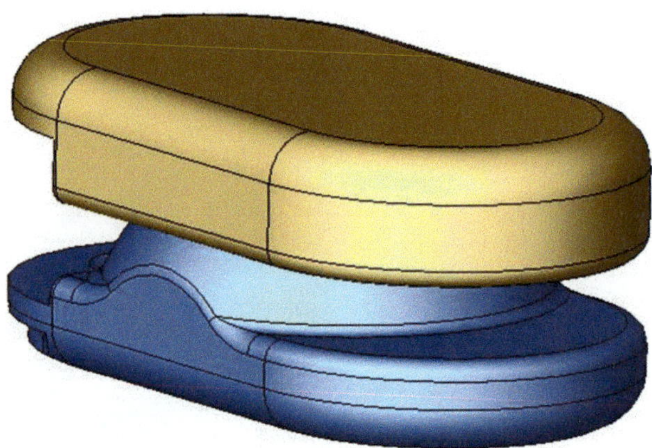

Fig. 11.2 Design of the NuBac prosthesis

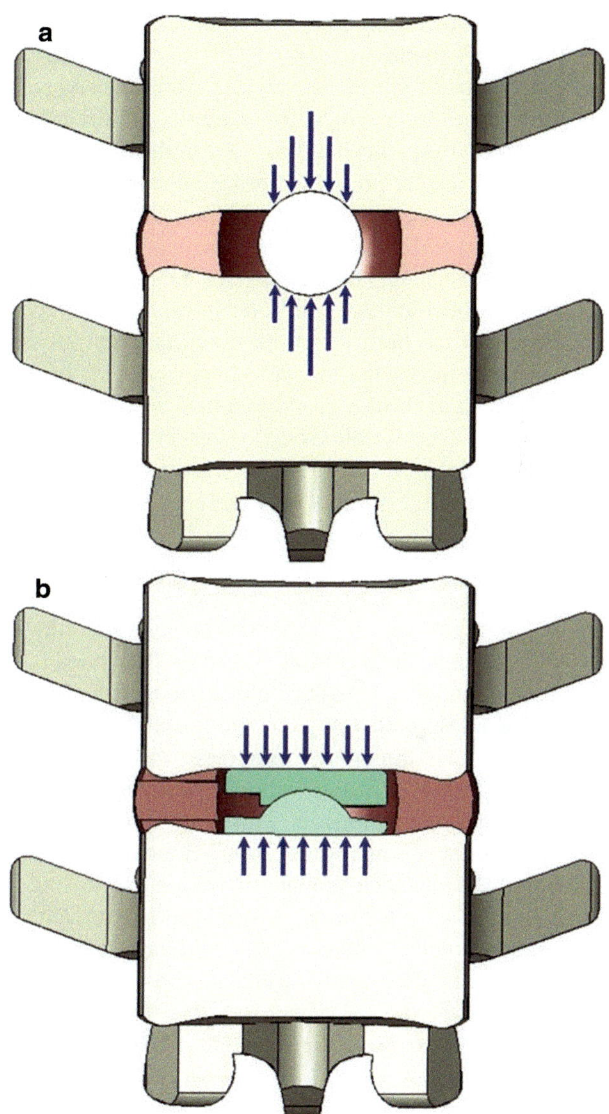

Fig. 11.3 (**a**, **b**) Load Distribution comparison between the Fernström ball (**a**) and the NuBac prosthesis (**b**)

Choice of Material

The NuBac is manufactured from polyetheretherketone (PEEK Optima, Invibio, Greenville, NC), a new bearing material for articulating spine devices where historically metal-on-ultra high molecular weight polyethylene (UHMWPE) is the most used, followed by metal-on-metal. PEEK is a thermoplastic with an elastic modulus close to that of bone, and it is radiolucent. Previously, biocompatibility and biodurability testing showed no significant material changes after aging and no cytotoxic or histopathologic responses or other inflammatory responses.

Four groups of six PEEK devices were investigated to determine the wear rate for different motion profiles, for example, unidirectional, multidirectional, multidirectional with frequency shifting, and multidirectional with accelerated aging.

All samples were presoaked in saline solution at 37 ± 2 °C for approximately 28 weeks. For the multidirectional testing, the conditions of ISO 18192-1 for TDA were followed with adjustment of the dynamic compressive magnitude to reflect the load-sharing mechanism of the device with the annulus. The single-directional testing was continued until 40 million cycles. A wear-in period up to one million cycles was observed for both the multidirectional test group and the group tested with frequency shifting, while no wear-in period was observed for the single-directional tested group and for the group that underwent accelerated aging. A bimodal wear rate was displayed for all groups tested multidirectionally, while the wear rate was consistently linear at 0.28 ± 0.02 mg/million cycles for the single-directional tested group. Articulation orientation softening is a known detrimental wear mechanism for UHMWPE due to molecular orientation of the polymer chains at the wear surface, leading to a decrease in shear strength and a significant increase in the wear rate [10]. For all tested groups, no increase of wear was observed, suggesting that PEEK does not undergo orientation softening at the wear surface. Also, for UHMWPE, exposure to radiation and oxidation lead to accelerated wear rates, susceptible to bond cleavage during irradiation [11].

For the accelerated aging test group for PEEK, no wear-in period was observed, suggesting that a thin cross-linked layer was developed during the aging process. In contrast to UHMWPE, the wear rate decreased significantly at five to ten million cycles and was not significantly different from the other test groups, suggesting that an oxidative layer was formed that is removed over time. For metal-on-UHMWPE articulation, it has been shown that frequency shifting can increase the wear rate by several orders of magnitude. A small but significant increase in the wear rate was observed as compared to the uni- and multidirectional testing as a result of the frequency shifting. The small variation in the wear rate suggests that PEEK is a consistent material with relatively low long-term wear properties and not subject to known major wear increasing factors of UHMWPE.

Reducing Risk for Expulsion and Subsidence

Unlike TDA nucleus, implants are not fixed to the vertebral bodies that challenge migration and expulsion of the implant. Although only one extrusion is reported for the Fernström ball, for the PDN device (Raymedica, Inc., Minneapolis, MN) extrusion rates between 8 and 36 % have been reported [12, 13].

This expulsion rate might be explained by the bulky properties of the device and the inability to adapt its shape to the changed angulation during bending. These characteristics can result in an uneven load distribution pattern during bending, with increased forces at the side of bending and decreased forces at the opposite side, pushing the implant to the opposite side. This might result in expulsion, especially when the implantation window of the annulus is at that specific place or if the annulus is, undesirably, in degenerative poor condition. The articulating properties of the NuBac device facilitate an even load distribution irrespective of the spinal position, for example, flexion-extension, lateral bending, and axial rotation. This feature may reduce the risk of implant extrusion during any condition. In addition, an even load distribution of the implant maintains an even load distribution on the end plates, while uneven load distribution may cause edema and fracture of the end plates resulting in subsidence.

To investigate the articulating characteristics of the device on expulsion risk, six adjacent pairs of human cadaver FSUs (L3–5) were tested. L3–4 served as intact control, and after nucleotomy the device was inserted via a right lateral approach at L4–5. Axial rotation, lateral bending and flexion/extension was tested by 100,000 cycles of unilateral left bending ranging from 2.5–7.5 Nm at 2 Hz with the compressive load ranging from 205–750 N. No expulsion occurred for any of the samples. There are no clinically validated standards for accessing the expulsion risk. The used scenario was the worst case scenario, as bending to the opposite side will open the annular window and might facilitate expulsion. The results demonstrated that the expulsion risk is low. This can be explained by the inner-articulating design that allows the upper and lower plate of the device to move along with the movement of the segment, resulting in keeping both plates of the device in full contact with the endplates. In addition, the height of the implant will be less at the bending side and higher at the opposite (window) side, which will also make it harder to expulse.

Multidirectional ROM and Load-to-Failure: An In Vitro Cadaveric Model

Multidirectional range of motion (ROM) and neutral zone were examined by Cunningham (Union Memorial Hospital, Baltimore) [14]. Eight human cadaveric spines (L2–3 and L4–5 segments) were evaluated with unconstrained intact movements of ±7.5 Nm for axial rotation, flexion-extension, and lateral bending testing. ROM and neutral zone at the operated level were quantified for the intact spine, spine with nucleotomy, and spine with NuBac implant.

After nucleotomy, multidirectional flexibility testing indicates significant increase in the segmental ROM and neutral zone (ANOVA, $p < 0.05$). In addition, both ROM and neutral zone for the device-reconstructed level returned to levels not statistically different from the intact condition (Fig. 11.5a, b), indicating that the device was able to reestablish the kinematics to the intact condition. The center-of-rotation is in the middle of the device, unlike for bulky devices where it is on the side of the device, facilitating both normal kinematics and preventing subsidence. After reconstruction, load-to-failure was investigated by axial compression. For seven specimens, the observed failure mechanism was fracture of the adjacent vertebral body without significant damage of the end plates. Observed mean failure load was $3,340 \pm 2,029$ N, which is comparable to the compressive failure load to that of an intact lumbar segment [15, 16].

Clinical Utility and Surgical Technique

The main indication for the NuBac intradiscal arthroplasty device is discogenic back pain caused by disc degenerative disease (DDD), similar to that for interbody fusion and total disc arthroplasty devices. The only indication difference between intradiscal arthroplasty and interbody fusion/total disc arthroplasty is the requirement for a certain minimal disc height for the former. The main reason for this minimal disc height requirement for intradiscal arthroplasty goes back to its clinical objectives mentioned previously: to restore/maintain the disc height and natural load sharing between the nucleus and annulus in order to achieve mechanical stability. If the disc has already collapsed too much, an intradiscal arthroplasty device has to over-stretch the annulus, leading to high tension in order to regain the normal disc height and therefore have the intradiscal arthroplasty device take all or the majority of the compressive load. By doing that, the contact stress between the device and the endplates would be unphysiologically high and lead to subsidence.

Using disc height as an indicator for the stage of disc degeneration cascade, significant disc height loss typically represents the late stage of disc degeneration. Therefore, intradiscal arthroplasty is more adequately indicated for patients at the early-to-moderate stage of the disc degeneration cascade, while fusion and total disc arthroplasty, due to their invasiveness and "bridge-burning" nature, are more appropriate for patients at the late stage of the cascade. The stage of degeneration should not be confused with the degree of pain. The early-to-moderate stage in the degeneration cascade does not have less pain than the late stage of the cascade. Patients with early-to-moderate disc degeneration can have as much pain, if not more, as patients at the late stage of degeneration.

In addition to being less invasive and less bridge-burning than total disc arthroplasty, intradiscal arthroplasty has another advantage of being compatible with different surgical approaches. In the limited clinical experience so far, the NuBac has been successfully implanted via all three common surgical approaches: posterior, straight lateral (ALPA), and retroperitoneal anterolateral.

Other than the differences in patient position and tissue dissection and retraction for these three different approaches, the general surgical procedure for the NuBac for the three approaches is similar. The following highlights some key issues related to each approach.

The posterior approach is often used for patients with sequestrated or large contained disc herniation. Patient position, skin incision, and the approach to the disc will be the same as that for discectomy. Depending on the pathology, the surgeon can approach the disc from either the left side or right side. Like a discectomy procedure, a partial laminectomy is often required, so that there will be enough window to conduct the discectomy and laminectomy. While it is acceptable to remove a small edge of the facet in the medial side, care should be taken not to dissect too much facet. A nerve retractor should be used during the discectomy and device implantation. For discs at L4/5 or above, the straight lateral approach can be used (Figs. 11.4a, b and 11.5a, b).

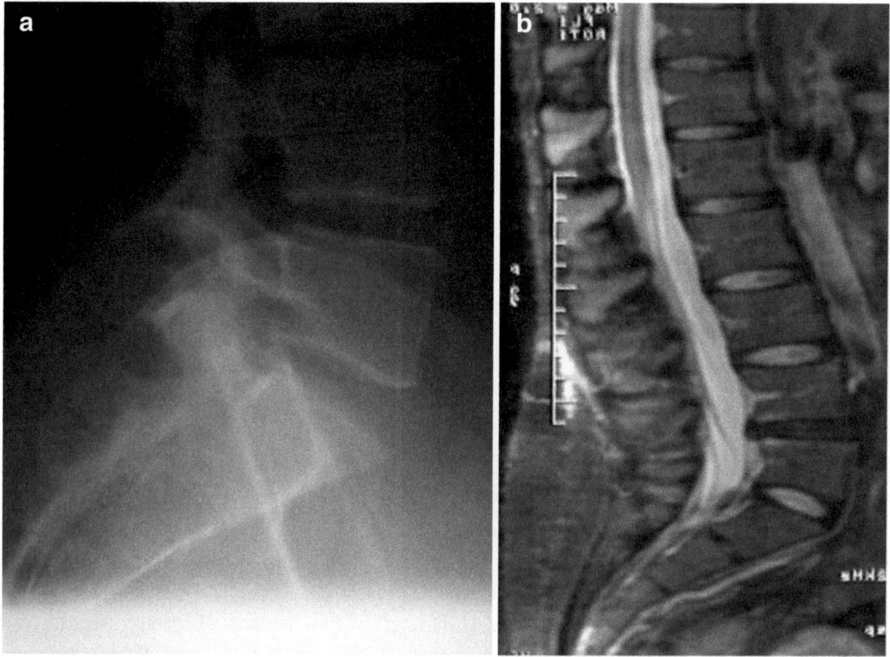

Fig. 11.4 (**a**, **b**) Images of a patient suffering of severe low-back pain, the consequence of a degenerated condition of the L4–L5 disc

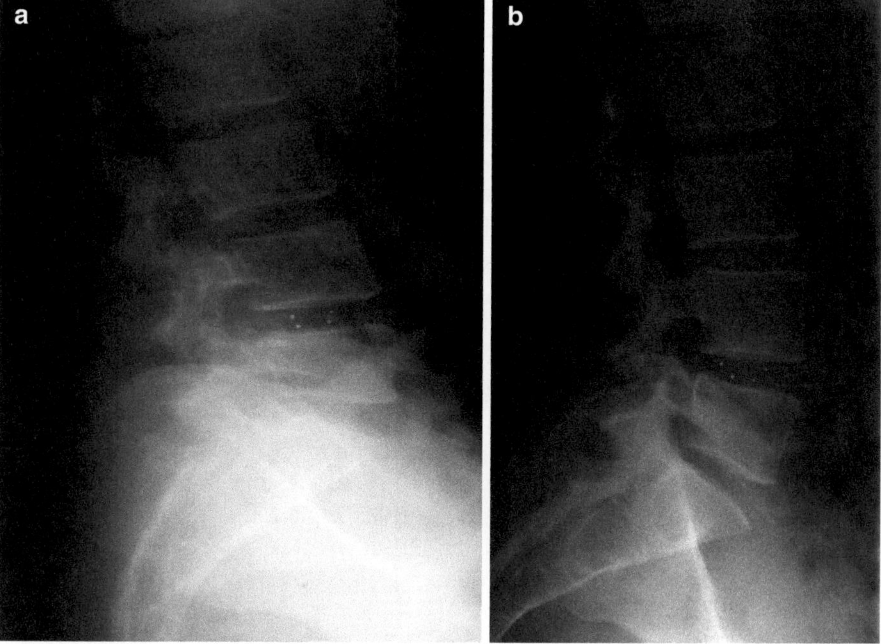

Fig. 11.5 (**a**, **b**) Restoration of disc height after NuBac implantation via ALPA approach (**a**); the clinical symptoms have dramatically improved after 1 year (**b**)

After positioning the patient in a lateral position, the disc is approached through a lateral retroperitoneal, trans-psoas pathway. Although this has not been a conventional approach in the past for discectomy and interbody fusion, this approach has gained some popularity recently for implanting nucleus devices [17] and interbody fusion [18]. As compared with the conventional retroperitoneal anterolateral approach, this approach has the advantages of allowing for anterior access to the disc space without an approach surgeon or the potential complications of an anterior intraabdominal procedure [18, 19]. It is suggested to use neuromonitoring of the lumbar plexus. Many devices are available on the market for this purpose.

For an intradiscal arthroplasty device, this approach also has the advantage of easy cleaning of the nucleus space. Alternatively, the conventional retroperitoneal anterolateral approach can be used. The disc can be approached from either side. Although the surgical approach is similar to that for total disc implantation and anterior interbody fusion, because of the small size of the NuBac implant, the area of disc exposure is much smaller than that for fusion and total disc replacement. With less tissue retraction and less bleeding, the risk of vascular injury and scar tissue formation should also be lower.

Because the NuBac procedure requires smaller disc exposure, less tissue dissection, and no endplate preparation, the surgical procedure and instrumentation for the NuBac are relatively simple and straightforward. After the disc exposure with one of these three approaches, a small 6×6 mm annular window is cut using a parallel cutter with a #11 blade. In cutting the annular window, care should be taken not to cut into the endplates. For a relatively narrow disc or during the posterior approach, the parallel cutter might be only used to cut the width of the annular window. The two vertical annular slits then can be connected by cutting two horizontal lines adjacent to the superior and inferior vertebrae. The box annular plug is then removed by pituitary rongeur. A complete discectomy is then performed with care not to damage the annulus and endplate. Up angle, down angle, and curved rongeurs are helpful to remove the nucleus in the corners or in the area that cannot be reached by a straight rongeur. After the discectomy, the annular window is then dilated with an annular dilator. The cavity size and location is then assessed with specially designed trials with different footprints, heights, and lordotic angles using fluoroscope. Care should be taken to make sure that the trial is positioned in the center of the disc in the AP fluoroscopic image. Because the trials may pack some loose nucleus toward the distal end of the cavity, it is advised to use the rongeur again to remove the packed nucleus material. The final implant size is then chosen based on the size and lordotic angle of the last trial. The NuBac implant is held by the implant inserter with the wedge angle in the distal end to facilitate the entry of the implant into the annular opening. After inserting the NuBac implant into the disc cavity, the AP and lateral fluoroscopic images should be taken to verify the implant position using the radiopaque markers before disengaging the inserter from the implant (Fig. 11.6a–c).

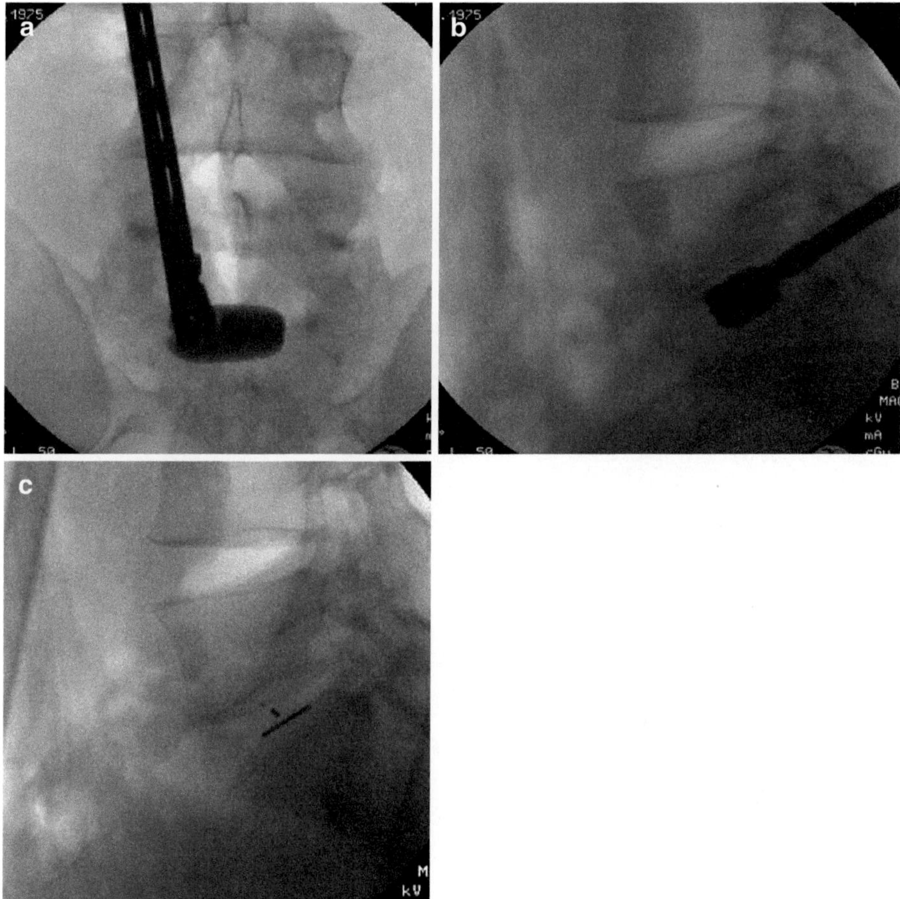

Fig. 11.6 (**a–c**) Sequences of correct trial positioning through the L5–S1 space, via posterior approach. (**a, b**); final NuBac positioning (**c**)

Clinical Results

A prospective, longitudinal, multicenter study to investigate safety and efficacy was initiated. The main patient inclusion criterion was symptomatic single- or double-level discogenic back pain. Depending on surgeon preferences and patient pathologies, anterolateral, lateral, or posterior approach was used for implantation. Function was measured with ODI and pain was measured with VAS. These self-administered patient questionnaires were collected preoperatively and at 6 weeks and 3, 6, 12, and 24 months postoperatively. The first patient was included in December 2004 and over 250 NuBac implants were implanted since then. One hundred and forty-four patients returned at least one patient questionnaire and were included in the

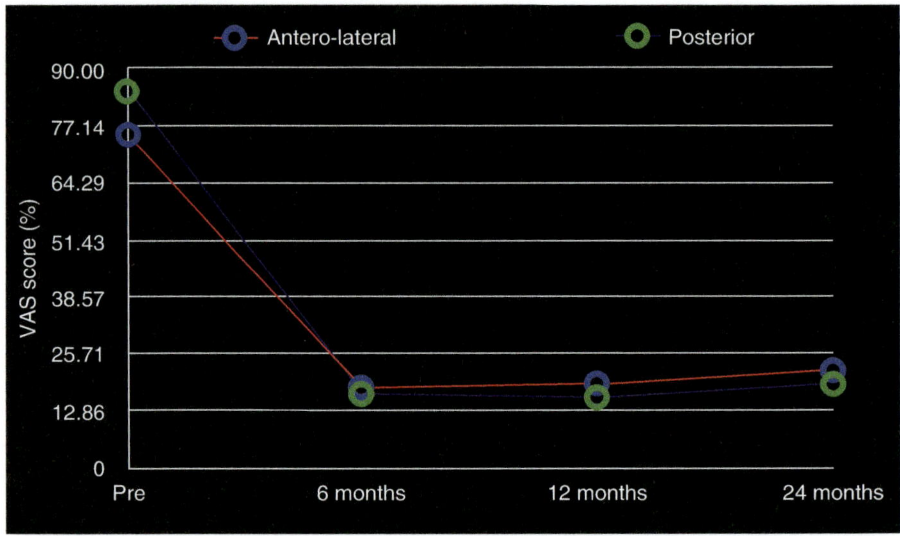

Fig. 11.7 VAS improvement score

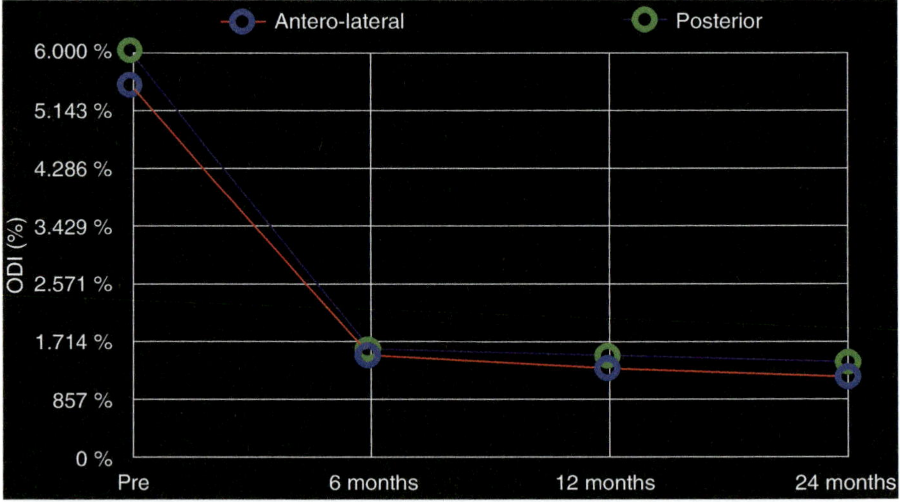

Fig. 11.8 ODI improvement score

study. The device has been implanted at L2-S1 with 2.0 % at L2–3, 4.7 % at L3–4, 52.7 % at L4–5, and 40.5 % at L5–S1. The mean operative time was 98 ± 49 min. The mean estimated blood loss was 60 ± 90 ml. The average ODI improved from 55 preoperatively to 30, 24, 22, 21, and 16, respectively, at 6 weeks and 3, 6, 12, and 24 months postoperatively. The average VAS decreased from 78 preoperatively to 33, 29, 25, 29, and 27, respectively, at 6 weeks and 3, 6, 12, and 24 months postoperatively [20] (Figs. 11.7 and 11.8). No major intraoperative or postoperative vascular or neurological complications have been reported. The main indication for the NuBac device is discogenic back pain secondary to Degenerative Disc Disease (DDD) and is similar to the indication for interbody fusion and TDA devices. It has been reported that surgical intervention shows better results in terms of patient satisfaction and function than conservative treatment. In addition, the literature reports a significant decrease in VAS and ODI for both fusion and TDAs, indicating that clinical results of TDAs are at least equivalent to fusion [21, 22].

References

1. Gillet P. The fate of the adjacent motion segments alter lumbar fusion. J Spinal Disord Tech. 2003;16:338–45.
2. Park P, Garton HJ, Gala VC. Adjacent segment disease after lumbar or lumbosacral fusion: review of the literature. Spine. 2004;29:1938–44.
3. Buettner-Janz K, Schellnack K, Zippel H. Biomechanics of the SB Charitè lumbar intervertebral disc endoprosthesis. Int Orthop. 1989;13:173–6.
4. Nachemson A. The load on lumbar disks in different positions of the body. Clin Orthop. 1965;45:107–22.
5. Brinckmann P, Grootenboer H. Change of disc height, radial disc bulge, and intradiscal pressure from discectomy. Spine. 1991;16(6):641–6.
6. Fernstrom U. Arthroplasty with intercorporal endoprothesis in herniated disc and in painful disc. Acta Chir Scand Suppl. 1966;357:154–9.
7. McKenzie AH. Fernstron intervertebral disc arthroplasty: a long-term evaluation. Orthop Int Ed. 1995;3(4):313–24.
8. Tan JS, et al. Interbody device shape and size are important to strengthen the vertebra-implant interface. Spine. 2005;30(6):638–44.
9. Lowe TG, et al. A biomechanical study of regional endplate strength and cage morphology as it relates to structural interbody support. Spine. 2004;29(21):2389–94.
10. Wang A. A unified theory of wear for ultra-high molecular weight polyethylene in multi-directional sliding. Wear. 2001;248(1–2):38–47.
11. Jahan MS, et al. Combined chemical and mechanical effects on free radicals in UHMWPE joints during implantation. J Biomed Mater Res. 1991;25(8):1005–17, 199.
12. Klara P, Ray C. Artificial nucleus replacement. Clinical experience. Spine. 2002;27(12):1374–7.
13. Shim CS, et al. Partial disc replacement with the PDN prosthetic disc nucleus device: early clinical results. J Spinal Disord Tech. 2003;16(4):324–30.
14. Bao QB, et al. Pioneer surgical technology: NUBAC artificial nucleus. In: Kim DH, editor. Dynamic reconstruction of the spine. 1st ed. New York: Thieme Medical; 2006. p. 128–36.
15. Bell GH, et al. Variations in strength of vertebrae with age and their relation to osteoporosis. Calcif Tissue Res. 1967;1(1):75–86.
16. Perry O. Fracture of the vertebral end-plate in the lumbar spine. Acta Orthop Scand. 1957;25(Suppl):34–9.
17. Bertagnoli R, Vazquez RJ. The anterolateral transPsoatic approach (ALPA): a new technique for implanting prosthetic disc-nucleus devices. J Spinal Disord Tech. 2003;16(4):398–404.
18. Ozgur BM, Aryan HE, Pimenta L. Extreme lateral interbody fusion (XLIF): a novel surgical technique for anterior lumbar interbody fusion. Spine J. 2006;6:435–43.
19. Berjano P, Balsano M, Buric J, Petruzzi M, Lamartina C. Direct lateral access lumbar and thoracolumbar fusion: preliminary results. Eur Spine J. 2012;21 Suppl 1:S37–42.
20. Balsano M, Zachos A, Ruggiu A, Barca F, Tranquilli-Leali P, Doria C. Nucleus disc arthroplasty with the NUBAC™ device: 2-year clinical experience. Eur Spine J. 2011;20 Suppl 1:S36–40.

21. Zigler J. Results of the prospective, randomized, multicenter food and drug administration investigational device exemption study of the ProDisc-L total disc replacement versus circumferential fusion for the treatment of 1-level degenerative disease. Spine. 2007;32(11):1155–62; discussion 1163.
22. Blumenthal S, Blumenthal S. A prospective, randomized, multicenter Food and Drug Administration investigational device exemptions study of lumbar total disc replacement with the CHARITE artificial disc versus lumbar fusion: part I: evaluation of clinical outcomes. Spine. 2005;30(14):1565–75; discussion E387–E9.

Chapter 12
Vertebral Body Augmentation in Osteoporotic Vertebral Compression Fractures

Roberto Postacchini and Gianluca Cinotti

Introduction

The procedures of vertebral body augmentation consist of the introduction of sub-stances, which are sometimes associated with metallic devices, into the vertebral body to increase its strength and stiffness when these mechanical properties are decreased as a result of fractures, primary tumors, or metastases.

The first procedure, called vertebroplasty, was performed by Galibert et al. [1] in 1987 in patients with a vertebral angioma. In the course of few years, the use of vertebroplasty has become increasingly frequent in patients with osteoporotic frac-tures of the vertebral body [2–5]. In the early 1990s, another technique, called kyphoplasty, was introduced with the goal of decreasing the complications of verte-broplasty and restoring the height of the fractured vertebral body. The first decade of the twenty-first century witnessed the advent of further techniques, including the so-called vertebral body stenting, in which a metallic device is used, with or without bone cement. However, many of the latter techniques never reached the popularity of the previous procedures and a few have occupied only a niche in the panorama of vertebral body augmentation procedures.

The advent of vertebral body augmentation has changed the therapeutic approach to osteoporotic compression fractures by replacing the traditional use of the corset, at least in a portion of patients with fractures.

R. Postacchini, MD (✉)
Italian University of Sport and Movement (IUSM),
Piazza Lauro de Bosis 6, Rome 00135, Italy

Israelitic Hospital Rome,
Piazza San Bartolomeo all'Isola 21, Rome 00186, Italy
e-mail: robby1478@hotmail.com

G. Cinotti, MD
Orthopedic Department, University Sapienza,
P.le Aldo Moro 5, Rome 00157, Italy

P.P.M. Menchetti (ed.), *Minimally Invasive Surgery of the Lumbar Spine*,
DOI 10.1007/978-1-4471-5280-4_12, © Springer-Verlag London 2014

Diagnosis of Osteoporotic Vertebral Fractures

In many cases, the clinical diagnosis of a recent osteoporotic vertebral compression fracture (VCF) is easy. Usually, the patient is a person aged over 65 years who, following a trauma of very mild severity or in the absence of any trauma, begins to complain of vertebral pain so severe as to compel them to bed rest or to limit considerably their activities of daily living. Many patients report having had episodes of back pain in their life, but in most cases there is no history of severe spine pain.

Initially, the vertebral pain is underestimated; however, it does not decrease in severity with increasing time despite bed rest and use of antiinflammatory and/or analgesic medication. Most patients seek an orthopedic visit after 2–3 weeks of the onset of pain. At clinical examination, the picture may be so typical as to allow, or strongly suspect, the diagnosis of vertebral fracture even in the absence of imaging studies. The elderly patient with an osteoporotic VCF moves with extreme caution and at times prefers to stand up rather than sit in a chair. When invited to lay down on the medical bed, the patient often has a different behavior compared to one with discogenic disease or vertebral osteoarthritis. The patient with osteoporotic fracture sits on the bed of the consulting room slowly and with evident effort, accompanied by pained grimaces. Often they state that they are unable to lay supine due to pain and when they agree to try it is done slowly, with grimaces and pained sighs. Then, when they are asked to turn in the prone position, at times there is a complete refusal; otherwise, this is done with considerable caution, slowness and clear evidence of pain. Again, when the patient is asked to lay on the flank to sit then on the bed, the movements are done slowly, with grimaces, sighs, and evident pain.

It is commonly believed that deep palpation on the spinous process of the fractured vertebra elicits severe pain so as to allow identification of the fractured vertebra. This is only partially true, because pain of similar severity can also often be evoked on palpation at different levels, particularly in elderly patients with vertebral osteoarthritis. It should be also borne in mind that the site of subjective pain may not correspond to the site of fracture. In fact, patients with fracture of the highest lumbar vertebrae or the lowest thoracic vertebrae often complain of pain in the lower lumbar spine.

In summary, the patient with a recent osteoporotic VCF often gives the impression, on clinical examination, of having much more pain than the patient with spine pain due to benign diseases, and this should lead to strong suspicion of a vertebral fracture. The site of fracture may not be determined or even suspected because either the reported pain is often in a different region than the fracture site, particularly for lesions in the thoracolumbar junction, and/or the deep palpation of spinous processes may not be diagnostic.

Radiographs of the spine may allow the diagnosis of recent fracture to be made, but usually only when recent radiographs are available showing the integrity of the fractured vertebra. It may be difficult or impossible, in fact, to distinguish on radiographs a recent from an old VCF, which is often visible in older patients who are not known to have had any previous fracture. The imaging study of choice is MRI, which permits a clear-cut distinction between a recent and an old fracture based on the presence or absence of changes of the signal intensity of the vertebral body on

T1- and T2-weighted sequences, that is, the hypointensity on T1 and hyperintensity on T2 images. In the course of few months from fracture, in fact, the signal intensity of the vertebral body becomes progressively normal, thus allowing identification of the fracture as an old injury.

Definitions

Vertebroplasty is the procedure in which bone cement or other materials are directly injected into a fractured vertebral body with no attempt to restore its height.

Kyphoplasty, or balloon kyphoplasty, is the procedure in which a balloon in inserted in the vertebral body and inflated to create a void in which bone cement or other material are injected.

Vertebral body stenting is a kyphoplasty procedure with the addition of an expandable titanium mesh implant to increase the mechanical strength and restore the height of the vertebral body.

Biomechanics

Several biomechanical studies on osteoporotic cadaveric vertebrae showed that the injection of bone cement or other materials increases the strength of bone to axial load. In most studies it was also found that there is an increase in stiffness of the injected vertebral body.

Dean et al. [6], by injecting a mean of 4 ml (range, 1–8 ml) of bone cement in autopsy specimens using a posterolateral approach, obtained an asymmetrical distribution of cement in the vertebral body. Then they measured the vertebral strength during constant rate axial compression. The strength was found to be significantly increased compared with the controls, and the increase did not appear to be correlated with the amount of cement injected. Similar results were obtained in a study of fractured vertebral bodies in which a varying amount of cement or a bio-active glass-ceramic composite had been inoculated [7]. Both materials restored the vertebral strength to the prefracture values using 2 ml of cement. However, restoration of the stiffness required a greater volume of material (4–8 ml), depending on whether the vertebra was thoracic or lumbar.

In a study on osteoporotic lumbar vertebrae [8], the bone cement was injected through the pedicles either unilaterally or bilaterally. In both instances the strength and stiffness of the vertebral bodies increased. The unilateral injection increased the strength to axial load by double, and the bilateral injection by three times, compared with that of untreated vertebral bodies.

Belkoff et al. [9], in an ex in vivo biomechanical evaluation of hydroxyapatite cement and standard cement for use with kyphoplasty, found that both cements significantly restored vertebral body height. Kyphoplasty with standard cement resulted in stronger repairs than did kyphoplasty with hydroxyapatite cement, but both treatments resulted in significantly less stiff vertebral bodies relative to their initial condition. Perry et al. [10], however, in a subsequent biomechanical evaluation of kyphoplasty with calcium sulfate cement (CSC, i.e., hydroxyapatite), in cadaveric osteoporotic vertebrae showed that CSC yielded similar vertebral body strength and stiffness as compared with standard bone cement. A biomechanical study [11] comparing polymethylmethacrylate (PMMA) and the biopolymer polypropylene fumarate cement (PPF-30) for kyphoplasty showed that strength restoration with PMMA and PPF-30 were 120 and 104 %, respectively, of the pretreatment strength. For stiffness, PMMA and PPF-30 restored vertebral bodies to 69 and 53 %, respectively, of the initial values.

The results of several experimental studies, including finite element analysis studies [12], indicate that it is unnecessary to inject high volumes of bone cement. In contrast, an exaggerated filling of the vertebral body may be detrimental because an excessive stiffness of a vertebral body may expose adjacent vertebrae to greater risk of subsequent fracture [13]. However, it is preferable to obtain a symmetrical distribution of the cement in the vertebral body.

A study [14] compared kyphoplasty to vertebral body stenting in cadaveric vertebrae after creating anterior wedge fractures. Vertebral bodies were repaired either with balloon kyphoplasty or with the titanium mesh implant and bone cement. Data for cement injection volume and height maintained following testing were compared between the groups. There was significantly less cement injected and significantly greater height maintained in the titanium implant group compared with the kyphoplasty group.

In another study [15] on human cadaveric vertebrae comparing kyphoplasty to vertebral body stenting after creating VCFs, it was found that after, deflating the balloon for kyphoplasty, there was a significant loss of reduction compared with vertebral body stenting (on average, kyphoplasty: 11.7 %; stenting: 3.7 %), and a significant total height gain in relation to preoperative height with the stenting procedure (on average, kyphoplasty: 8.0 %; stenting: 13.3 %).

A novel system for treatment of VCFs has recently been compared with balloon kyphoplasty in cadaveric vertebrae [16]. It is the Kiva® System, consisting of a stacked coil implant made of polyetheretherketone (PEEK) and delivered over a guide-wire. The system is designed to provide height restoration and mechanical stabilization while improving cement containment. Kiva® exhibits similar biomechanical performance to balloon kyphoplasty but may decrease the risk of extravasation through the containment mechanism of the implant design and by reducing the cement volume.

Indications

Vertebral body augmentation is usually indicated for recent osteoporotic VCFs, that is, not more than 3–4 months duration, in patients with pain unresponsive to conservative treatments such as bed rest and pain medication. As for the corset, at the time of diagnosis, the orthopedic surgeon, together with the patient, should make a choice between the use of a corset or a surgical procedure, based on several factors, such as the time elapsed from the fracture, the severity of pain, the amount of decrease in height of the vertebral body, and the patient's willingness to undergo a surgical procedure. Once the use of corset has been chosen, it should be worn for at least 2 months without changing the decision, unless the patient does not tolerate the corset, the pain is not enough controlled by the conservative management, or the vertebral body undergoes a significant decrease in height in the first few weeks after fracture as shown by sequential imaging studies. It should be considered, in fact, that the decrease in height usually does not occur until after 1 month of the occurrence of the fracture.

If an augmentation procedure is envisaged, a CT scan, following MRI, may be indicated when there are any doubts about the integrity of the anterior, and particularly the posterior, wall of the vertebral body. CT, in fact, may show better than MRI the presence of clefts through which the material injected can leak out the vertebral body. This holds particularly true when a vertebroplasty is planned.

Vertebral body augmentation may not be indicated in the first 3 weeks after the fracture because there can be a greater risk of leakage of cement through small clefts of the cortical bone of the vertebral body. This holds particularly true for vertebroplasty in which the cement is injected directly into the cancellous bone of the vertebra. After 3 months from the fracture, kyphoplasty or vertebroplasty are seldom indicated because pain is usually decreased in severity and the healing process may make it difficult to inject enough cement in the vertebral body. For the same reason, despite the different opinion of other authors [17, 18], our personal experience indicates that, in the vast majority of cases, there is no indication for vertebral body augmentation beyond 4 months from the injury. One of the main reasons is that it is difficult or impossible to inject bone cement, or an adequate amount of cement, in a fractured vertebral body when the injury has healed. A marked decrease in height of the vertebral body is not a contraindication for vertebroplasty or kyphoplasty, even if in this case the procedure may be technically more difficult [19].

The most appropriate indications for vertebral body stenting are represented by fractures of less than 1 month duration that show a collapse not greater than one-third of the original height of the vertebra and at least 15° of wedge deformity (evaluated on an adjacent uninjured vertebra) [20]. The vertebral deformity should also be correctable, as demonstrated by the increase of height loss in standing radiographs compared with those in the supine position. Older fractures in which the healing process has already begun or those needing no significant correction do not represent a good indication. Personal experience also indicates that the stenting procedure has a high ability of restoring vertebral height, but severely osteoporotic patients may not be good candidates because the high strength provided by both the cement and the metallic mesh expose them to higher risks of adjacent vertebral fractures. Furthermore, since the procedure is a combination of kyphoplasty and vertebroplasty, the risk of cement leakage is higher than for

Table 12.1 Prerogatives and drawbacks of the three most frequently performed procedures of vertebral body augmentation

	Vertebroplasty	Kyphoplasty	Stenting
Duration of surgery	Short for unilateral approach	Long (bilat. approach)	Long (bilat. approach)
Restorations of VBH[a]	None or very little	Moderate	High
Leakage of cement	High rate	Low rate	High rate
Adjacent fractures	Moderate rate	High rate	Probably high rate
Clinical outcome	Very good	Good	Very good
Limitations of indications	Partial	None	High
Cost	Low	Medium	High

[a]Vertebral body height

kyphoplasty alone. The prerogatives and drawbacks of the three procedures are listed in Table 12.1.

Vertebral body augmentation is not indicated when MRI or CT scan show a clear-cut interruption of the posterior wall of the vertebral body due to the risk of leakage of cement in the spinal canal. The procedure is also contraindicated in pregnant women and in the presence of nerve root or the spinal cord compression.

Operative Techniques and Materials

The procedure should be carried out in the operating theatre because of greater guarantee of sterility. Usually it is performed under local anesthesia, associated with patient sedation. Local anesthesia is preferred by most patients and allows the procedure to be carried out even in older subjects with general comorbidities. Furthermore, it permits the patient to be checked with regard to the possible appearance of leg symptoms due to compression of neural structures by either the trocar(s) used to penetrate into the vertebral body or the cement during injection.

A single or double fluoroscope can be used. If two fluoroscopes are available, which allow the procedure to be performed much more rapidly, one is employed for the AP and the other for the lateral view.

Usually the material injected in the vertebral body is PMMA, the standard bone cement, or a mixture of PMMA and hydroxyapatite. The adjunct of hydroxyapatite, which is osteoconductive and bioabsorbable, decreases the amount of PMMA, and thus the stiffness of the material injected. The cement is introduced by a "dedicated" syringe or thin cannula with a piston that pushes the cement slowly and intermittently into the vertebra under frequent fluoroscopic control for immediate detection of possible leakage of cement out of the vertebral body. The cement should have a slow polymerization rate and be injected when it is viscous enough not to leak through clefts of the cortical bone; however, it should not be too solid to risk that the injection has to be interrupted because of too precocious polymerization.

Khyphoplasty

Kyphoplasty is usually carried out by a transpedicular approach. The patient is placed prone on the operating table. The local anesthesia is carried out using a spinal needle introduced at 5 cm from the midline under AP view and advanced obliquely to reach the lateral border of the pedicle on the side that is initially approached if a bilateral procedure is performed. The skin incision, made at the entry point of the needle, is a few millimeters long. A trocar is introduced under AP view with an oblique direction to reach the lateral border of the pedicle. It is advanced for a short distance into the pedicle and then a lateral view of the spine is obtained to check the distance of the tip of the trocar from the vertebral body. The trocar is deepened into the pedicle using alternately the AP and lateral view, until its tip reaches the medial wall of the pedicle in AP view and the junction of the pedicle with the vertebral body in the lateral view. The trocar is then introduced for a short distance into the vertebral body. A Kirshner wire is inserted in the trocar and pushed into the body for about two-thirds of its sagittal diameter. The trocar is removed and replaced by the working cannula under the guide of the Kirschner wire, which is then removed and a drill is inserted. This is advanced in the vertebra until the tip is in proximity of the anterior cortex to create the space for balloon. The latter is inserted and inflated with contrast medium. If the kyphoplasty is performed bilaterally, the same procedure is carried out on the opposite side while deflating the first balloon when the Kirschner wire is inserted into the vertebral body. A thin cannula filled with cement is introduced in the working cannula of each side and the cement is injected alternately on the two sides, thus creating two roundish blocks of cement inside the vertebral body (Fig. 12.1). If the approach is unilateral, the Kirschner wire, the drill, and the balloon are introduced as close as possible to the central area of the body in both the AP and lateral view.

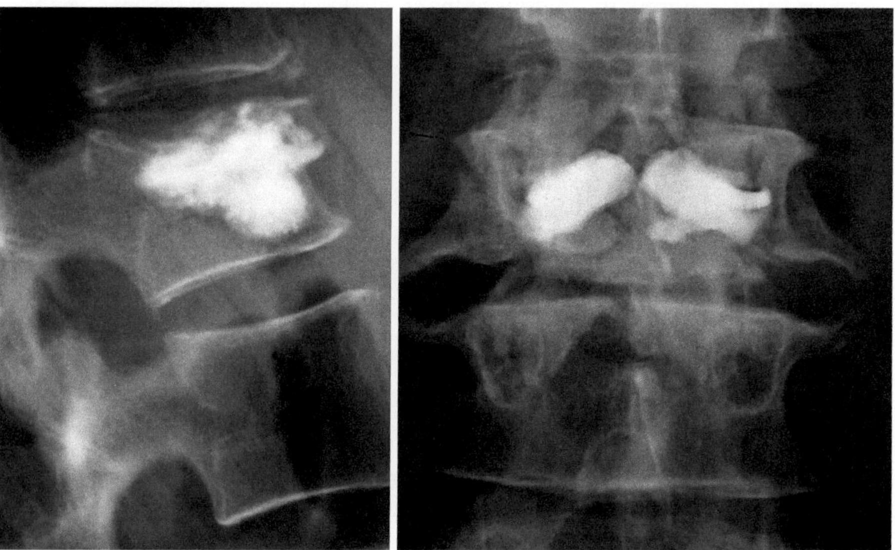

Fig. 12.1 Lateral and AP view of a patient undergoing kyphoplasty for an osteoporotic VCF of L1. In the AP view, two roundish blocks of cement are visible in the vertebral body

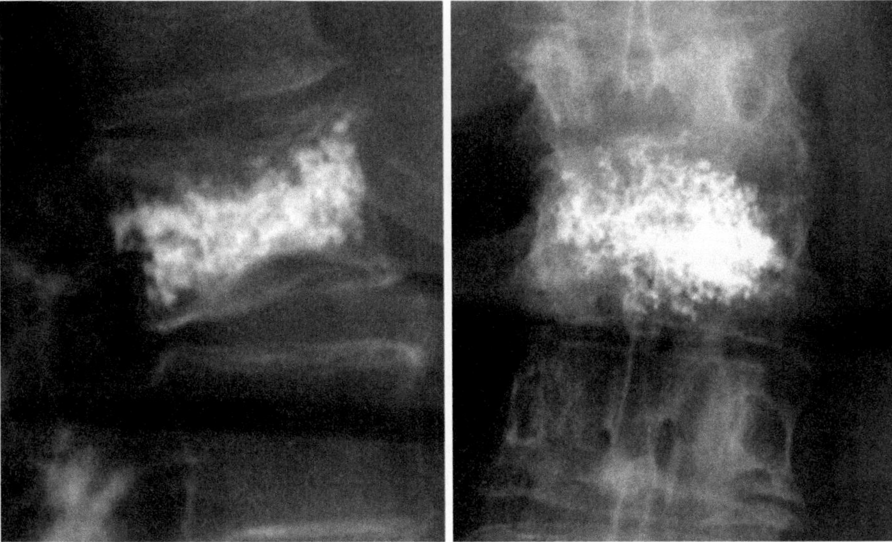

Fig. 12.2 Vertebroplasty of a lumbar vertebra. The cement infiltrates a large part of the intertrabecular spaces of the cancellous bone of the vertebral body

Vertebroplasty

The approach can be transpedicular, as for the kyphoplasty or, more often, a posterolateral approach is used. For the latter approach, the patient may be placed prone or in the lateral decubitus position. When using the latter position, as we prefer, the procedure is carried out unilaterally. The spinal needle used for the anesthesia is introduced at 10 cm from the midline at the level of the pedicle of the involved vertebra. With the fluoroscope set up for lateral image, the needle is advanced obliquely at an angle of 50–60° to the sagittal plane towards the lateral aspect of the posterior portion of the vertebral body at the junction of the latter with the pedicle. The trocar is introduced in the same direction as the anesthesia needle and inserted in the vertebral body until it reaches the central part of the body in AP and lateral view. The stylet of the trocar is removed and a small amount of contrast medium is injected to check whether it leaks out the body ventrally, or posteriorly into the spinal canal. The cement that is then injected infiltrates the intertrabecular spaces of a large part of, or the entire, vertebral body (Fig. 12.2).

Vertebral Body Stenting

This procedure, also called stentoplasty, is performed by a bilateral transpedicular approach, as previously described. The difference with kyphoplasty is that the balloon is placed inside a stent consisting of a titanium mesh. When inflating the balloon, the stent expands and reaches the cancellous bone located in proximity of the

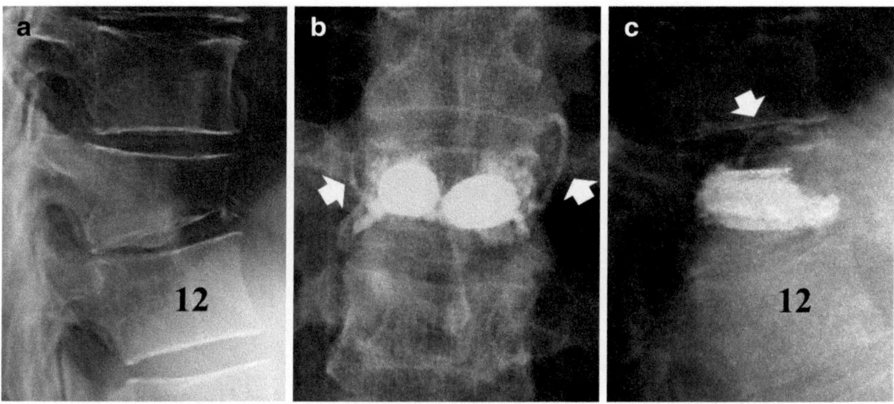

Fig. 12.3 Wedge-shaped fracture of T11 in a 54-year-old woman. (**a**) Pre-treatment radiograph. (**b**) Vertebral body stenting carried out with almost complete restoration of the anterior height of the vertebral body. (**c**) Cement leakages occurred in the paravertebral tissue (*arrows*) with no clinical sequelae

vertebral end-plates. The shape and height of the fractured vertebra may thus be restored better than with kyphoplasty because, when the balloon is deflated and retrieved, the metallic mesh remains on site with little or no loss of the correction (Fig. 12.3). After extraction of the balloon, the injected cement fills the void and infiltrates the adjacent cancellous bone through the holes of the stent.

Complications

Complications of vertebral body augmentation procedures my occur during the approach to the vertebral body or during the injection of PMMA or similar materials into the vertebra, the latter event being by far the most frequent. The most common complication is the leakage of cement out of the vertebral cortex directly, or through the basivertebral vein, in the adjacent disc, the spinal canal, or the intervertebral foramen (Fig. 12.4). Less frequent complications are extravasations of cement into the extravertebral venous system with or without pulmonary embolism. In this instance, pulmonary embolism may occur.

Bono et al. [21] reported on four complications in a series of 375 patients treated with kyphoplasty. Of these complications, two occurred during the approach, which was extrapedicular in one case and pedicular in the other. Both complications were neurological in nature, that is, an anterior cord syndrome and a paraparesis. The recovery was complete in one case and partial in the other case. Recently, two cases have been reported of leakage of cement into the spinal canal through a breach in the medial wall of the pedicle during kyphoplasty [22]. The leakage, which caused paraparesis, was detected by postoperative CT scan. Retrospectively looking at stored fluoroscopic images, it was found that improper position of the trocar in AP and lateral view simultaneously while taking entry caused the pedicle wall violation.

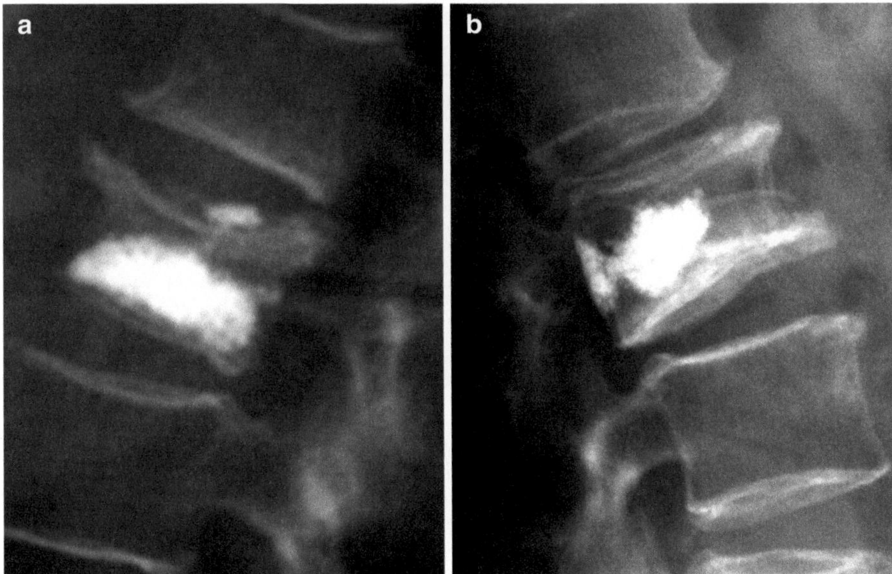

Fig. 12.4 Two examples of leakage of cement during vertebroplasty. (**a**) Leakage in the disc above. (**b**) Asymptomatic leakage in the concavity of the posterior wall of the vertebra body

Phillips et al. [23] obtained cinefluoroscopic images in patients undergoing kyphoplasty to compare the amount of leakage of the contrast medium out of the vertebral body before introducing the balloon (mimicking vertebroplasty injection) and after inflating the balloon to create the intravertebral void. Transcortical leakage of contrast medium and filling of epidural vessels and inferior vena cava was significantly greater when mimicking a vertebroplasty than while injecting the kyphoplasty void.

In a series [24], 40 patients were treated with kyphoplasty (57 vertebrae) and 66 patients (124 vertebrae) underwent vertebroplasty. There were 18 % of patients in the kyphoplasty group and 49 % in the vertebroplasty group that showed cement leakage into the paravertebral soft tissues or veins. Cement leakage into the disk space occurred in 12 % of the kyphoplasty group and 25 % of the vertebroplasty group. However, no complications related to cement leakage were noted.

In another series [25], cement leakage occurred in 17 (9.94 %) of 71 patients undergoing kyphoplasty. There were 7 paravertebral leaks, 6 leaks into the disc space, 3 leaks into the channel of needling insertion, and 1 spinal canal leak. Four patients (5.63 %) developed pulmonary complications postoperatively, one of them with confirmed diagnosis of pulmonary embolism directly caused by cement leakage.

A questionnaire study [26] aimed at detecting the incidence of complications of vertebroplasty and kyphoplasty obtained details of 3,216 vertebroplasties and 5,139 kyphoplasties. The risk of cement extrusion from the vertebra (odd ratios 2.64, $p<0.01$) and into the spinal canal (odd ratios 435, $p<0.01$) was markedly higher for vertebroplasty. Instead, the odds ratio for neurologic complications (odd ratios 2.56, $p=0.1$) did not indicate significant predisposition for either procedure.

A systematic review of English-language and German-language articles published between 2002 and 2009 revealed that the rate of relevant complications was significantly higher for vertebroplasty than kyphoplasty [27]. Another literature review [28] showed a rate of about 9 % for cement leakage during kyphoplasty compared with up to 41 % rate for vertebroplasty, the leakage being mainly into the disc space. For kyphoplasty, the probability for symptomatic cement leakage averaged 1.3 %; complications due to the surgical technique, postoperative infections, bleeding, or cardiovascular complications were rare, with less than 1 % incidence. A review of 12 studies [29] (each including more than 15 cases) in which kyphoplasty was used revealed that severe complications such as pulmonary embolism, spinal stenosis, radiculopathy, and epidural hematoma occurred in 13 of the 737 patients. Leakage of cement occurred in 133 out of 1,205 treated vertebrae.

Several single case reports of rare complications have been published, such as a case in which CT scan revealed a cement embolus inside the right ventricle due to right ventricle perforation during a kyphoplasty procedure [30], or the case of a patient who had embolization of the right T9 segmental artery with penetration of cement into the radicular artery beneath the pedicle during vertebroplasy [31].

In one of our patients, a pneumothorax occurred after a thoracic vertebroplasty performed through a posterolateral approach, and another patient had a fracture of the sternum due to the supine position on a special square frame.

In a series of patients undergoing vertebral body stenting, 26 % had an asymptomatic cement leakage, mostly in the paravertebral tissues or veins [20].

Clinical Outcomes

Innumerable studies including less than 100 patients have reported on the clinical results of vertebroplasty or kyphoplasty. The vast majority of them report satisfactory results in terms of pain relief and improvement of physical function and quality of life. However, only few studies dealt with a high number of cases, were systematic reviews of the literature, or prospective randomized controlled trials.

One study [32] reported on an institutional experience of 1,634 patients with a mean age of 73 years who underwent vertebroplasty for painful osteoporotic fractures of ≥ 2 months duration. The patients were prospectively evaluated with a mean follow-up of 25 months (range, 11–44). The VAS, ODI, use of analgesic medication, and external brace were recorded before and after treatment. The mean VAS score decreased from 7.94 to 1.12 points and the mean ODI value diminished from 82 to 6 %. A brace was worn by 1,279 patients before surgery and only112 after vertebroplasty.

In a systematic review of the literature [33], 1,587 articles were found on vertebroplasty and kyphoplasty, of which only 27 were prospective (randomized or non-randomized) multiple-arm studies with cohorts of ≥ 20 cases. In these studies, overall, the mean VAS score (0–10) decreased by 5.07 points after kyphoplasty and

4.55 points after vertebroplasty, while the decrease was −2.1 in the conservatively treated patients. Quality of life improvement was greater after kyphoplasty than vertebroplasty. It was found that a greater pain relief was obtained by patients operated within 7 weeks of the onset of the fracture.

Based on a literature review associated to retrospective chart/case review for clinical data, Garfin and Reilley [34] reported that 95 % of patients undergoing kyphoplasty or vertebroplasty have significant improvement in pain and function. They also stated that kyphoplasty improves vertebral body height when performed within 3 months of the onset of the fracture.

In 2009, these triumphant results were contradicted by two prospective, randomized, multicenter studies published in the *New England Journal of Medicine* [35, 36]. Both studies compared a cohort of patients treated with vertebroplasty to a similar cohort undergoing a sham procedure. The conclusions of both studies were that improvements in pain and pain-related disability associated with VCF in patients treated with vertebroplasty were similar to the improvements in the control group. These studies, however, stirred up numerous criticisms. One of them concerned the volume of cement injected. Only one of the investigations provided information on the amount of cement inoculated, which was on average 2.8 ± 1.2 ml, an amount too small for restoration of vertebral strength, particularly for the lowest thoracic and lumbar vertebrae [37]. Another criticism concerned the time elapsed from the onset of the fracture [38]. Both trials, in fact, enrolled patients who have had pain for ≤12 months, a duration too long by far for a vertebroplasty investigation, resulting in both trials of an intervention on healed fractures.

As regards the increase in height of the vertebral body, in two comparative studies of vertebroplasty and kyphoplasty, in which a total of 347 patients were treated, it was found that the correction of the kyphotic deformity and restoration of the anterior vertebral body height was significantly better in the patients undergoing kyphoplasty [39, 40]. The posterior vertebral body height was marginally restored in one study and not restored in the other. On the other hand, Garfin and Reilley expressed the opinion that only kyphoplasty is effective in increasing the anterior vertebral body height [34].

In an article on the clinical experience with 34 cases of vertebral body stenting, the authors [20] report that the average kyphosis angle, which preoperatively was 23° (13–32°), was corrected to 12° (0–16°) postoperatively. As for the increase in height of the vertebral body, in five cases there was no height restoration, while in the remaining patients the height gain was 50 % in 12, 75 % in 14, and 100 % in 3.

New Vertebral Fractures Following Vertebral Body Augmentation

New vertebral compression fractures may occur in a vertebra distant from that previously treated or one adjacent to that injected with cement (Fig. 12.5). In the latter

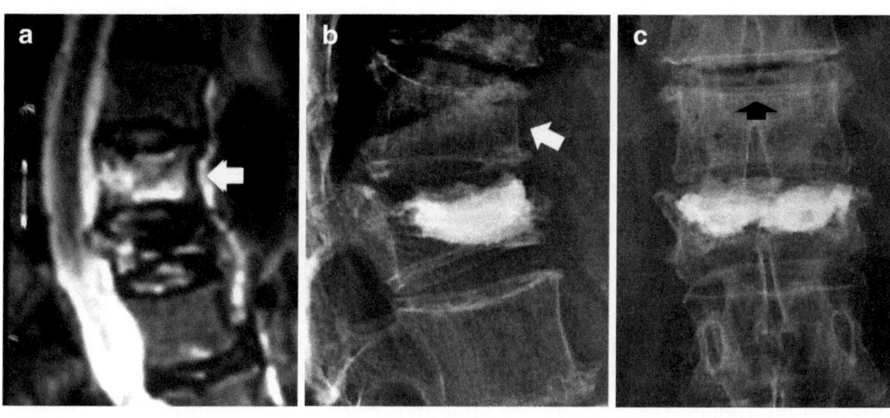

Fig. 12.5 Fracture of a vertebra adjacent to one previously undergoing kyphoplasty in a 61-year-old woman. (**a**) MRI T2 weighted image showing hyperintensity of T12 vertebral body (*arrow*) with a recent fracture and an old fracture of the L1 vertebra filled with cement. (**b**) Lateral radiograph showing the moderate wedge shape deformity of T12 (*arrow*). (**c**) AP view. Only a slight collapse of the upper end-plate of T12 is visible (*arrow*)

instance, there are high chances that the new fracture is somewhat related to greater strength and stiffness of the treated vertebra.

A retrospective study [41] was performed on 36 patients who underwent 46 augmentation procedures (20 fractures treated with kyphoplasty and 26 with vertebroplasty). The mean patient's age was similar in the two groups. The mean cement injection per vertebral body was 4.65 and 3.78 ml for the kyphoplasty and vertebroplasty group, respectively. Ninety-five percent of the kyphoplasty procedures were performed bilaterally, whereas only 19 % of the vertebroplasties were bilateral. Within a 3-month period, there were five new adjacent level fractures seen in three patients who underwent a kyphoplasty (5/20 [25 %]) and none in the vertebroplasty group. The authors attributed the higher incidence of new fractures in the kyphoplasty group to the higher volume of cement injected and the bilateral approach.

A study [42] analyzed 98 patients with a mean age of 70.6 years who underwent kyphoplasty for postmenopausal VCF. Age, body mass index, history of tobacco use, number of initial vertebral fractures, intradiscal cement leakage, history of non-spinal fractures, use of antiosteoporotic medications, bone mineral density, bone turnover markers, and 25(OH)D levels were assessed. Nine patients (11 levels) (22.5 % of patients; 11.2 % of levels) developed a new fracture. Cement leakage was identified in seven patients (17.5 %). The patients without recurrent fractures demonstrated higher levels of 25(OH)D (22.6 ± 5.51 vs. 14.39 ± 7.47; $p = .001$) and lower N-terminal cross-linked telopeptide values (17.11 ± 10.20 vs. 12.90 ± 4.05; $p = .067$) compared with the patients with recurrent fractures. The authors conclude that bone metabolism and 25(OH)D levels seem to play a role in the occurrence of post-kyphoplasty recurrent vertebral fractures. A similar study was performed by Rho et al. [43], who retrospectively analyzed the occurrence of new VCF in 147 patients treated with vertebroplasty or kyphoplasty. Possible risk factors, such as age, gender, body mass index, bone mineral density (BMD), location of treated vertebra, treatment modality, amount of bone cement injected, anterior-posterior ratio of the fractured vertebra, cement leakage into the disc space, and pattern of cement distribution, were assessed. New VCF occurred in 18.4 % of patients at a median time of 70 days from the original treatment. The adjacent vertebra was involved in 66.7 % of the patients. Significant differences were found between the new VCF and control groups with regard to age, treatment modality, BMD, and the proportion of cement leakage into the disc space. Disc cement leakage and low BMD were the most important risk factors.

A systematic review of the literature [44] was performed to assess the potential risk of new vertebral fractures following vertebroplasty and kyphoplasty versus conservative treatment. A high degree of heterogeneity was found among the results, which made it impossible to state that cement augmentation is as safe as conservative treatment with respect to new fractures. The combined odds ratio of vertebroplasty and kyphoplasty versus conservative treatment gave a hint that there might be little difference. Similar results were obtained in another systematic review of the literature [45] in which the authors found few large-sample, randomized controlled trials specifically performed to investigate new fractures as an outcome of vertebroplasty or kyphoplasty. Pooled results from only two randomized controlled trials were reported, showing no significant increase of the secondary fracture rate after vertebral augmentation therapy compared with that of conventional treatment.

There is no precise information on the rate of new fractures after vertebral body stenting, but the rate is probably similar to that of kyphoplasty or even higher.

Personal Experience

Few published studies make a clear-cut distinction between the results at very short-term (first 4 weeks) from those at medium-term (third to fifth month) and long-term (more than 1 year). Such a distinction is of paramount importance because it is well known that the natural evolution, in the vast majority of osteoporotic fractures, is toward the resolution of pain or its considerable decrease in severity in the course of 5–8 months.

In the first few days after vertebroplasty or kyphoplasty, a portion of patients have a considerable decrease in pain while some still have moderate or even severe pain. In most cases, however, the pre-treatment pain is decreased. Our personal experience indicates that the clinical improvement at very short term is related to the volume of cement injected as well as the site and type of fracture. Patients who have received a volume of cement of less than one-third of the size of the vertebral body have a lower decrease in pain than those in whom at least half of the vertebral body appears filled with cement on fluoroscopy. For the thoracic vertebrae that have received a proportionally equal amount of cement, the result tends to be better than for the lumbar, but particularly the thoracolumbar, vertebrae.

At medium-term, most patients in whom the vertebral body is filled with cement by at least 40 % have a satisfactory result. That is, they have no significant pain or

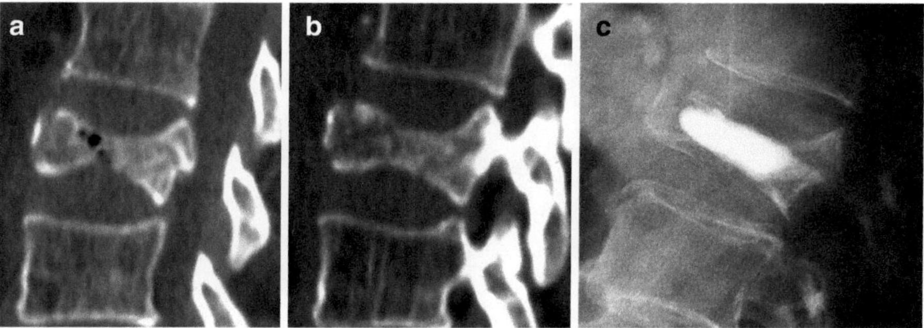

Fig. 12.6 A 63-year-old man with a T11 fracture of 2 months duration still complained of considerable pain. (**a** and **b**) CT scans show a severely collapsed vertebral body with intravertebral vertical and oblique clefts. (**c**) Lateral radiograph after kyphoplasty. Despite the severe collapse, a large part of the vertebral body could be filled of cement with excellent clinical outcome

only moderate pain, less than that complained of by many patients treated with a corset. Patients with thoracic or lumbar fracture tend to have a better result than those with thoracolumbar injury, particularly when the latter caused a significant segmental kyphosis.

At long-term, almost all patients have at least a fair outcome, similar to those treated conservatively.

Patients with severe collapse of the vertebral body may have a good clinical outcome, even when treated after 1 month of the onset of fracture (Figs. 12.6 and 12.7). However, the outcome may be poor if the collapse is associated with a wedge shape deformity or a vacuum phenomenon, particularly when it has a great extent [7].

Vertebroplasty appears to provide better clinical results than kyphoplasty, probably because the cement infiltrates a large part of the intertrabecular spaces rather than creating two blocks of cement in a region of the vertebra as occurs with kyphoplasty, which, however, exposes the patient to significantly lower risks of cement leakage than vertebroplasty (Table 12.1).

After vertebroplasty it is highly unusual to observe a significant increase in height of the vertebral body (Table 12.1). However, it is also unusual to find an increase in height and kyphotic alignment by 50 % or even more after kyphoplasty, as stated by a few authors [34, 46], although a mild to moderate increase may often be obtained. Vertebral body stenting is more effective in restoring vertebral height, but it involves a relatively high rate of cement leakage (Fig. 12.3).

As regards new VCFs, the severity of osteoporosis and the degree of stiffness of the treated vertebral body, resulting from the amount of bone cement injected, are the main factors exposing the patient to the risk of a new fracture, particularly in a vertebra adjacent to that previously treated. Because kyphoplasty usually involves the injection of a greater amount of cement by bilateral approach, this technique appears to expose the patient to higher risks of new fractures of adjacent vertebrae. Thus, a large amount of cement in the vertebral body gives higher chances of good result at short term, but also higher probabilities to favor a fracture in adjacent vertebrae. It is up to the surgeon to choose the right compromise based on the age,

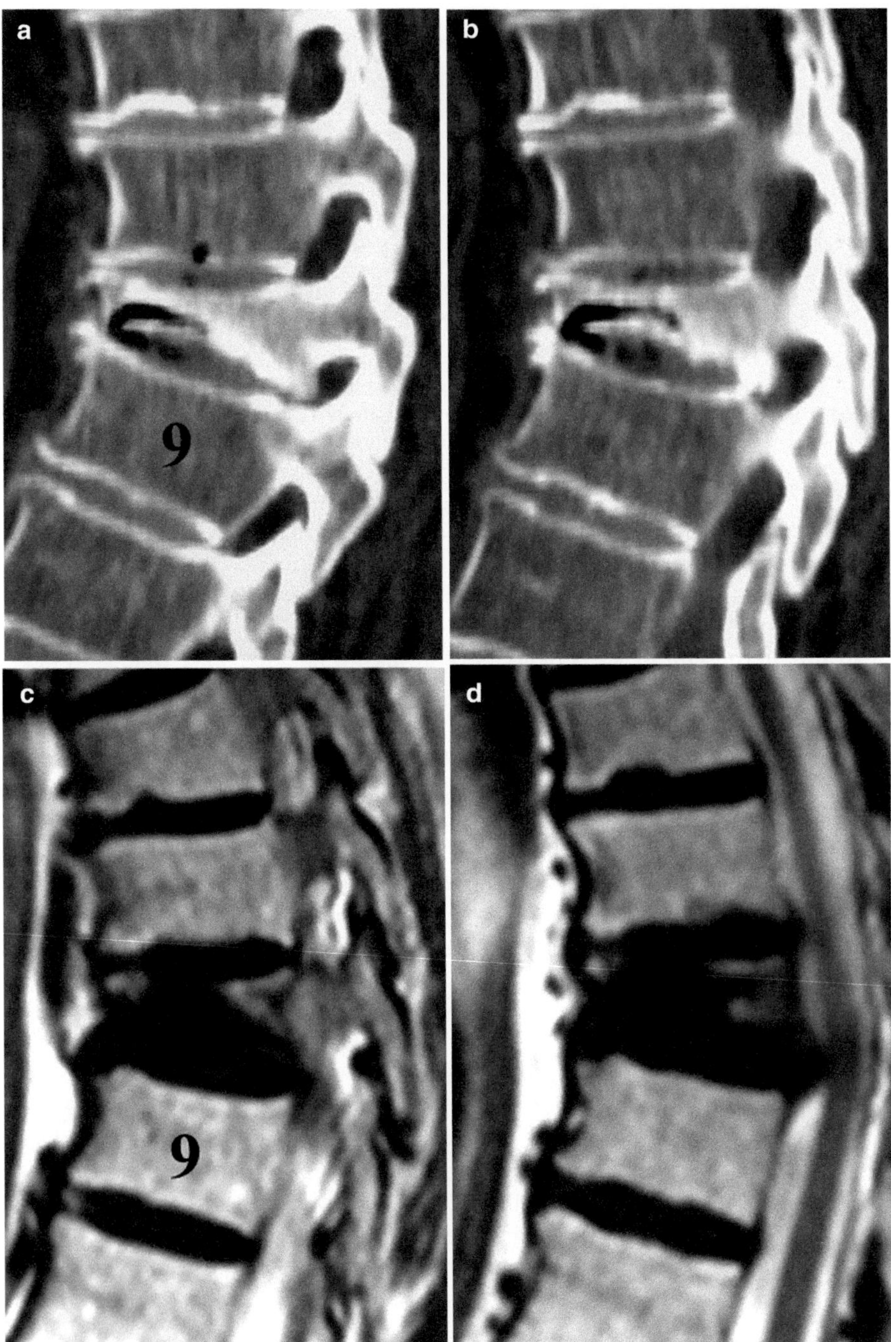

Fig. 12.7 A 74-year-old woman sustained a fracture of T8. CT scans (**a** and **b**) showed severe collapse and wedge-shaped deformity of the vertebral body in which a long cleft was present. The patient, who had severe pain, underwent kyphoplasty with mild correction of the deformities as shown by MR images (**c** and **d**). Postoperatively, she continued to complain of severe pain for several months after surgery

severity of osteoporosis, number and site of previous fractures, and severity of pain of the individual patient.

In our experience, the leakage of cement in the adjacent disc space does not play a relevant role, because very rarely was a new vertebral fracture observed in patients who had evidence of cement leakage in the adjacent disc.

Conclusions

In most cases, the presence of an osteoporotic VCF of recent onset can be strongly suspected, or even generically diagnosed, based on the behavior of the patient on clinical examination. MRI, which should often be carried out at both the thoracic and lumbar level, is the most useful diagnostic tool to discriminate a recent from an old fracture.

The vertebral augmentation procedures currently performed are vertebroplasty, kyphoplasty, and, though less frequently, vertebral body stenting. The former can be carried out by a posterolateral approach and unilaterally, while the latter two are routinely carried out by a transpedicular bilateral approach. All procedures should generally be done not later than 4 months of the onset of fracture. The volume of cement to inject should be at least half of the size of the vertebral body.

Kyphoplasty can restore vertebral body height, but only to a mild or moderate extent, while vertebral body stenting has the highest ability to increase the vertebral height and correct a kyphotic deformity, provided it is performed within 4–6 weeks of the onset of injury. Vertebroplasty has no or little ability to change the shape of the vertebra.

The most common complication is the leakage of cement out the vertebral body, a complication that can be potentially devastating when the cement leaks into the spinal canal. The leakage occurs more frequently with vertebroplasty and vertebral body stenting than with kyphoplasty.

The clinical outcomes are related, particularly at short term from vertebral augmentation, to the amount of cement injected. This is because the greater the volume of cement injected, the better the outcome. However, the injection of a great amount of cement into the vertebral body appears to predispose to fracture of adjacent vertebrae, which would appear to be more frequent with kyphoplasty than vertebroplasty. The clinical results can be poor in patients with very severe collapse or wedge-shape deformity of the vertebral body and in the presence of a large intravertebral vacuum phenomenon.

References

1. Galibert P, Deramond H, Rosat P, Le Gars D. Preliminary note on the treatment of vertebral angioma by percutaneous acrylic vertebroplasty. Neurochirurgie. 1987;33:166–8.
2. Barr JD, Barr MS, Lemley TJ, McCann RM. Percutaneous vertebroplasty for pain relief and spinal stabilization. Spine. 2000;25:923–8.
3. Deramond H, Depriester C, Toussaint P, Galibert P. Percutaneous vertebroplasty. Semin Musculoskelet Radiol. 1997;1:285–96.

 4. Gangi A, Kasler B, Dietman J-L. Percutaneous vertebroplasty guided by a combination of CT and fluoroscopy. AJNR Am J Neuroradiol. 1994;15:83–6.
 5. Postacchini F, Cinortti G, Di Virgilio R. Vertebroplastica e cifoplastica nelle fratture vertebrali osteoporotiche. Spine News. 2001;10:288–90.
 6. Dean JR, Ison KT, Gishen EM. The strengthening effect of percutaneous vertebroplasty. Clin Radiol. 2000;55:471–6.
 7. Belkoff SM, Mathis JM, Jasper LE, Deramond H. The biomechanics of vertebroplasty. The effect of cement volume on mechanical behavior. Spine. 2001;26:1537–41.
 8. Tomeh AG, Mathis JM, Fenton DC, Levine AM, et al. Biomechanical efficacy of unipedicular versus bipedicular vertebroplasty for the management of osteoporotic compression fractures. Spine. 1999;24:1772–6.
 9. Belkoff SM, Mathis JM, Deramond H, Jasper LE. An ex vivo biomechanical evaluation of a hydroxyapatite cement for use with kyphoplasty. AJNR Am J Neuroradiol. 2001;22:1212–6.
10. Perry A, Mahar A, Massie J, Arrieta N, Garfin S, Kim C. Biomechanical evaluation of kyphoplasty with calcium sulfate cement in a cadaveric osteoporotic vertebral compression fracture model. Spine J. 2005;5:489–93.
11. Kim C, Mahar A, Perry A, Massie J, Lu L, Currier B, Yaszemski MJ. Biomechanical evaluation of an injectable radiopaque polypropylene fumarate cement for kyphoplasty in a cadaveric osteoporotic vertebral compression fracture model. J Spinal Disord Tech. 2007;20:604–9.
12. Liebschner MAK, Rosenberg WS, Keaveny TM. Effect of bone cement volume and distribution on vertebral stiffness after vertebroplasty. Spine. 2001;26:1547–54.
13. Berlemann U, Ferguson SJ, Nolte L-P, Heini PF. Adjacent vertebral failure after vertebroplasty: a biomechanical investigation. J Bone Joint Surg Br. 2002;84B:748–52.
14. Upasani VV, Robertson C, Lee D, Tomlinson T, Mahar AT. Biomechanical comparison of kyphoplasty versus a titanium mesh implant with cement for stabilization of vertebral compression fractures. Spine. 2010;35:1783–8.
15. Rotter R, Martin H, Fuerderer S, Gabl M, et al. Vertebral body stenting: a new method for vertebral augmentation versus kyphoplasty. Eur Spine J. 2010;19:916–23.
16. Wilson DC, Connolly RJ, Zhu Q, Emery JL, Kingwell SP, Kitchel S, Cripton PA, Wilson DR. An ex vivo biomechanical comparison of a novel vertebral compression fracture treatment system to kyphoplasty. Clin Biomech (Bristol, Avon). 2012;27:346–53.
17. Perez-Higueras A, Alvarez L, Rossi RE, Quinones D, et al. Percutaneous vertebroplasty: long-term clinical and radiological out come. Neuroradiology. 2002;44:950–4.
18. Nieuwenhuijse MJ, van Erkel AR, Dijkstra PD. Percutaneous vertebroplasty for subacute and chronic painful osteoporotic vertebral compression fractures can safely be undertaken in the first year after the onset of symptoms. J Bone Joint Surg Br. 2012;94:815–20.
19. Phe WCG, Gilula LA. Percutaneous vertebroplasty: indications contraindications and technique. Br J Radiol. 2003;76:69–75.
20. Heini PF, Teuscher R. Vertebral body stenting/stentoplasty. Swiss Med Wkly. 2012;142:w13658.
21. Bono CM, Kauffmann CP, Garfin SR. Chapter 72. Surgical options and indications: kyphoplasty and vertebroplasty. In: Herkowitz HN, Dvorak J, Bell G, Nordin M, Grob D, editors. The lumbar spine. 3rd ed. Philadelphia: Lippincott Williams & Wilkins; 2004. p. 672–82.
22. Park SY, Modi HN, Suh SW, Hong JY, et al. Epidural cement leakage through pedicle violation after balloon kyphoplasty causing paraparesis in osteoporotic vertebral compression fractures – a report of two cases. J Orthop Surg Res. 2010;5:54.
23. Phillips FM, Wetzel FT, Lieberman I, Campbell-Hupp M. An in vivo comparison of the potential for extravertebral cement leakage after vertebroplasty and kyphoplasty. Spine. 2002;27:2173–9.
24. Hiwatashi A, Westesson PL, Yoshiura T, Noguchi T, et al. Kyphoplasty and vertebroplasty produce the same degree of height restoration. AJNR Am J Neuroradiol. 2009;30:669–73.
25. Ren H, Shen Y, Zhang YZ, Ding WY, et al. Correlative factor analysis on the complications resulting from cement leakage after percutaneous kyphoplasty in the treatment of osteoporotic vertebral compression fracture. J Spinal Disord Tech. 2010;23:e9–15.

26. Zarghooni K, Siewe J, Kaulhausen T, Sobottke R, Eysel P, Röllinghoff M. Complications of vertebroplasty and kyphoplasty in the treatment of vertebral fractures: results of a questionnaire study. Acta Orthop Belg. 2012;78:512–8.
27. Felder-Puig R, Piso B, Guba B, Gartlehner G. Kyphoplasty and vertebroplasty for the management of osteoporotic vertebral compression fractures: a systematic review. Orthopade. 2009;38:606–15.
28. Bula P, Lein T, Strassberger C, Bonnaire F. Balloon kyphoplasty in the treatment of osteoporotic vertebral fractures: indications-treatment strategy-complication. Z Orthop Unfall. 2010;148:646–56.
29. Sietsma MS, Heerspink FO, Ploeg WT, Jutte PC, Veldhuizen AG. Kyphoplasy as treatment for osteoporotic vertebral compression fractures: relatively safe, but still no evidence of functional improvement; a review of the literature. Ned Tijdschr Geneeskd. 2008;152:944–50.
30. Tran I, Gerckens U, Remig J, Zintl G. First report of a life threatening cardiac complication after percutaneous balloon kyphoplasty. Spine. 2012;38:E316–8.
31. Matouk CC, Krings T, Ter Brugge KG, Smith R. Cement embolization of a segmental artery after percutaneous vertebroplasty: a potentially catastrophic vascular complication. Interv Neuroradiol. 2012;18:358–62.
32. Anselmetti GC, Manca A, Hirsch J, Montemurro F, et al. Percutaneous vertebroplasty in osteoporotic patients: an institutional experience of 1,634 patients with long-term follow-up. J Vasc Interv Radiol. 2011;22:1714–20.
33. Papanastassiou ID, Phillips FM, Van Meirhaeghe J, Berenson JR, et al. Comparing effects of kyphoplasty, vertebroplasty, and non-surgical management in a systematic review of randomized and non-randomized controlled studies. Eur Spine J. 2012;21:1826–43.
34. Garfin SR, Reilley MA. Minimally invasive treatment of osteoporotic vertebral body compression fractures. Spine J. 2002;2:76–80.
35. Buchbinder R, Osborne RH, Ebeling PR, Wark JD, et al. A randomized trial of vertebroplasty for painful osteoporotic vertebral fractures. N Engl J Med. 2009;361:557–68.
36. Kallmes DF, Comstock BA, Heagerty PJ, Turner JA, et al. A randomized trial of vertebroplasty for osteoporotic spinal fractures. N Engl J Med. 2009;361:569–79.
37. Boszczyk B. Volume matters: a review of procedural details of two randomised controlled vertebroplasty trials of 2009. Eur Spine J. 2010;19:1837–40.
38. Gangi A, Clark WA. Have recent vertebroplasty trials changed the indications for vertebroplasty? Cardiovasc Intervent Radiol. 2010;33:677–80.
39. Kim KH, Kuh SU, Chin DK, Jin BH, et al. Kyphoplasty versus vertebroplasty: restoration of vertebral body height and correction of kyphotic deformity with special attention to the shape of the fractured vertebrae. J Spinal Disord Tech. 2012;25:338–44.
40. Yan D, Duan L, Li J, Soo C, et al. Comparative study of percutaneous vertebroplasty and kyphoplasty in the treatment of osteoporotic vertebral compression fractures. Arch Orthop Trauma Surg. 2011;13:645–50.
41. Frankel BM, Monroe T, Wang C. Percutaneous vertebral augmentation: an elevation in adjacent-level fracture risk in kyphoplasty as compared with vertebroplasty. Spine J. 2007;7:575–82.
42. Zafeiris CP, Lyritis GP, Papaioannou NA, Gratsias PE, et al. Hypovitaminosis D as a risk factor of subsequent vertebral fractures after kyphoplasty. Spine J. 2012;12:304–12.
43. Rho YJ, Choe WJ, Chun YI. Risk factors predicting the new symptomatic vertebral compression fractures after percutaneous vertebroplasty or kyphoplasty. Eur Spine J. 2012;21:905–11.
44. Bliemel C, Oberkircher L, Buecking B, Timmesfeld N, et al. Higher incidence of new vertebral fractures following percutaneous vertebroplasty and kyphoplasty – fact or fiction? Acta Orthop Belg. 2012;78:220–9.
45. Zou J, Mei X, Zhu X, Shi Q, et al. The long-term incidence of subsequent vertebral body fracture after vertebral augmentation therapy: a systemic review and meta-analysis. Pain Physician. 2012;15:E515–22.
46. Garfin SR, Yuan HA, Reilley MA. Kyphoplasty and vertebroplasty for the treatment of painful osteoporotic compression fractures. Spine. 2001;26:1511–5.

Chapter 13
The Sacroiliac Joint: A Minimally Invasive Approach

Bengt Sturesson

Introduction

In antiquity, the Greek physician Hippocrates discussed the function of the sacroiliac joint (SIJ). On the basis of his study of animals, he concluded that the SIJ was normally immobile but that some mobility was possible during pregnancy [1]. In the early twentieth century, the SIJs were believed to be the main source of low-back pain [2–9]. However, this belief went out of fashion during the 1930s when interest became focused on the intervertebral disc, after the herniated disc was demonstrated to be a source of sciatic pain [10]. In the 1950s, Weisl [11, 12] and Solonen [13], using different approaches, shed new light on the knowledge concerning the SIJs. Weisl demonstrated movement of the SIJ; Solonen [13] made an anatomical and biomechanical analysis of the SIJ and also described its innervation.

Currently, in the fields of manual medicine, physiotherapy, and chiropractic, the consideration of SIJ dysfunction plays a fundamental role in diagnostics and treatment. Various clinical tests that evaluate position, movement, tenderness, and pain provocation are regarded as essential for diagnosis. The terminology used to discuss the SIJ includes such terms as *locking* and *hypo-* and *hypermobility*.

In the debate on the role of the SIJs as a source of back pain, the crucial questions to be answered are: Do the SIJs move? How can a sacroiliac disorder be diagnosed? If SIJ dysfunction is diagnosed, what treatment can be recommended?

B. Sturesson, MD
Department of Orthopedics, Ängelholm County Hospital, Ängelholm, Sweden
e-mail: sturesson.bengt@gmail.com

P.P.M. Menchetti (ed.), *Minimally Invasive Surgery of the Lumbar Spine*,
DOI 10.1007/978-1-4471-5280-4_13, © Springer-Verlag London 2014

Background and Etiology

Development of the Sacroiliac Joint

The cartilage that lines the sacral and iliac joint surfaces develops from the pelvic mesenchyme around the eighth intrauterine week. At that time, a layer of mesenchymal cells forms cavities from which the SIJs develop [14]. In the eighth month, the SIJs are fully developed and differences can be seen between the smooth, white, and shining cartilage of the sacrum and the dull, gray, and irregular cartilage of the iliac side [15].

During the first decade of life, the articular surfaces of the SIJ are flat and even. In the second decade, congruent irregularities develop on both the iliac and sacral articular surfaces [15, 16]. In the third decade, running centrally along the entire length of the iliac surface is a convex ridge, which fits into a corresponding sacral groove [15]. The elevations on the iliac side become about 10 mm high in the fourth decade of life. Contemporaneously, sacral margin osteophytes appear and the joint surface becomes more "yellowish and roughened" [15]. Symmetry between the right and left SIJ is now an exception rather than a rule [13–15].

Over the age of 50, osteophytes are more frequent and ankylosis occurs. Brooke [5] found that 77 % of all men over the age of 53 had an ankylosis. However, Stewart [17] found that only 3 of 308 cases had ankylosis, Vleeming [18] found ankylosis in 2 of 13 men, and Resnick [19] in 4 of 46 specimens.

Biomechanics

The function of the SIJ is to transfer the force of the upper part of the body through the pelvis to the legs [20]. It has also a shock-absorptive function in walking, running, and jumping with a reciprocal movement in the SIJ [21]. The location and the vertical position of the SIJ make it vulnerable to extensive loading by daily activities [22]. Solonen [13] used a purely mathematical model where the SIJ angle in the frontal plane was the essential factor determining the load over the SIJ. He estimated that with an angle of 10° in the frontal plane, the load over each SIJ in standing and slow walking was three times the weight of the upper body. This load increases to four times the weight of the upper body in rapid walking.

The movement of the SIJs is small and varies between individuals and according to the load applied [12, 21, 23–25]. Different techniques for analyzing sacroiliac movement in living persons have been used. Radiostereometric analysis (RSA) is currently the most exact procedure. This technique is widely used to measure small movement in orthopedic research [26, 27] and is used independently by different groups measuring SIJ movements [21, 23, 24, 27–29]. Tantalum markers with a diameter of 0.8 mm are implanted into the pelvic bones. At least three, but usually four to six markers are placed geometrically well spread into each ilium and into the sacrum. In various studies, Sturesson et al. [21, 23, 24] demonstrated that the sacrum is rotated forwards (nutation) when patients change from a supine position to a sitting or standing position. Between the supine and standing positions the average nutation is 1.2°, and 90 % of the movement is located around the x-axis [23]. Sturesson also demonstrated that movements do not differ between symptomatic and asymptomatic joints. Also, SIJ movements were reduced when standing on one leg with the other leg flexed, as additional muscle force was applied to the joint. The largest movement, averaging 2°, occurred when changing from standing to lying prone with forced hyperextension of a leg. SIJ mobility in men is on average 30–40 % less than in women [23].

In another study, an external Hoffman Slätis frame was used and a slight compression applied. The movement in the SIJ that occurred from lying supine to standing was reduced by half, on average 0.6°; there was also a reduction in pain [30]. This finding is in agreement with studies that use pelvic belts to normalize SIJ movement [31–33]. In a mathematical model, Snijders et al. [34] showed that the muscle force needed at the anterior iliac spine to stabilize the SIJ is relatively low. The SIJ can effectively be stabilized with the low force exerted by the oblique and transverse muscles at the anterior pelvis, combined with a long lever from the SIJ to the anterior iliac spine. Tullberg et al. [29] studied the effect of successful manipulation of the SIJ. The patients ($n = 10$) were examined both clinically and with RSA, before and after manipulation. Manipulation did not alter the position of the sacrum in relation to the ilium. The result seems to indicate that effective manipulation is not dependent on positional change of the joints [35].

The theory of form and force closure [16, 18, 35–37] is a biomechanical model that takes the friction in the SIJ as well as the muscle forces exerted on the SIJ into consideration [38]. The shear forces applied on the SIJ in the standing position would create creep if friction did not exist in the SIJ. The theory assumes that to stabilize the SIJ, it is necessary that the forces of the trunk, pelvis, and leg muscles be effectively coupled.

Form closure refers to a stable situation with closely fitting joint surfaces, where no extra forces are needed to maintain the state of the joints, irrespective of the load situation. If the sacrum fits perfectly between the iliac bones, no additional forces are needed to maintain the position. However, in this situation mobility is almost impossible (Fig. 13.1).

Force closure is described as the opposite situation: a bilateral force exerted on the iliac bones is needed to keep the sacrum in place (Fig. 13.1). The force needed is to increase friction between the elements so no movement occurs. Force closure can be exerted by muscle forces [34, 38–41] or by a pelvic belt [39] or an external fixator [30].

In reality, a combination of the irregularities in the SIJs, the wedge shape of the SIJ (form), and the compression forces generated by muscles and ligaments (force) stabilize the joint in the loaded situation. This combination of form and force closure, preventing shear forces, is also called the self-locking mechanism (Fig. 13.1).

The strong ligaments around the SIJ cannot alone effect the stability of the SIJ. However, according to the theory of form and force closure, a dynamic stabilization of the pelvis is necessary. It is proposed that the posterior muscles, such as the

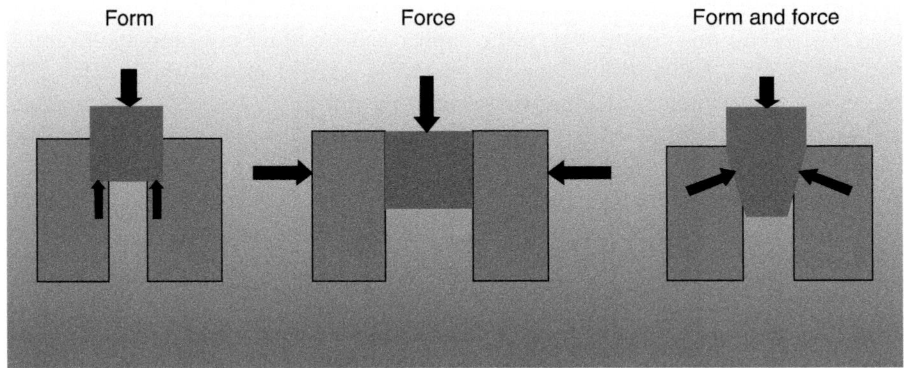

Fig. 13.1 Model of form and force closure (Adapted after Vleeming et al. [16])

latissimus dorsi, erector spinae, gluteus maximus, and biceps femoris muscles, together with the anterior transverse and oblique muscles generate forces that are effective in compressing the SIJ and inducing friction [42].

Various electromyography (EMG) studies [34, 38–41] indicate that the transverse and oblique abdominal muscles take part in the stabilization of the pelvis and the SIJ. In the biomechanical model, Snijders et al. [38] proposed that the transverse and oblique muscles, together with stiff dorsal sacroiliac ligaments, exert a stabilizing effect with gentle contraction on the iliac wing. A comparison of EMG activity in the transverse and oblique muscles with and without a pelvic belt in ten healthy volunteers showed that the muscle activity was significantly lower with a belt. In another study, the same research group examined the differences in EMG recordings of the same muscle groups between sitting on an office chair with and without crossed legs [34]. The results show that sitting with crossed legs leads to a significant decrease in the EMG activity in the muscles studied, indicating that sitting with crossed legs provides a stabilized situation in the SIJ. Hodges and Richardson [40] showed that the transverse abdominal muscles are activated in advance by reflexes in the central nervous system prior to limb movement in either the upper or of lower extremities. Moreover, they showed that this function is disturbed in patients with chronic low-back pain [39, 41]. This supports the position that these individuals are unable to stabilize the pelvis and thus need treatment.

Etiology

The SIJ undergoes degenerative changes from the third decade [15]. Why some individuals experience pain from degeneration is poorly understood. The same situation exists with all joints and is well studied in knee arthritis [43, 44]. Sacroiliac pain during pregnancy is well described [45–48], and some women develop chronic sacroiliac pain [49]. The incidence of different etiologies is not fully described. The combination of cartilage degeneration, lack of stability, and pain sensitization exists with all different causes of sacroiliac pain.

- Degeneration of the SIJ, *degenerative sacroiliitis,* occurs as earlier described. It is possible that movement increases with age [23] and together with reduced ability of stabilization, pain occurs.
- Posttraumatic degenerative sacroiliitis can occur after a disruption to the SIJ after a low-energy fall, a direct high-energy hit, a compression of the pelvis from side to side, or an extreme rotation of the joint without visible fracture. The mechanism behind this is probably that either the cartilage or the strong sacroiliac ligaments are injured. The pain can start immediately or slowly increase after the trauma.
- Posttraumatic sacroiliitis also occurs after pelvic fractures where the SIJ is clearly torn but no posttraumatic fusion in the SIJ occurs. The most usual case is the open book fracture, but posttraumatic pseudarthrosis can also occur after more severe pelvic fractures.
- Persistent sacroiliac pain after pregnancy – pelvic girdle pain (PGP) – occurs after about 0.1 % of all pregnancies. During pregnancy, around 25 % of women experience PGP with different severity. Most women recover during the first week after delivery, but in some cases the recovery can take up to 18 months. After that, about 0.1 % continue to experience severe pain and disability.
- Inflammation of the SIJ: Ankylosing spondylitis can be seen with sacroiliitis many years before factors are visible in blood tests. Sacroiliitis can occur together with psoriasis and inflammatory bowel disease and can also be seen in reactive arthritis after infection (Reiter's syndrome).
- Acute bacterial infection can occur in the SIJ.
- Congenital abnormalities with variations in the lumbosacral transition are not unusual. For example, an enlarged transverse process from L5 can articulate in the SIJ. The differences in the movement pattern in the SIJ and in the lumbosacral disk increase the chances of local degeneration

Presentation, Diagnosis, and Treatment Options

Diagnosis

Several clinical diagnostic SIJ tests were reviewed in the European Guidelines for Pelvic Girdle Pain [50]. The authors reviewed a wide variety of examinations, procedures, and tests that have been used to investigate pregnant and nonpregnant patients. It has been stated that position or movement tests have no diagnostic value, and that the widely used standing hip flexion test (Gillet test or "rücklauf") [51] is an illusion [24].

In the studies where the examination procedures of pregnant women are described, a combination of methods for diagnosis has been used: inspection of walking, posture and pelvic tilt, palpation of ligaments and muscles, tests for a locked SIJ, and pain provocation tests for the SIJ and the symphysis. The early studies focused more on the inspection and palpatoric findings, whereas the later studies have focused more on pain provocation tests, probably due to the higher reliability and specificity of these latter tests. The pain provocation tests with the highest reliability and most frequently used for SIJ pain are the P4/thigh thrust test and Patrick's FABER (*f*lexion, *ab*duction, and *e*xternal *r*otation) test. For pain in the symphysis, these tests include palpation of the symphysis, and the modified Trendelenburg test is used as a pain provocation test [50].

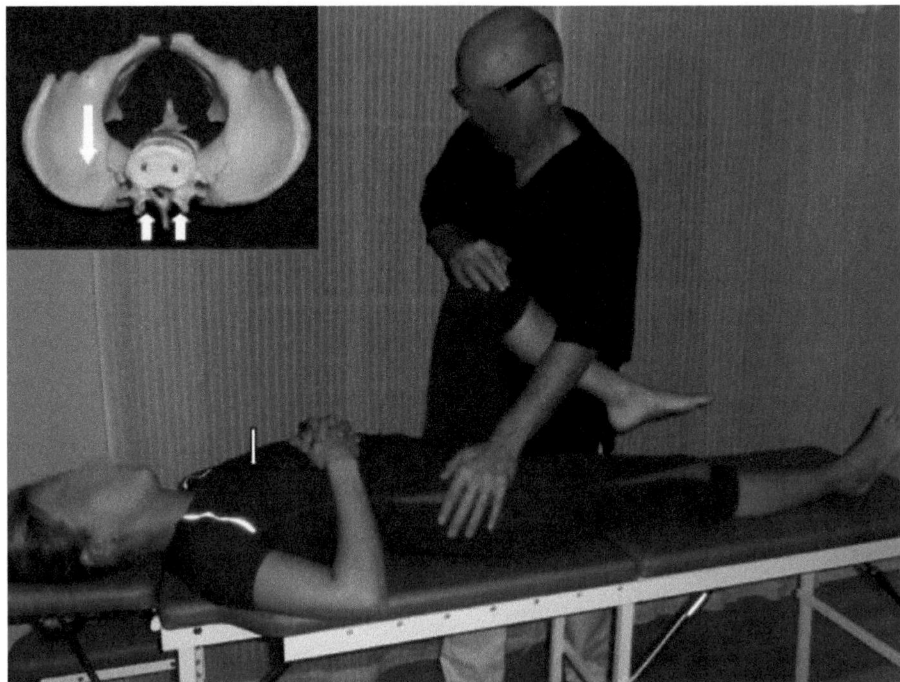

Fig. 13.2 Posterior pelvic pain provocation test (P4/thigh thrust test)

The recommendations from the European guidelines for clinical examination tests of PGP are as follows.

For SIJ pain:

- Posterior pelvic pain provocation test (P4/thigh thrust test) [52] (Fig. 13.2)
- Patrick's FABER test (Fig. 13.3)
- Palpation of the long dorsal SIJ ligament [53]
- Gaenslen's test [54] (Fig. 13.4)

For symphysis pain:

- Palpation of the symphysis
- Modified Trendelenburg function test of the pelvic girdle

Functional pelvic test

- Active straight leg raise test (ASLR) [40] (Fig. 13.5).

Functional pain history

- It is strongly recommended that a pain history be taken with special attention paid to pain arising during prolonged standing, walking, and/or sitting. To ensure that the pain is in the pelvic girdle area, it is important that the precise area of pain be indicated: the patient should either point out the exact location on his/her body, or preferably shade-in the painful area on a pain location diagram [50].

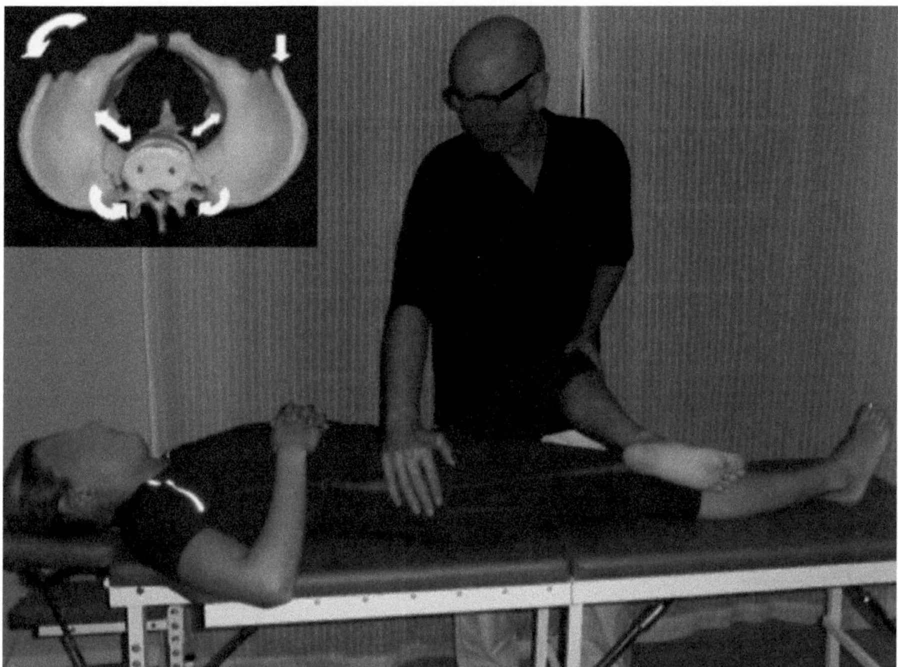

Fig. 13.3 Patrick's FABER test

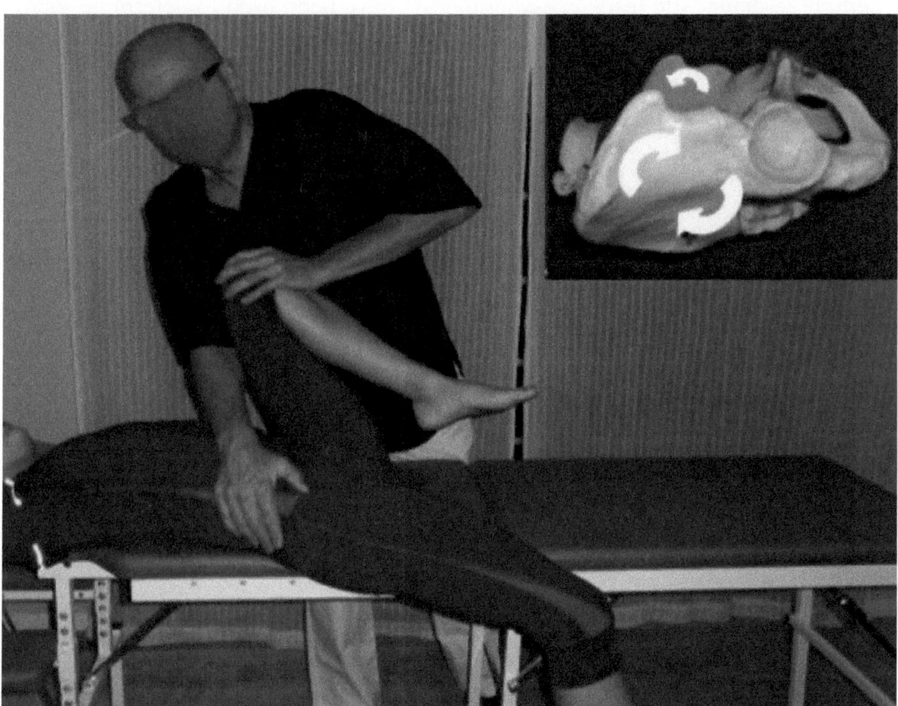

Fig. 13.4 Gaenslen's test

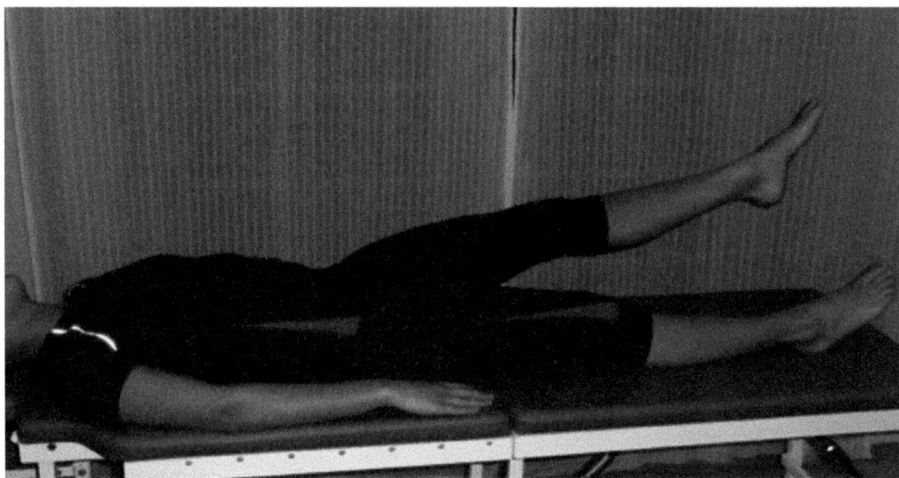

Fig. 13.5 Active straight leg raise test (ASLR)

Diagnostic Blocks

A sacroiliac intraarticular block has been proposed as the gold standard in diagnosing SIJ pain [55, 56]. This has also been proven in a double-blind trial where three diagnostic tests assessing the SIJ have been used to determine sacroiliac pathology [57]. A recent clinical review of SIJ interventions concluded that the evidence for the diagnostic accuracy of SIJ injections is good [58].

Physical Treatment

Different physical exercise programs have been proposed for sacroiliac pain, but the level of evidence is low. In the European guidelines [50] the recommendation is to use an individualized training program with specific stabilizing exercises as a part of a multimodal treatment program [59, 60]. The exercise program is recommended to start with activation and control of local deep lumbopelvic muscles. Gradually, the program can be enlarged to include the training of more superficial muscles in dynamic exercises to improve control mobility, strength, and endurance capacity. A pelvic belt can be fitted to test for symptomatic relief. The risk of using a pelvic belt for a longer period is subcutaneous fat hypotrophy. There is no evidence for the effect of manipulation or mobilization. Water gymnastics, acupuncture, and massage might be helpful as part of a multidisciplinary individualized treatment.

Surgical Techniques

Surgical Treatment

Surgical treatment for the SIJ was described early in the last century [54, 61]. In all reports of sacroiliac fusion, the preoperative evaluation was thorough and surgery was performed only on patients for whom nonoperative treatment had been unsuccessful [54, 61–74]. The studies include from 2 to 78 patients and the results were assessed by the authors as fair to excellent in 48–89 % of the patients. In a case report by Berthelot et al. [67], two patients who underwent surgery experienced total pain relief. Different techniques are described, but the transiliac technique described by Smith-Petersen and Rogers [61] with some modifications was the most widely used. The different surgical techniques are demanding for both surgeon and patient and the pseudarthrosis rate is around 10 %. The perioperative bleeding can be quite considerable, as the surgical access is through the cancellous bone in the posterior iliac wing. The hospital stay is long (5–7 days) and the rehabilitation is demanding for the patient.

Minimally Invasive Techniques

Following the development of minimally invasive surgery in the lumbar spine, several new techniques for sacroiliac fusion have been proposed. Transiliac screw fixation without fusion has been used, but no clinical studies are reported for degenerative sacroiliac disorders. Different new procedures with minimally invasive fusion techniques are proposed [75–78] but still no evidence for surgical treatment exists. A minimally invasive technique that fits well with the theory of form and force closure is the iFuse® implant system from SI-BONE [78]. However, before any surgical technique is offered, at least 6 months of physical exercise that follows an individualized and specifically tailored exercise program should be prescribed.

The iFuse® Technique

The iFuse® technique is an easy procedure, but it presupposes good knowledge of the iliosacral anatomy. Necessary imaging before surgery consists of either an MRI of a CT scan of the pelvis. If a sacral MRI does not reveal any abnormalities in the lumbosacral transition, no additional imaging is needed preoperatively. The main reason for the MRI examination is to rule out red flags prior to any surgery. However, if a sacral anomaly is shown on the MRI examination, a CT is recommended.

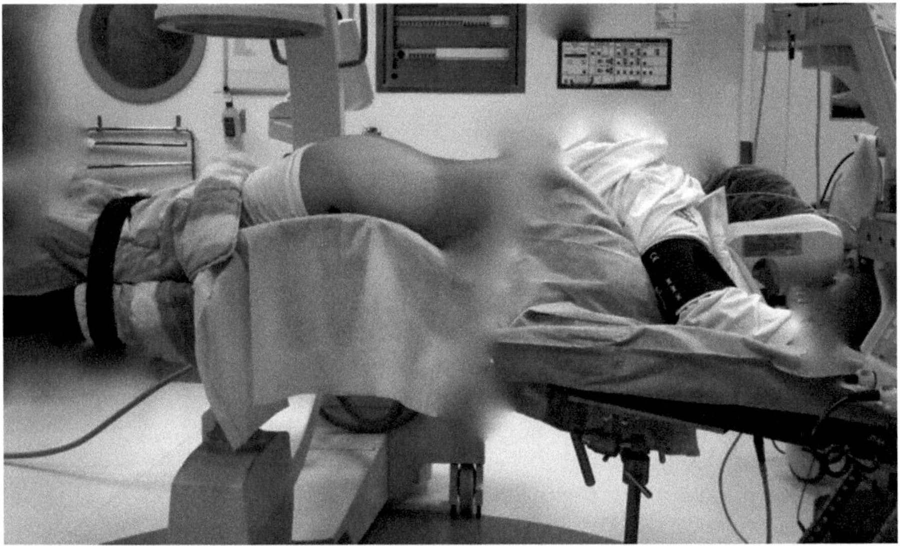

Fig. 13.6 C-arm that can be moved to obtain optimal images of patient on table

Patient Positioning

The patient is placed on a Jackson table or a flat table allowing a C-arm to be freely moved to obtain optimal images in lateral, inlet, and outlet views (Fig. 13.6). These positions are necessary to get an optimal result and reduce the risk of surgical complications. Three implants are recommended to achieve enough contact between bone and implants. The iFuse® implant is a titanium plasma-coated triangular rod with the similar coating used for joint implants with noncemented techniques.

The first implant is directed to the first sacral body. The technique used is similar to implanting an iliosacral screw. The main surgical risk is of injury to the L5 nerve, though care must be taken to avoid injuring all neural structures and vessels in and around sacrum. The L5 nerve is located anterior to the sacral ala. If the sacral ala is well visible with the C-arm, a skin mark for the incision can be made (Fig. 13.7). A 3-cm incision is made 1 cm caudal to the ala line along the sacral line down to the fascia.

Pin

A 3 mm Steinmann pin is introduced just anterior to the sacral line and 1 cm caudal to the ala line in the lateral view of the fluoroscopy. The Steinmann pin is advanced with care, taking the pin position in the outlet and inlet view into consideration. The tip of the pin has to be advanced to the position below the sacral ala and superior to the first foramen, and just in the middle of the sacrum in the lateral view (Fig. 13.8).

Fig. 13.7 Skin mark for incision caudal to the ala line

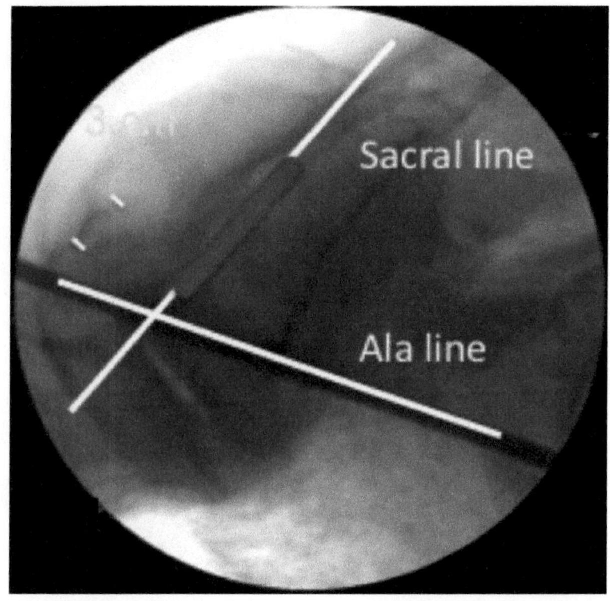

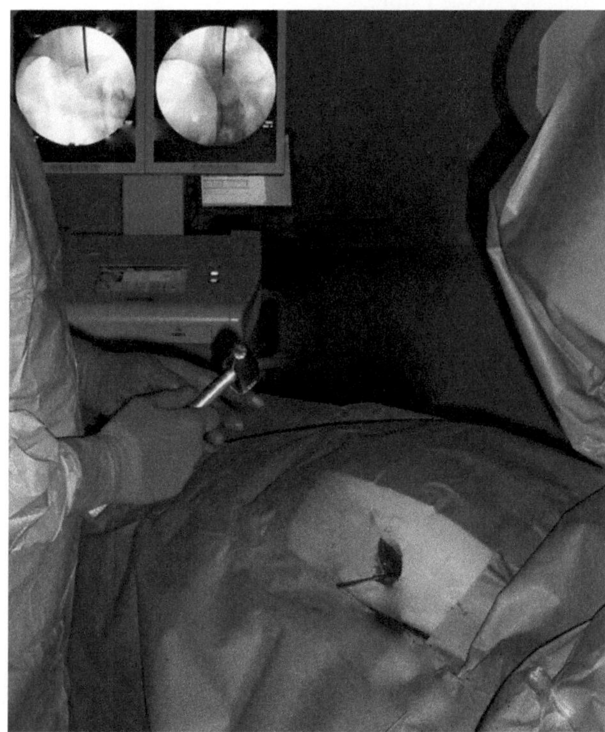

Fig. 13.8 Introduction of Steinmann pin

Fig. 13.9 Drill penetrating
the ilium and SIJ

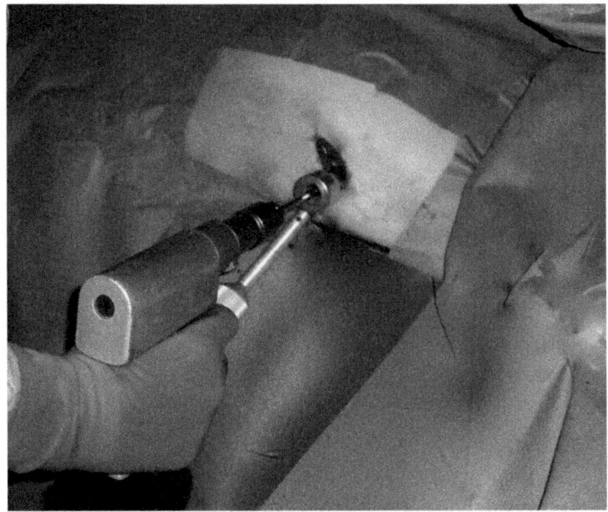

The first implant located in the S1 area should be as long as is practical so it will
have as much contact with sacral bone as possible. This is important for bone fusion
to the implant. The length of the first implant also has to be selected so it will be
possible to introduce a posterior lumbosacral screw if lumbar spine surgery becomes
necessary in the future.

Drill

The pin sleeve is removed and a cannulated drill is introduced over the Steinmann
pin. The drill is advanced through the iliac bone and the SIJ. The sacral bone, being
softer than the SIJ, does not need to be drilled (Fig. 13.9).

Broach

The drill sleeve is removed and a triangular broach is introduced, one flat side of its
profile being parallel to the sacral ala line. The broach has to be tapped deep enough
that the last teeth pass the SIJ (Fig. 13.10).

Implant

The broach is removed and an in appropriate length implant is introduced
(Fig. 13.11). The position and depth is checked in all three views (lateral, inlet,

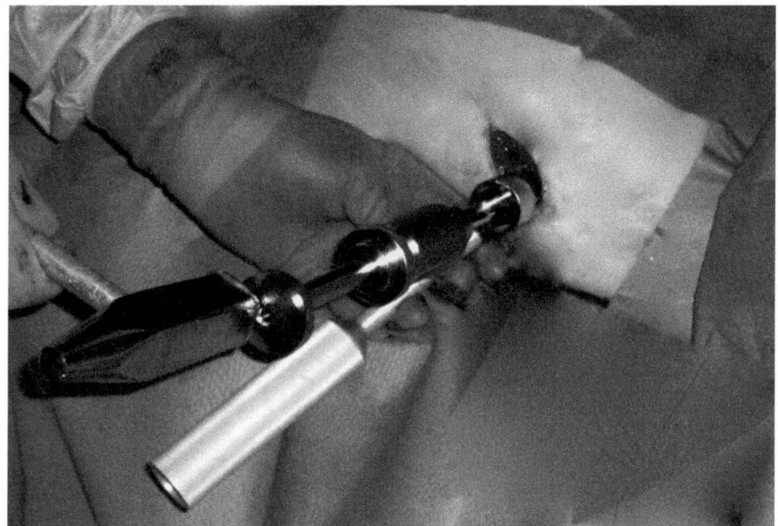

Fig. 13.10 Tapping the broach

Fig. 13.11 Introduction of implant

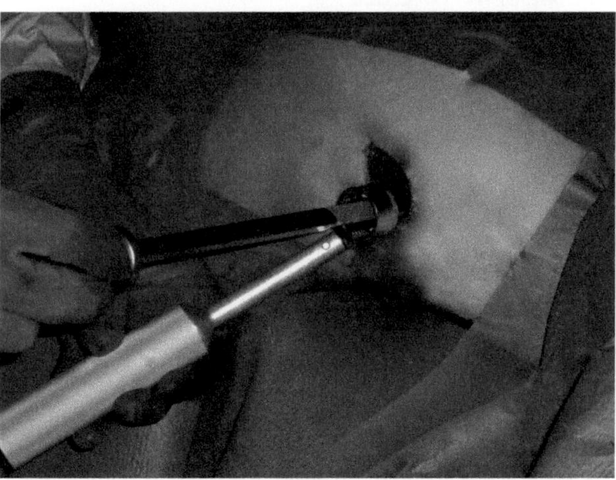

outlet). The tip of the implant lateral to the iliac wall has to be 2–5 mm proud. This is easiest done with a finger in the wound, feeling the lateral end of the implant. After that the second and third implants are introduced with the same procedure, taking care of the anatomy. It is recommended that the implants be more or less parallel to each other. This is easily achieved with the help of the parallel guide. It is also recommended that the second implant be placed somewhat more anterior in the lateral view than the first, and that bridge the cartilaginous joint rather than the ligamentous part of the SIJ.

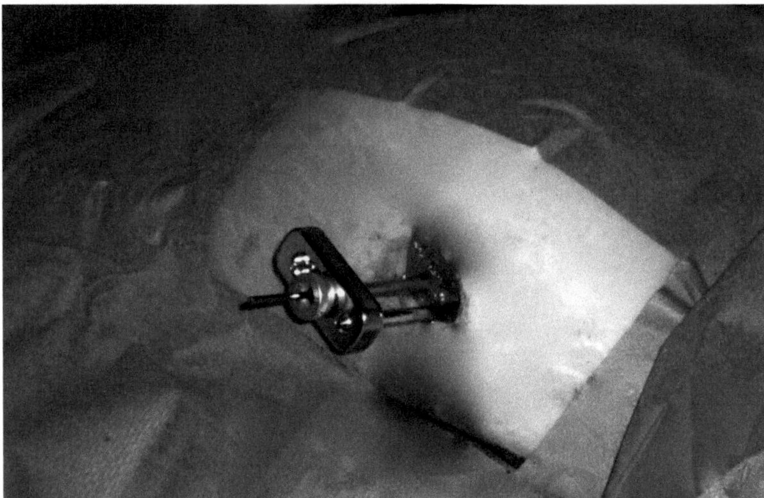

Fig. 13.12 Introduction of second implant after device positioning, in order to obtain a parallel positioning

Postoperative Care

Partial weight bearing with crutches and with the affected side bearing only half the body weight is immediately allowed and is recommended for 3–6 weeks. Postoperative low-dose computer tomography is recommended for monitoring the implant positioning. The healing period is the same as with fusion healing, which is roughly 5 months. During this period, the patient should not undertake heavy physical work. The follow-up is mainly clinical, checking pain and function. The ASLR test is recommended as a functional test during the healing period. At a 5-month follow-up, clinical diagnostic tests can be used to assess the outcome. If the patient is still in pain at the 5-month follow-up, a plain outlet view X-ray and/or a CT is recommended to look for radiolucent zones.

Complications

So far, neither infection nor implant breakage has been reported. Revisions have been performed because of malpositioning of the implant in about 1 % of cases and because of healing disturbances in about 1 %. Compared with the 10 % pseudarthrosis rate reported from the open procedures, the iFuse® complication rate is low. No serious nerve or vascular damage has been reported.

Conclusions and Personal View

The author has more than 25 years of experience with patients with pain that originates from the SIJs. Around 50 patients have undergone surgery with a modified Smith-Peterson technique, with about 80 % good or excellent results [73]. In most cases, an external fixator was used as a postoperative stabilizer. However, this technique was demanding for both patient and surgeon, and the soft tissue exploration persistently resulted in a reduced muscle condition in the greater gluteal muscle, even in patients with optimal bone healing. The minimally invasive technique with iFuse® offers the patient a procedure that results in minimal harm to the muscles and soft tissues, a short hospital stay, and a relatively fast recovery. For the surgeon, this technique is easy to learn and less demanding than any open technique. The personal impression after the performance of about 50 iFuse® procedures is that the patient outcome is more than 90 % excellent. Nonetheless, differentiating the SIJ as the pain source in patients with low or lowest lumbar pain is challenging. As with many therapeutic procedures, the technique is still not evidence based. Scientific reports of the outcomes of this method have begun to appear [78–80], and longitudinal studies as well as randomized controlled studies are in progress.

References

1. Lynch FW. The pelvic articulations during pregnancy, labor, and the puerperium: an x-ray study. Surg Gynecol Obstet. 1920;30:575–80.
2. Goldthwait JE, Osgood RB. A consideration of the pelvic articulations from an anatomical, pathological and clinical standpoint. Boston Med Surg J. 1905;152(21):593–601.
3. Albee FH. A study of the anatomy and the clinical importance of the sacroiliac joint. JAMA. 1909;53(16):1273–6.
4. Smith-Petersen MN. Clinical diagnosis of common sacroiliac conditions. Am J Roentgenol Radium Ther. 1924;12:546–50.
5. Brooke R. The sacro-iliac joint. J Anat. 1924;58:299–305.
6. Yeoman W. The relation of arthritis of the sacro-iliac joint to sciatica with an analysis of 100 cases. Lancet. 1928;212(5492):1119–22.
7. Chamberlain WE. The symphysis pubis in the roentgen examination of the sacroiliac joint. Am J Roentgenol Radium Ther. 1930;24(6):621–5.
8. Sashin D. A critical analysis of the anatomy and the pathologic changes of the sacro-iliac joints. J Bone Joint Surg Am. 1930;12(4):891–910.
9. Cyriax E. Minor displacements of the sacro-iliac joints. Br J Phys Med. 1934;8:191–3.
10. Mixter WJ, Barr JS. Rupture of the intervertebral disc with involvement of the spinal canal. N Engl J Med. 1934;211(5):210–5.
11. Weisl H. The ligaments of the sacro-iliac joint examined with particular reference to their function. Acta Anat (Basel). 1954;20(3):201–13.
12. Weisl H. The movements of the sacro-iliac joint. Acta Anat (Basel). 1955;23(1):80–91.

13. Solonen KA. The sacroiliac joint in the light of anatomical, roentgenological and clinical studies. Acta Orthop Scand Suppl. 1957;27:1–127.
14. Schunke GB. The anatomy and development of the sacro-iliac joint in man. Anat Rec. 1938;72(3):313–31.
15. Bowen V, Cassidy JD. Macroscopic and microscopic anatomy of the sacroiliac joint from embryonic life until the eighth decade. Spine. 1981;6(6):620–8.
16. Vleeming A, Stoeckart R, Volkers ACW, Snijders CJ. Relation between form and function in the sacroiliac joint. Part I: clinical anatomical aspects. Spine. 1990;15(2):130–2.
17. Stewart TD. Pathologic changes in aging sacroiliac joints: a study of dissecting-room skeletons. Clin Orthop Relat Res. 1984;183:188–96.
18. Vleeming A. The sacro-iliac joint; an anatomical, biomechanical and radiological approach. Thesis. Erasmus University Rotterdam; 1990.
19. Resnick D, Niwayama G, Goergen TG. Degenerative disease of the sacroiliac joint. Invest Radiol. 1975;10(6):608–21.
20. Lovejoy CO. Evolution of human walking. Sci Am. 1988;259(5):118–25.
21. Sturesson B, Uden A, Vleeming A. A radiostereometric analysis of the movements of the sacroiliac joints in the reciprocal straddle position. Spine. 2000;25(2):214–7.
22. Snijders CJ, Vleeming A, Stoeckart, Kleinrensink GJ, Mens JMA. Biomechanics of sacroiliac joint stability: validation experiments on the concept of self-locking. In: Vleeming A, Mooney V, Dorman T, Snijders C, editors. Proceedings of the second interdisciplinary world congress on low back pain: the integrated function of the lumbar spine and sacroiliac joint. San Diego; 1995. p. 77–91.
23. Sturesson B, Selvik G, Udén A. Movements of the sacroiliac joints. A roentgen stereophotogrammetric analysis. Spine. 1989;14(2):162–5.
24. Sturesson B, Udén A, Vleeming A. A radiostereometric analysis of movements of the sacroiliac joints during the standing hip flexion test. Spine. 2000;25(3):364–8.
25. Jacob HAC, Kissling RO. The mobility of the sacroiliac joints in healthy volunteers between 20 and 50 years of age. Clin Biomech (Bristol, Avon). 1995;10(7):352–61.
26. Selvik G. Roentgen stereophotogrammetry: a method for the study of the kinematics of the skeletal system. Acta Orthop Scand Suppl. 1989;232:1–51.
27. Selvik G. Roentgen stereophotogrammetric analysis. Acta Radiol. 1990;31(2):113–26.
28. Egund N, Olsson TH, Schmid H, Selvik G. Movements in the sacroiliac joints demonstrated with roentgen stereophotogrammetry. Acta Radiol Diagn (Stockh). 1978;19(5):833–46.
29. Tullberg T, Blomberg S, Branth B, Johnsson R. Manipulation does not alter the position of the sacroiliac joint. A roentgen stereophotogrammetric analysis. Spine. 1998;23(10):1124–8.
30. Sturesson B, Udén A, Önsten I. Can an external frame fixation reduce the movements in the sacroiliac joint? A radiostereometric analysis of 10 patients. Acta Orthop Scand. 1999;70(1):42–6.
31. Vleeming A, Buyruk M, Stoeckart R, Karamursel S, Snijders CJ. An integrated therapy for peripartum pelvic instability: a study of the biomechanical effects of pelvic belts. Am J Obstet Gynecol. 1992;166(4):1243–7.
32. Mens JM, Vleeming A, Snijders CJ, Stam HJ, Ginai AZ. The active straight leg raising test and mobility of the pelvic joints. Eur Spine J. 1999;8(6):468–73.
33. Mens JM, Damen L, Snijders CJ, Stam HJ. The mechanical effect of a pelvic belt in patients with pregnancy-related pelvic pain. Clin Biomech (Bristol, Avon). 2006;21(2):122–7.
34. Snijders CJ, Slagter AHE, van Strik R, Vleeming A, Stam HJ, Stoeckart R. Why leg-crossing? The influence on common postures on abdominal muscle activity. Spine. 1995;20(18):1989–93.
35. Snijders CJ, Vleeming A, Stoeckart R. Transfer of lumbosacral load to iliac bones and legs. Part 2: loading of the sacroiliac joints when lifting a stooped posture. Clin Biomech. 1993;8:295–301.
36. Vleeming A, Volkers ACW, Snijders CJ, Stoeckart R. Relation between form and function in the sacroiliac joint. Part II: biomechanical aspects. Spine. 1990;15(2):133–6.

37. Snijders CJ, Vleeming A, Stoeckart R. Transfer of lumbosacral load to iliac bones and legs. Part 1: biomechanics of self-bracing of the sacroiliac joints and its significance for treatment and exercise. Clin Biomech. 1993;8:285–94.
38. Snijders CJ, Ribbers MT, de Bakker HV, Stoeckart R, Stam HJ. EMG recordings of abdominal and back muscles in various standing postures; validation of a biomechanical model on sacroiliac joint stability. J Electromyogr Kinesiol. 1998;8:205–14.
39. Hodges PW, Richardson CA. Inefficient muscular stabilization of the lumbar spine associated with low back pain: a motor control evaluation of transversus abdominis. Spine. 1996; 21(22):2640–50.
40. Hodges PW, Richardson CA. Feedforward contraction of transversus abdominis is not influenced by the direction of arm movement. Exp Brain Res. 1997;114(2):362–70.
41. Hodges PW, Richardson CA. Delayed postural contraction of transversus abdominis in low back pain associated with movement of the lower limb. J Spinal Disord. 1998;11(1):46–56.
42. Vleeming A, Snijders CJ, Stoeckart R, Mens JMA. A new light on low back pain. In: Vleeming A, Mooney V, Dorman T, Snijders C, editors. Proceedings of the second interdisciplinary world congress on low back pain: the integrated function of the lumbar spine and sacroiliac joint. San Diego; 1995. p. 147–68.
43. Dieppe P, Cushnaghan J, Tucker M, Browning S, Shepstone L. The Bristol 'OA500 study': progression and impact of the disease after 8 years. Osteoarthritis Cartilage. 2000;8(2):63–8.
44. Paradowski PT, Englund M, Roos EM, Lohmander LS. Similar group mean scores, but large individual variations, in patient-relevant outcomes over 2 years in meniscectomized subjects with and without radiographic knee osteoarthritis. Health Qual Life Outcomes. 2004;2:38.
45. Östgaard HC, Andersson GBJ, Karlsson K. Prevalence of back pain in pregnancy. Spine. 1991;16(5):549–52.
46. Östgaard HC, Andersson GBJ, Schultz AB, Miller JAA. Influence of some biomechanical factors on low-back pain in pregnancy. Spine. 1993;18(1):61–5.
47. Mantle MJ, Greenwood RM, Currey HL. Backache in pregnancy. Rheumatol Rehabil. 1977;16(2):95–101.
48. Sturesson B, Udén G, Udén A. Pain pattern in pregnancy and "catching" of the leg in pregnant women with posterior pelvic pain. Spine. 1997;22(16):1880–3; discussion 1884.
49. Albert H, Godskesen M, Westergaard J. Prognosis in four syndromes of pregnancy-related pelvic pain. Acta Obstet Gynecol Scand. 2001;80(6):505–10.
50. Vleeming A, Albert HB, Östgaard HC, Sturesson B, Stuge B. European guidelines for the diagnosis and treatment of pelvic girdle pain. Eur Spine J. 2008;17(6):794–819.
51. Kirkaldy-Willis WH, Hill RJ. A more precise diagnosis for low-back pain. Spine. 1979;4(2):102–9.
52. Östgaard HC, Zetherström G, Roos-Hansson E. The posterior pelvic pain provocation test in pregnant women. Eur Spine J. 1994;3(5):258–60.
53. Vleeming A, Pool-Goudzwaard AL, Annelies L, Hammudoghlu D, Stoeckart R, Snijders CJ. The function of the long dorsal sacroiliac ligament: its implication for understanding low back pain. Spine. 1996;21(5):556–62.
54. Gaenslen FJ. Sacro-iliac arthrodesis: indications, author's technic and end-results. JAMA. 1927;89(24):2031–5.
55. Maigne JY, Aivaliklis A, Pfefer F. Results of sacroiliac joint double block and value of sacroiliac pain provocation tests in 54 patients with low back pain. Spine. 1996;21(16):1889–92.
56. Maigne JY, Planchon CA. Sacroiliac joint pain after lumbar fusion: a study with anesthetic blocks. Eur Spine J. 2005;14(7):654–8.
57. Broadhurst NA, Bond MJ. Pain provocation tests for the assessment of sacroiliac joint dysfunction. J Spinal Disord. 1998;11(4):341–5.
58. Simopoulos TT, Manchikanti L, Singh V, Gupta S, Hameed H, Diwan S, Cohen SP. A systematic evaluation of prevalence and diagnostic accuracy of sacroiliac joint interventions. Pain Physician. 2012;15(3):E305–44.

59. Stuge B, Lærum E, Kirkesola G, Vøllestad N. The efficacy of a treatment program focusing on specific stabilizing exercises for pelvic girdle pain after pregnancy. A randomized controlled trial. Spine. 2004;29(4):351–9.

60. Stuge B, Veierød MB, Lærum E, Vøllestad N. The efficacy of a treatment program focusing on specific stabilizing exercises for pelvic girdle pain after pregnancy. A two-year follow-up of a randomized clinical trial. Spine. 2004;29(10):E197–203.

61. Smith-Petersen MN, Rogers WA. End-result study of arthrodesis of the sacro-iliac joint for artritis – traumatic and non-traumatic. J Bone Joint Surg Am. 1926;8(1):118–36.

62. Olerud S, Walheim GG. Symphysiodesis with a new compression plate. Acta Orthop Scand. 1984;55(3):315–8.

63. Waisbrod H, Krainick JU, Gerbershagen HU. Sacroiliac joint arthrodesis for chronic lower back pain. Arch Orthop Trauma Surg. 1987;106(4):238–40.

64. Moore MR. Surgical treatment of chronic painful sacroiliac joint dysfunction. In: Vleeming A, Mooney V, Snijders C, Dorman T, Stoeckart R, editors. Movement, stability, and low back pain: the essential role of the pelvis. New York: Churchill Livingstone; 1997. p. 563–72.

65. Keating JG, Avillar MD, Price M. Sacroiliac joint arthrodesis in selected patients with low back pain. In: Vleeming A, Mooney V, Snijders C, Dorman T, Stoeckart R, editors. Movement, stability, and low back pain: the essential role of the pelvis. New York: Churchill Livingstone; 1997. p. 573–86.

66. Belanger TA, Dall BE. Sacroiliac arthrodesis using a posterior midline fascial splitting approach and pedicle screw instrumentation: a new technique. J Spinal Disord. 2001;14(2): 118–24.

67. Berthelot JM, Gouin F, Glemarec J, Maugars Y, Prost A. Possible use of arthrodesis for intractable sacroiliitis in spondylarthropathy: report of two cases. Spine. 2001;26(20):2297–9.

68. van Zwienen CM, van den Bosch EW, Snijders CJ, van Vugt AB. Triple pelvic ring fixation in patients with severe pregnancy-related low back and pelvic pain. Spine. 2004;29(4):478–84.

69. Giannikas KA, Khan AM, Karski MT, Maxwell HA. Sacroiliac joint fusion for chronic pain: a simple technique avoiding the use of metalwork. Eur Spine J. 2004;13(3):253–6.

70. Buchowski JM, Kebaish KM, Sinkov V, Cohen DB, Sieber AN, Kostuik JP. Functional and radiographic outcome of sacroiliac arthrodesis for the disorders of the sacroiliac joint. Spine J. 2005;5(5):520–8.

71. Schütz U, Grob D. Poor outcome following bilateral sacroiliac joint fusion for degenerative sacroiliac joint syndrome. Acta Orthop Belg. 2006;72(3):296–308.

72. Ebraheim NA, Ramineni SK, Alla SR, Ebraheim M. Sacroiliac joint fusion with fibular graft in patients with failed percutaneous iliosacral screw fixation. J Trauma. 2010;69(5):1226–9.

73. Sturesson B. Pelvic girdle pain – indication for surgery? In: Szpalski M, Gunzburg R, Rydevik B, Le Huec J-C, Mayer HM, editors. Surgery for low back pain. Heidelberg: Springer; 2010. p. 165–8.

74. Kibsgård TJ, Røise O, Sudmann E, Stuge B. Pelvic joint fusions in patients with chronic pelvic girdle pain: a 23-year follow up. Eur Spine J [Internet]. 2012; Available from: http://www. springerlink.com/index/10.1007/s00586-012-2512-8.

75. Al-Khayer A, Hegarty J, Hahn D, Grevitt MP. Percutaneous sacroiliac joint arthrodesis: a novel technique. J Spinal Disord Tech. 2008;21(5):359–63.

76. Wise CL, Dall BE. Minimally invasive sacroiliac arthrodesis: outcomes of a new technique. J Spinal Disord Tech. 2008;21(8):579–84.

77. Khurana A, Guha AR, Mohanty K, Ahuja S. Percutaneous fusion of the sacroiliac joint with hollow modular anchorage screws: clinical and radiological outcome. J Bone Joint Surg Br. 2009;91(5):627–31.

78. Sembrano J, Reiley MA, Polly Jr DW, Garfin SR. Diagnosis and treatment of sacroiliac joint pain. Curr Orthop Pract. 2011;22(4):344–50.

79. Rudolf L. Sacroiliac joint arthrodesis—MIS technique with titanium implants: report of the first 50 patients and outcomes. Open Orthop J. 2012;6(1):495–502.

80. Sachs D, Capobianco R. One year successful outcomes for novel sacroiliac joint arthrodesis system. Ann Surg Innov Res. 2012;6(1):13.

Chapter 14
Image and Robotic Guidance in Spine Surgery

Yair Barzilay, Eyal Itshayek, Josh E. Schroeder,
Meir Liebergall, and Leon Kaplan

Introduction

The advent of spinal instrumentation allowed spine surgeons to treat complex spinal pathologies while maintaining or correcting alignment and maintaining or restoring spinal stability. Pedicle screws became an integral part of these complex procedures [1]. As spinal procedures progressed and became more complex, misplacement of pedicle screws, with the attendant risk of injury to the spinal cord, nerve roots, great vessels, or visceral tissue, or loss of mechanical stability, became a factor influencing surgical outcome.

Risk factors related to screw misplacement include the surgeon's experience, anatomic variables (level in the spine, i.e., cervical, thoracic, lumbar, or sacral, and size of the pedicle), congenital anomalies or variances, deformity, and revision surgery (notably posterolateral bone fusion mass) [2–16]. In the literature detailing free hand or fluoroscopy-assisted pedicle screw instrumentation, misplacement rates of 7.4–65.5 % have been reported in the cervical spine [17, 18], 5–41 % in the lumbar spine, and 3–55 % in the thoracic spine [2–16, 19–27]. Implant-related nerve damage has been reported in 0–8 % of cases, while the reported incidence of dural laceration caused by screws is 0–16 % [2–16, 28]. Screw-related injuries to viscera and blood vessels have also been reported sporadically [29, 30]. However, these complications may be underreported, and they represent the experience in large centers with high patient volumes, which are assumed to have lower complication rates compared with centers with smaller patient volumes [28].

Y. Barzilay, MD (✉) • J.E. Schroeder, MD • M. Liebergall, MD • L. Kaplan, MD
Spine Unit, Department of Orthopedic Surgery, Hadassah-Hebrew University
Medical Center, Jerusalem, POB 12000, 91120, Israel
e-mail: dbar@hadassah.org.il

E. Itshayek, MD
Department of Neurosurgery, Hadassah-Hebrew University
Medical Center, Jerusalem, Israel

P.P.M. Menchetti (ed.), *Minimally Invasive Surgery of the Lumbar Spine*,
DOI 10.1007/978-1-4471-5280-4_14, © Springer-Verlag London 2014

Over the last 20 years, surgeons' efforts to consistently achieve perfect screw placement have been paralleled by technological advances leading to the introduction of new tools aimed at reducing the rate of screw misplacement, reducing complication rates, and improving clinical outcomes. Screw placement was once verified with intraoperative X-ray, but this technique has clear drawbacks–it is retrospective and does not allow real time verification. It is also time consuming and increases the risk of infection. Later, real-time two-dimensional (2D) fluoroscopy was introduced to guide and verify screw placement. The drawbacks to 2D fluoroscopy include lower accuracy compared with techniques offering three-dimensional (3D) visualization and guidance [31], increased risk of infection due to repeated fluoroscopy machine movement between AP and lateral trajectories [32], and exposure of the patient, operating room staff, and surgeon to ionizing radiation.

Radiation exposure has become an important issue in the recent years. Both patients [33] and surgeons [34, 35] are at risk for radiation-induced malignancies. The risk for cancer among orthopedic surgeons has been estimated to be 5.37 times greater than risk in the general population [35], and the risk for breast cancer in female orthopedic surgeons is 2.88 times higher [34]. One study estimated that up to 29,000 future cancers could be related to CT scans performed in the US in 2007 [36]. The risk of developing a radiation-related cancer may be higher in the young, especially young females, and in cases where radiation exposure focuses on areas rich in viscera [33]. Radiation exposure has also been linked to other health problems, such as cataracts in the young and dermatological conditions. For all of these reasons, the US Food and Drug Administration (FDA) launched an initiative to reduce unnecessary radiation exposure from medical imaging in February 2010 [37].

Radiation exposure during fluoroscopy-guided spine surgery is estimated at 3.4–66 s per screw [38–42], depending on fluoroscopy technique (check fluoroscopy versus real-time continuous fluoroscopy) and whether the surgeon uses open freehand or percutaneous fluoroscopy-guided implantation. Surgeons performing vertebral body augmentation and minimally invasive spine surgery (MISS) under fluoroscopy guidance are exposed to higher doses of ionizing radiation [43–45].

Well-placed pedicle screws have a biomechanical advantage over misplaced screws. One cadaver study demonstrated that pedicle breaching reduces pullout strength by 11 % [46]. Another cadaver study found that medially misplaced screws had slightly greater mean pullout strength compared with well-placed pedicle screws, and that laterally misplaced screws had less mean pullout. "Airball" screws had only 66 % of the mean pullout strength of well-placed screws [47].

For all these reasons, navigation and robotic systems were developed, with the goals of reducing patient and staff exposure to radiation, as well as achieving greater accuracy and enhanced stability, and thus reducing surgical complications and the need for revision surgeries. The aim of this chapter is to discuss the different navigation and robotic systems, and to summarize the data regarding their accuracy and the radiation associated with their use. We will also raise questions that may need to be addressed in future studies.

Systems and Registration Processes
for Image-Guided Spine Surgery (IGSS)

Two-Dimensional (2D) Fluoroscopy-Based
Image Guidance (Virtual Fluoroscopy)

A calibration grid is attached to the C-arm. A series of fluoroscopy images in AP, lateral, and sometimes the pedicle oblique view are acquired with a reference frame attached to a stable anatomical landmark, often a spinous process in the vicinity of the vertebrae that will be operated. These images are transferred to the navigation workstation and this data set is used to navigate implants on the virtual anatomy viewed on the screen. An infrared camera aimed at the reference arc and navigation tools allows continuous recognition of the navigation tools in relation to the relevant anatomy. A continuous "line of sight" must be kept between the infrared camera, the reference arc, and the navigation tools. The accuracy of the system will be maintained as long as the stability of the reference arc is maintained, motion segments do not change their position compared to acquired images, and the navigation tools are kept in line with the desired trajectory.

Two-dimensional-fluoroscopy guidance has the advantage of a simple registration process. In addition, patients are spared the requirement of obtaining preoperative CT examinations, reducing their radiation exposure. However, it does not provide 3D visualization of the spinal anatomy during navigation; thus, the risk of navigation errors is increased and abnormal axial anatomy is more likely to remain unrecognized. Errors may also be greater in cases of poor bone quality, excess intraabdominal gas, morbid obesity, spinal deformity, prior surgery, and congenital anomalies [48]. Furthermore, image resolution is typically best in the center of the field and any structures around the periphery may appear distorted secondary to parallax, so to maintain the accuracy of navigation across several spinal segments the process of data acquisition and anatomic registration may need to be repeated several times [49].

CT-Based Image Guidance

Navigation systems based on CT guidance use preoperative thin-slice scans and one of several registration processes to create a data set, which forms the basis for intraoperative navigation. Preoperative CT scans are obtained with the patient in a supine position, while patients are in the prone position during surgery, usually on a Jackson frame, allowing a free abdomen. The resulting vertebral shift and realignment creates a risk for navigation errors; thus, each vertebra must be registered separately to accurately plan and perform the surgery.

Registration for Preoperative CT-Based Navigation

Point-Matching Technique

Chosen anatomical points on reconstructed views of the preoperative CT scan are registered intraoperatively to the patients' carefully dissected anatomy and viewed on the navigation screen. This procedure is time consuming, requires careful dissection of the relevant anatomy to the bony landmarks and matching of 4–8 points to allow adequate registration [50, 51]. Previous laminectomy that has left little posterior bony anatomy may leave a patient with an inadequate set of anatomical points for registration [52]. The registration process must be repeated for each vertebra separately to compensate for motion between the preoperative CT (supine) and the intraoperative anatomy (prone) [53–55].

Surface-Matching Technique

Multiple randomly chosen anatomical points on the patients' surface anatomy are touched to increase the number of data points. Selection of multiple points reduces the chance of error in the -point matching technique but adds to procedure time [51].

CT-to-Fluoroscopy Merging Systems

Intraoperative AP and lateral fluoroscopy images are taken with a grid connected to a C-arm and a reference arc attached to the patients' anatomy. These images are merged to the preoperative CT scan, allowing registration of more than one vertebra [56–58].

Electromagnetic Registration Systems

Electromagnetic (EM) systems have been developed as another method for tracking the location of instruments during surgical navigation to address the disadvantages of optical devices, mainly. cables and the requirement to maintain a "line of sight" between the infrared camera, the reference arc, and the surgical instruments. Three orthogonal electromagnetic fields are generated by a transmitter attached to a fixed anatomic reference point. The positional data of these instruments are collected by a receiver and integrated to facilitate navigation. Since a line of sight is not required, the surgeon and nursing staff are able to work freely within the operative field. However, EM image guidance may be compromised by metal artifacts, including surgical implants, as well as by any electromagnetic fields originating from other equipment in the operating room such as monopolar electrocautery, electrocardiogram monitoring, and cell phones. Given the limited area of these EM fields, the transmitter may also need to be repeatedly transferred to additional anatomic structures to obtain sufficient tracking information for multilevel procedures [40, 41, 59, 60].

Another EM investigational system combined a needle with an EM tip and a robotic arm-based flat panel CT to guide interventional pain clinic procedures, such as facet injections and selective nerve root blocks [61].

Intraoperative Cone Beam CT-Based Systems

The advent of cone-beam CT (cbCT) registration systems is considered a breakthrough compared with navigation systems based on preoperative CT studies (Fig. 14.1). During the scan, multiple (usually 50–100) fluoroscopy images are taken as the cbCT automatically rotates around the patient for 190–360°, covering a variable range of motion segments. These properties vary from one system to another. The scan is performed after the patient is positioned for surgery to prevent positional changes in anatomy. A reference arc is attached close to the surgical target to allow automatic registration and transfer of the data set to the navigation system. Two-dimensional images are reconstructed in the axial, coronal, and sagittal planes, similar to a CT scan. These reconstructions allow intraoperative planning of implant trajectory, size, and length, as well as intraoperative navigation. A second intraoperative scan may be performed to confirm implant position and may lead to immediate intra-operative correction of misplaced implants, thereby avoiding early revision surgery.

Intraoperative CT

The use of standard CT equipment within the operating theater provides higher image quality compared with cbCT. Patient radiation exposure is significant; however, the surgeon and OR staff are not exposed [62]. The capital expense is greater,

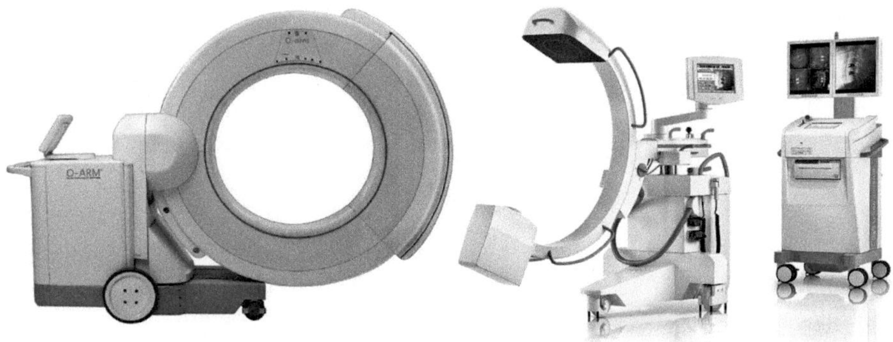

Fig. 14.1 Cone beam CT (cbCT) used for spine surgery. The Ziehm Vision Vario 3D (Ziehm Imaging, Nuremberg, Germany) and O-Arm (Medtronics, Minneapolis, MN, USA) are representative of a range of cbCT products that are currently available

the process of scanning and registration is longer, and intraoperative CT (iCT) does not allow the use of a Jackson frame. The system cannot be mobilized between different operating rooms [62–65].

Robotic Guidance in Spine Surgery

In recent years, a variety of robots for different surgical applications have been introduced [66, 67]. Surgical robots can be divided into three broad categories: (1) Supervisory-controlled systems enable the surgeon to plan the operation offline, specifying motions that the robot must follow to perform the operation. The robot then performs the procedure autonomously with the surgeon supervising closely. (2) Telesurgical systems allow the surgeon to directly control surgical instruments held by the robot via a joystick or hand controls, with either passive or active task execution. (3) Shared-control systems allow both the surgeon and the robot simultaneous direct control of surgical instruments [68]. To date, the majority of robotic-assisted spine operations have involved a shared-control system.

A recent review [69] discussed 18 robotic systems, of which five are clinically available. One is dedicated to spine surgery, one aimed at needle interventions, two are focused on radiosurgery, and one was tested for spine surgery but is used primarily in other surgical specialties. The authors concluded that the field of spine surgical robots "is still at an early stage of development but with great potential for improvement."

A Robotic System in Clinical Use

To the authors' best knowledge, only one robotic system dedicated to spine surgery is clinically used [70–76]. The system consists of a grid attached to a C-arm, a workstation containing a miniature robot, a computer running dedicated software that allows preoperative planning and intraoperative execution, and a screen (Fig. 14.2a). The bone-mounted miniature robot is a semi-active system offering surgical tool guidance while leaving performance of the actual surgical operation, such as drilling, in the surgeon's hands (Fig. 14.2b). The concept was first published in 2003 and 2004 [77, 78], followed by lab testing [79, 80], and a clinical developmental phase [81, 82].

The robotic procedure consists of five steps:

1. Preoperative planning–DICOM images of a dedicated protocol CT scan are imported by the robotic workstation software. This software can be installed on a standard laptop or desktop computer and allows for preoperative planning. The software creates 2D reconstruction images of each vertebra in the region of interest with planning for virtual implant placement in the optimal position. This is a crucial step that allows for detection of abnormal anatomy, absent pedicles, and deformity, as well as determination of implant diameters and lengths (Fig. 14.3).

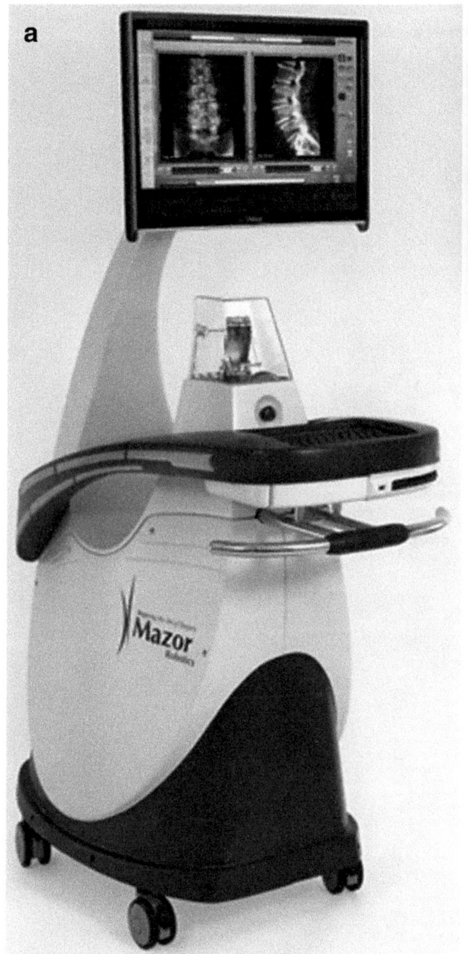
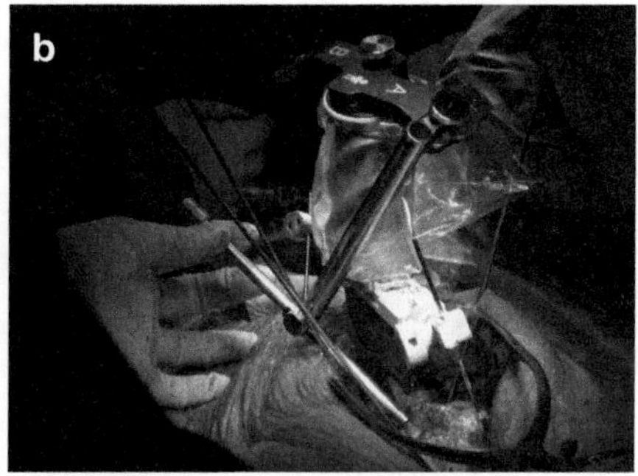

Fig. 14.2 (**a**) A robotic workstation (Renaissance, Mazor Robotics, Caesarea, Israel). The computer runs software allowing preplanning, image acquisition, registration, and control of robot execution; a touch screen and a 250 g 6 DF miniature robot. (**b**) The robot is mounted on a clamp, which is connected to a posterior fusion mass in a revision surgery (Photo courtesy Dr. I.H. Lieberman, Texas Back Institute, Plano TX, USA)

2. Platform attachment–One of three platforms is used. The unilateral bed mount device or the bilateral multidirectional bed mount device are attached to the surgical frame caudally and to the patients' anatomy through a K-wire or a miniclamp cranially. The Hover-T Bridge is attached to Steinmann pins drilled into the posterior iliac crests and to a K-wire drilled into a spinous process. Both platforms are designed for minimally invasive surgery. A clamp may be connected to a spinous process in open procedures after subperiosteal dissection is completed (Fig. 14.4).

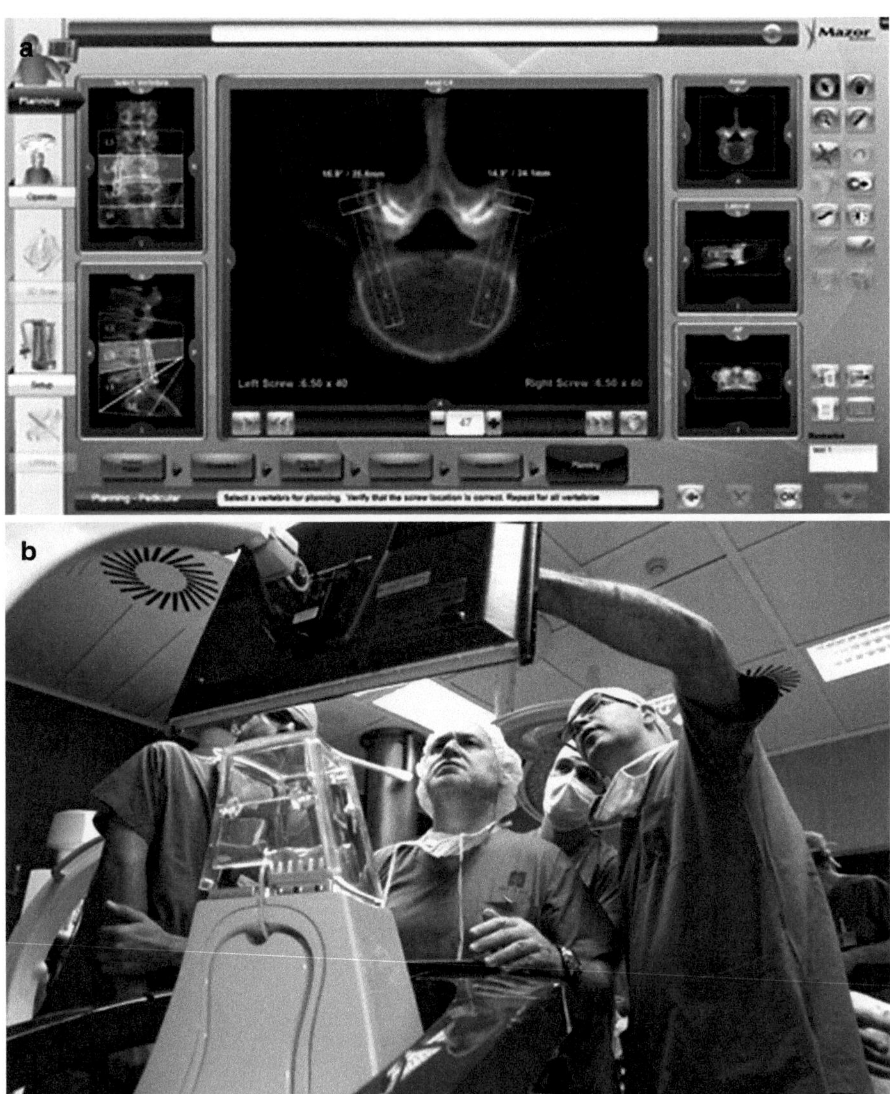

Fig. 14.3 Preoperative planning allows recognition of patients' unique anatomy, and allows preoperative measurement of implant length and size. (**a**) The summary window allows preoperative assessment of implant alignment and the estimated rod length. (**b**) Surgical team at the workstation during preoperative planning

3. Image acquisition and registration–Targets for image acquisition are connected to the robotic platform, and AP and 60° oblique fluoroscopic images are semi-automatically registered to the preoperative CT images. The surgeon must visually verify the accuracy of the registration process before going forward.

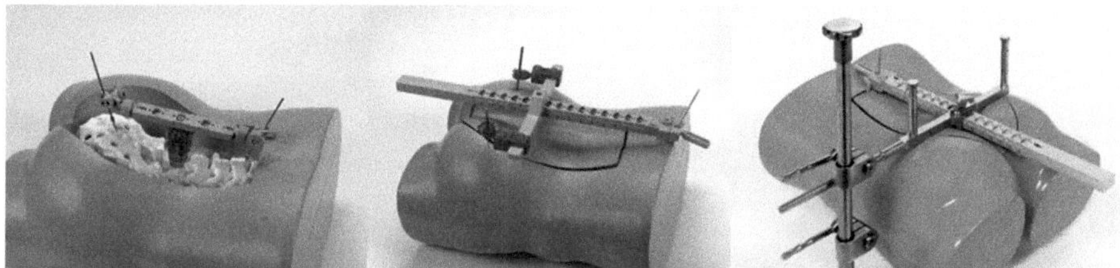

Fig. 14.4 Three platforms allow robotic guidance: a clamp (*left*), the Hover T frame (*center*), and a bed-mount device (*right*). The latter two are for use in minimally invasive spine surgery, while the clamp is used in open procedures

4. Robot assembly and motion–The miniature robot is attached to the mounting frame and one of three arms is connected to it, according to the software guidance. It is then instructed to move and lock into position, so that a guiding tube at the distal end of its arm is aligned with the planned screw/tool trajectory. The guiding tube, with trocar inserted, is then advanced percutaneously or through the open wound until contact with the pedicle entry point is felt. The trocar is withdrawn and replaced with a working channel. The toothed end of the working channel is gently tapped into the bony surface anatomy of the spine.
5. Trajectory execution–Drilling through the working channel along the planned trajectory is performed. Following drilling, a fiducial may be tapped into the pedicle in open procedures. In percutaneous procedures, a hollow reduction tube is placed through the working channel and advanced into the pedicle and through the posterior vertebral wall. A K-wire is then placed into the vertebral body and the reduction tube is withdrawn. This procedure is repeated until trajectories are drilled and fiducials or K-wires (KW) are placed at all levels to be treated. Instrumentation may then be placed. At this point robotic guidance is complete. In minimally invasive procedures, the mounting system may be left attached to allow repeat robot guidance in case one of the trajectories is lost.

Robotic Systems Under Development

In 2010, a Korean group published a cadaver study on an investigational system combining a bi-planar fluoroscopy machine, a computerized workstation, and an assistive robot for percutaneous KW and pedicle screw insertion [83]. The system does not use a target device or a reference frame, and therefore does not need a secondary procedure to attach these structures to the patient's anatomy. Two registration processes are required. The first registration matches the coordinates of the robot manipulator and the bi-planar images based on point matching; the second registration is between preoperative CT or MRI and intraoperative bi-planar fluoroscopy. The researcher reported a distance of error of 1.38 ± 0.21 mm, $2.45° \pm 2.56°$ deviation in the axial plane, and $0.71° \pm 1.21°$ deviation in the sagittal plane when comparing post-op CT to planning. The system has not reached clinical usage.

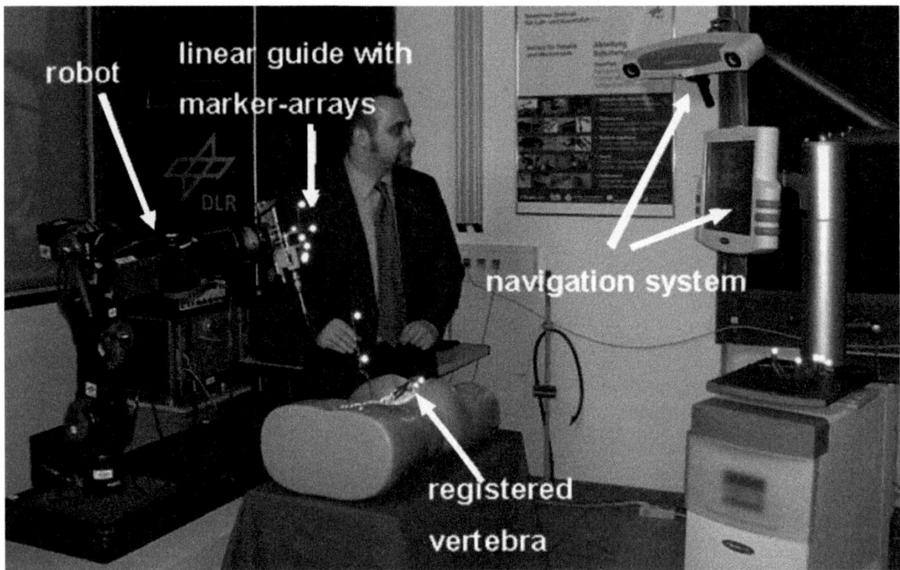

Fig. 14.5 Experimental setup for the placement of pedicle screw with robotic assistance in a prototype robotic system (German Aerospace Centre [DLR e.V.] Institute of Robotics and Mechatronics, Wessling, Germany), shown here with a VectorVision navigation system (BrainLab, Feldkirchen, Germany) (Used with permission from John Wiley and Sons. Ortmaier et al. [85])

In 2012, a Swiss group published their results on an investigational robotic navigated system developed for cervical applications [84]. The system consists of a compact robot with four degrees of freedom, suspended over the operative field by a passive supporting structure. Additional components include an optical tracking system, a surgical input device, and a workstation with software for planning and navigation. The data set is generated by point-to-point and surface matching of each vertebra registered to a preoperative thin-slice CT. The robot is positioned by the surgeon over the operative field. After locking the passive supporting structure, the robot guides the surgeon to the planned trajectory using guiding tools, and KW is drilled and is replaced by a screw.

In 2006, a team in a German aerospace center published a trial on a navigation system and an impedance-controlled light-weight robot holding a surgical instrument [85]. The navigation system was used to position pedicle screws in artificial bone and bovine spine and to compensate for pose errors during machining. The robot "floats" over the spine, and occupies a significant space (Fig. 14.5). The authors concluded that milling was more accurate than drilling, that the robot should withstand higher milling forces (30 N) than the tested design (15 N), and that the accuracy of the tracking system is a critical parameter, as it is used to close the position control loop. In the set-up used, tracking accuracy seemed to be a limiting factor. Additionally, the latency of the tracking system would have been minimized. This project did not reach clinical usage in spine surgery. The robot under current development by this group is planned for other fields of surgery.

In 2009, South Korean scientists published an investigational system for fusion procedures [86]. The system consisted of a human-guided robot for the spinal fusion surgery with a dexterous end-effector that is capable of high-speed drilling, and is position-controlled by a five degrees-of-freedom robot body that has a kinematically closed structure to withstand strong reaction forces. The robot allows the surgeon to control the position and orientation of the end-effector. Incorporated for improved safety is a "drill-by-wire" mechanism wherein a screw is tele-drilled by the surgeon in a mechanically decoupled master/slave system. The system has haptic properties, imitating the sensation during screw insertion. A tracking system has not been yet developed for the system.

A Clinically Available Tele-Surgical Robotic System

A tele-surgical system (Fig. 14.6) has been in clinical use for urological, gynecological, and surgical procedures for over the last decade [87–94] with an impressive penetration into the market in these specialties. This system has been tested for spinal applications on a healthy pig. In preliminary studies, laminotomy, laminectomy, excision of disc material, and repair of a dural tear were performed [91]. The authors concluded that with proper robotic tools, the system can be used for posterior spinal procedures. The same system has also been tested in a swine model for laparoscopic anterior lumbar interbody fusion (ALIF) using a retroperitoneal approach [88]. The authors reported little retraction of the great vessels and a very clear view of the operative field, allowing successful ALIF. In humans, only case

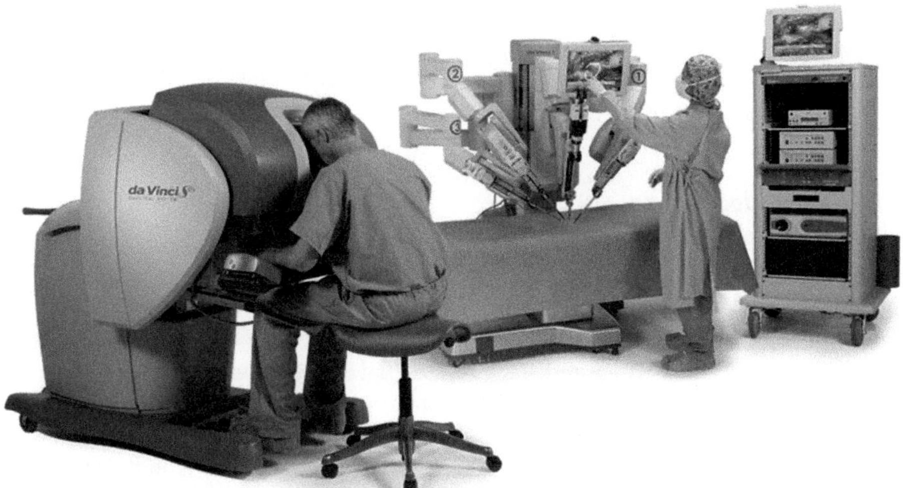

Fig. 14.6 Tele-surgical robotic system (da Vinci, Intuitive Surgical, Sunnyvale CA, USA). The system has been tested for spine surgery in an animal model and used in cases of soft tissue tumor removal in different areas of the spine (Copyright Intuitive Surgical, used with permission)

reports were published, including robot-assisted transoral odontoidectomy for decompression of the craniocervical junction [87], resection of paraspinal schwannoma [93], and resection of a thoracolumbar neurofibroma [90].

Review of the Literature Regarding Image and Robotic Guidance in Spine Surgery

Image guidance has been used in spine surgery for about three decades, while robotic-guided spine surgery emerged only in the past decade. In addition, several companies have developed fluoroscopy-based 2D and 3D systems, and preoperative or intraoperative cbCT based image-guided systems, leading to competition and continuous improvement in these products, but only one company has developed a commercially available robotic system for spine surgery. Other robotic systems are still in the developmental phases or were abandoned. For these reasons, the published data regarding IGSS [2, 11, 17, 19, 21, 40, 41, 52, 95–127] are far more extensive than the body of literature regarding robotic-guided spine surgery [69, 75, 87–94].

In our review of the literature, we have chosen to focus on specific questions related to the effect of image or robotic guidance on spine surgery:

1. Is there a learning curve? How long is it?
2. Do these systems improve the accuracy of implant placement?
3. Do these systems reduce the frequency of nerve damage or damage to other important organs?
4. Do these systems reduce radiation exposure to the patient, operating room staff, and surgeon?
5. Do these systems lead to superior mechanical properties through improved accuracy; if so, does this affect the need for revision surgery?

Image-Guided Spine Surgery

Learning Curve

A learning curve in image-guided spinal surgery has been documented [128–131]. In virtual fluoroscopy, one study suggested that the learning curve extends for approximately 6 months, after which guidance resulted in fewer breaches of the pedicles and shorter operating time [128]. Another study documented a decrease in the rate of thoracic pedicle cortex perforation from 37.5 % to 4.2 % in new users as they gained experience on cadavers practicing 3D point-matching techniques based on preoperative CT images [129].

It is thought that, during the learning curve period, surgeons adopt a new work flow. They must achieve acceptable registration of the patients' anatomy to the imaging studies while positioning the infrared camera where it enables consistent recognition of the reference arc and navigation tools. The surgeon must become accustomed to looking at a computer screen instead of the operative field. In addition, operative instruments must be held in line with the planned trajectory, without tilting them, once the bone trajectory has been set; tilting the tools would create a "false-accurate trajectory" on screen and end in deviation [52].

Accuracy

How does IGSS compare to non-navigated pedicle screw instrumentation? In the growing mass of published data [2, 11, 17, 19, 21, 40, 41, 52, 95–127], most studies point to higher accuracy when using image guidance; only two studies concluded that image guidance is not superior to non-navigated instrumentation in spine surgery [95, 109].

The first meta-analysis comparing image-guided pedicle screw placement with non-navigated placement was published in 2007 [132]. The median accuracy of screw placement with assistance from navigation was 95.2 % versus a 90.3 % median accuracy for screws placed without navigation assistance. In 2010, another meta-analysis reported 93.3 % accuracy for the placement of pedicle screws with navigation, compared to 84.7 % without. In 2009, another meta-analysis reported 85.48 % accuracy for screw placement with 2D navigation and 90.76 % accuracy using 3D navigation [31]. The same authors published a newer meta-analysis in 2011 comparing accuracy using conventional methods of pedicle screw placement to accuracy using three types of image guidance (3D point matching, virtual fluoroscopy, and cbCT) [21]. They concluded that image guidance resulted in higher accuracy across the board. In comparisons between the three image guidance systems, no system was found to be more accurate for in vivo (clinical) studies; however, CT-based systems were more accurate in cadaver studies.

Two meta-analyses were published in 2012 [19, 133]. Gelalis et al. included only prospective clinical studies and omitted cadaver studies. The authors were in agreement with the conclusion of previous meta-analyses, and found greater accuracy with CT-based navigation compared to virtual fluoroscopy [19]. The authors also noted that screws inserted freehand tend to breach the pedicle medially, while CT-navigated screws tend to breach laterally. According to this meta-analysis, neurological complications were similar in image-guided and non-navigated procedures. The second meta-analysis reported the pooled breach rate to be 6 % in image-guided procedures versus 15 % using non-navigated techniques [133].

Five randomized controlled studies compared image-guided spine surgeries and conventional techniques. Four of these studies reported higher accuracy with IGSS [11, 117, 134, 135]. One study comparing 3D cbCT image guidance to conventional technique for the placement of thoracic pedicle screws for deformity correction reported much higher breach rates with the conventional technique (23 %) when compared to 3D cbCT IGSS (2 %) [117]. A second comparative study reported

95.3 % accuracy in procedures performed under 3D cbCT guidance versus 84.1 % in those performed freehand [135]. A third study evaluating 3D cbCT reported accurate placement in 95.65 % of the cases operated under guidance with breaches under 2 mm in 4.35 % and no breaches over 2 mm. With fluoroscopy control, accuracy fell to 83.33 % overall, with breaches under 2 mm in 13.1 % and over 2 mm in 3.57 % [134]. In a study comparing point-matching CT IGSS to non-navigated technique, the breach rate was 13.4 % using the conventional technique versus 4.6 % with CT guidance [11].

One randomized controlled trial reported no benefit using a preoperative CT-based navigation system compared to a conventional technique [136].

Radiation Exposure

Using fluoroscopy control for pedicle screw instrumentation in open procedures, radiation exposure time ranges from 3.4–66 s per screw [38–42, 137]. Exposure during pedicle screw insertion is 10–12-fold higher than in non-spinal procedures [137].

During fluoroscopy-controlled vertebral body augmentation procedures, the average fluoroscopy exposure time per level ranges between 2.9 min±23 s [138] and 10.1 min±22 s [33].

In a study measuring radiation exposure to the surgeon performing percutaneous one- and two-level transforaminal lumbar interbody fusion (TLIF) under fluoroscopy control [43], the mean exposure time per case was 1.69 min, with 76 mrem exposure to the surgeon's dominant hand. At this rate, the maximal annual occupational exposure allowance would be reached after 194 procedures. Since pulsed fluoroscopy was used in the study, TLIF cages were inserted without fluoroscopy control and running electromyography (EMG) was also used; thus, one can assume that in other set-ups the radiation exposure may be higher.

In a cadaver study testing radiation exposure to the surgeon during percutaneous screw placement [139], all screws were within the bone confines, with acceptable trajectory. Total fluoroscopy time for placement of ten percutaneous pedicle screws was 4 min 56 s (29 s per screw). The protected dosimeter recorded less than the reportable dose. The ring dosimeter recorded total radiation exposure of 103 mrem, or 10.3 mrem per screw placed. Exposure to the eyes was 2.35 mrem per screw. The authors concluded that a surgeon would exceed occupational exposure limit for the eyes and extremities with percutaneous placement of 4,854 and 6,396 screws, respectively.

In cadaver studies [38, 41, 140, 141], image-guided procedures were associated with less radiation exposure to the surgeon when compared with conventional use of fluoroscopy. With the use of navigation systems based on preoperative CT with point-matching registration, or iCT-based image guidance, the surgeon is exposed to no intraoperative radiation [64]. In image-guided procedures that require intraoperative acquisition of fluoroscopy images or an intraoperative 3D fluoroscopy study as well as cbCT, the surgeon's radiation exposure depends on both the amount of radiation used and distance from the radiation source. In these procedures, the operating room staff can step back behind a leaded wall or stay out of the room during periods of active radiation.

From the patient's perspective, preoperative CT-based IGSS is associated with higher levels of radiation exposure compared with fluoroscopy [42, 142]. Intraoperative cbCT scan is equivalent to 40 s of fluoroscopy, or about half of a CT scan of the same region-of-interest (ROI) [143]. A patient undergoing two intraoperative cbCT scans, for example, prenavigation for registration and post instrumentation to validate screw position, is thus exposed to a radiation dose that is equivalent to a CT scan of the same ROI, or 80 s of fluoroscopy. This is a similar level of exposure to the reported radiation dose during percutaneous fluoroscopy-controlled one- and two level TLIF [43], and less than the dose associated with one-level fluoroscopy-controlled vertebral body augmentation [138].

Procedure Duration

Several studies investigated the effect of image guidance on operative time. Image guidance was associated with longer operative time in some studies [11, 53, 115, 136, 144, 145], while surgeries were shorter in others [117, 131, 134, 146].

Several investigators described a reduction in procedure duration as they moved down their learning curve, suggesting that the relationship between use of image guidance and operative time depends on how well navigation systems are assimilated in a specific hospital. How effective is the setup? Is the infrared camera positioned properly for undisturbed navigation? How far down the curve have the surgeons traveled? And how good is the coordination between X-ray technicians and the surgical team?

Robotic Guidance in Spine Surgery

Accuracy

In a cadaver study, 2 experienced spine surgeons inserted pedicle screws to the thoracolumbar spine of a cadaver with fluoroscopy control (control group), while 13 surgeons instrumented cadaver thoracolumbar spine with robotic guidance (study group). A total of 234 pedicle screws were implanted in 12 cadavers. Screw placement accuracy was measured according to the Gertzbein and Robbins classification [10]. Screw placement deviations in the group using the robotic guidance averaged 1.1 ± 0.4 mm versus 2.6 ± 0.7 mm in the control group. Pedicle wall breaches of 4 mm or more occurred in 1.5 % of the study group placements versus 5.4 % of control group placements [147].

In the early clinical phases, robotic guidance performed successfully in 93 % of the cases in which it was used, and 96 % of the screws were assessed as accurate [76].

In a case series of 31 patients undergoing robotic-guided percutaneous posterior lumbar interbody fusion (PLIF) with posterior fixation, 133 pedicle screws were placed [73]. According to the Gertzbein and Robbins scoring system [10], in the axial plane, 91.7 % of the screws were evaluated as group A and 6.8 % were evaluated as group B. In the sagittal plane, 81.2 % of the screws were evaluated as group A and 9.8 % were evaluated as group B. One screw was evaluated as group C in the axial plane, and one as group D in the longitudinal plane.

A retrospective multinational-multicenter study summarized placement of 3,271 pedicle screws and guide-wires inserted in 635 patients; 49 % were inserted percutaneously [70]. The series included diverse clinical entities, from simple degenerative cases to severe deformities. Accuracy was assessed in 646 pedicle screws inserted in 139 patients using postoperative CT scans, and in the remaining patients assessment was by intraoperative fluoroscopy. Clinically acceptable screw placement was recognized in 98 % of the cases. Postoperative CT scans demonstrated that 98.3 % of screws (635/646) fell within the safe zone; 89.3 % were completely within the pedicle, 9 % had a breach of <2 mm, 1.4 % breached 2–4 mm, and only two screws (0.3 %) deviated by more than 4 mm from the pedicle wall. Transient neurologic deficits were observed in four cases, but following revision, no permanent nerve damage was encountered.

In a retrospective analysis [72], patient records and CT scans were analyzed in a cohort of 57 conventional open screw placement performed in 2006, 20 open robotic-guided placements performed in 2007, and 35 percutaneous robotic-guided pedicle screw placements performed in 2008–2010. A total of 94.5 % of robot-assisted and 91.4 % of conventionally placed screws were within the pedicle or encroaching the cortical pedicle wall. Percutaneous robotic and open robotic-guided subgroups did not differ. The revision rate for misplaced screws was 1 % for robotic guided surgery and 12.2 % for conventional open surgery.

In a retrospective analysis of prospective data in a series of 102 consecutive patients undergoing robotic-guided spine surgery [71], robotic-guided screw placement was executed in 95 patients. The robot was not used as planned in seven patients for the following reasons: severe deformity (one patient), very high body mass index (one patient), extremely poor bone quality (one patient), registration difficulty caused by previously placed loosened hardware (one patient), difficulty with platform mounting (one patient), and technical issues with the device (two patients). In the 95 executed cases, 949 screws (87.5 % of 1,085 planned screws) were successfully implanted, and 98.9 % of executed screws were in clinically acceptable position. Eleven screws (1.0 %) were misplaced (all presumably due to "skiving" of the drill bit or trocar off the side of the facet). Ten misplacements were recognized intraoperatively and corrected manually; one diagnosed postoperatively resulted in a revision surgery for screw removal. In 110 screws (10.1 %), robotic guidance was aborted and screws were manually placed, generally due to poor registration and/or technical trajectory issues (the trajectory was out of the working volume of the robot).

Only one randomized controlled trial was conducted to compare freehand and robotic-guided lumbar and sacral pedicle screw insertion [74], including 60 patients who were randomly allocated into the two groups. A total of 298 screws were implanted; 93 % had good positions in the freehand group (Gertzbein and Robbins A or B), and 85 % in the robotic-guidance group. Ten robot-guided screw placements required intraoperative conversion to freehand. One misplaced screw that had been placed freehand needed surgical revision.

The authors felt the bed mount device, which was connected to the operative bed on the caudal side and to a spinous process via a KW on the cranial side, was unstable, leading to motion and incorrect trajectories, and that "cannula skidding" (skiving of the working channel on the side of the facet) led to lateral screw misplacement in some cases.

The authors of this chapter, who are experienced robotic-guided spine surgeons, feel that these misplacements are suggestive of surgeons who are still on a learning curve. Skiving (skidding) occurs for one of several reasons: (1) planning on a steep slope or on a ridge, leading to loss of entry point; (2) the entry point is not prepared or is insufficiently prepared (nibbling in open procedures or using a specific tool in percutaneous procedures), leading to slippage of the guiding tool; or (3) the guiding tool is inserted too forcefully or too deep, leading to skiving (Fig. 14.7). The authors have made all of these errors themselves, and teach others how to avoid them, but would not have initiated a randomized controlled trial while at a relatively early point on the learning curve.

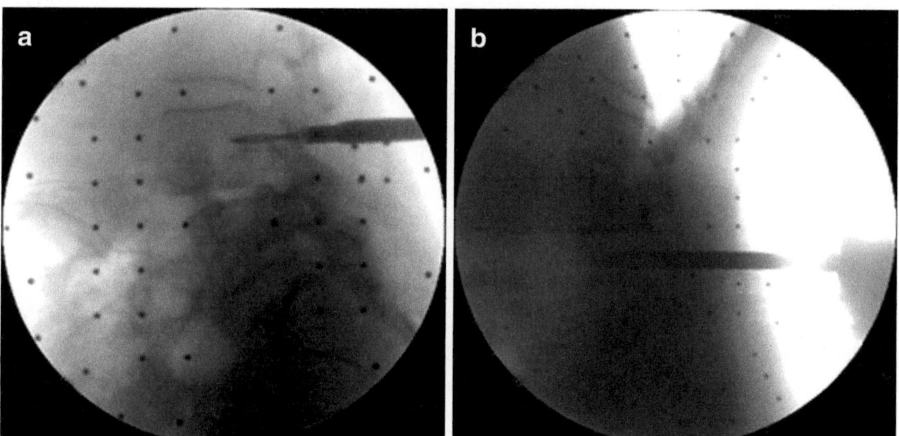

Fig. 14.7 There are three main reasons for pedicle screw misplacement in robotic-assisted spine surgery: planning errors, an unstable robotic platform, and skiving of the drill bit or trocar off the working channel. (**a**) Good surgical technique resulted in a well-placed fiducial and pedicle screw. (**b**) In this procedure, the trocar and the guiding tube were pushed too deep, resulting in slippage on the lateral border of the facet and lateral misplacement of the fiducial. This trajectory was corrected manually

Radiation Exposure

In a cadaver study comparing robotic-guided (study group) pedicle screws to fluoroscopy-controlled (control group) pedicle screw instrumentation, surgeons' radiation exposure in the study group averaged 4.2 mrem versus 136 mrem in the control group [147]. In a retrospective study comparing robotic-guided to fluoroscopy-controlled pedicle screws, the average fluoroscopy exposure per screw was 34 s in robotic-guided compared to 77 s in conventional cases [72]. In the only randomized controlled trial comparing fluoroscopy control to robotic guidance, intraoperative radiation did not differ between the two study groups (1.9 min), while preoperative CT in the robotic guided group added 411 mGy cm to patient exposure [74]. Radiation exposure in robotic-guided surgery reflects the confidence of the surgeon in the system. Exposure levels in the cadaver study [147] reflect the best scenario each surgeon should strive to reach.

Early in the learning curve, every step in robotic-guided procedures is monitored under fluoroscopy; however, as surgeons gain experience and adopt proper surgical technique, less radiation is needed. In the authors' institution, fluoroscopy images are taken for registration, after drilling is performed for all planned trajectories (with KW placed in minimally invasive procedures or metal fiducials placed in the drilled pedicles in open procedures), and at the end of the procedure, before closure. Fluoroscopy to assess placement during surgery is taken only if the guiding tube is felt to skive, before drilling is performed (unpublished data). These measures resulted in reduction in fluoroscopy time in vertebral body augmentation (manuscript under revision) and in spinal fusion surgery (unpublished data).

Procedure Time

In a cadaver study comparing fluoroscopy to robot guidance, 234 pedicle screws were implanted in 12 cadavers. Robot guidance resulted in an average procedure time of 1.23 h, compared with an average 1.98 h in the control group [147]. In a randomized controlled trial comparing robotic guidance with fluoroscopy [74], surgical time for screw placement was shorter with the freehand technique (84 min) compared with robotic guidance (95 min), however preparation time in the operating room and overall OR time were not different for the two groups.

The authors of this chapter agree that during the learning curve, screw-related procedure time is longer with robot guidance, as reported above in the discussion of the learning curve in image-guided procedures; however, in our experience, when the procedure is well assimilated in OR routines, the time required for robotic guidance will become comparable to fluoroscopy guidance in short-segment fixation and will be shorter for long-segment fixation. This notion is especially true for percutaneous pedicle screws.

Tele-Surgical Robotic Systems and Spine Surgery

Tele-surgical robotic systems allow the surgeon to directly control the surgical instruments held by the robot via a joystick or hand controls. Task execution can be either passive or active. To date, only one tele-surgical robotic system is in clinical use. While the system has been used primarily in urology, it has also been used for ALIF procedures via the retroperitoneal approach in two porcine models [88, 94]. It was also tested on laminotomy, laminectomy, disc incision, and dural suturing procedures on the thoracolumbar spine of a porcine model [91]. The authors concluded that with the development of appropriate surgical tools, this system may be used clinically. A cadaveric study has shown the technical feasibility of trans-oral robotic surgery for decompression of the craniocervical junction as well as resection of both intra- and extradural tumors of this region [89].

In humans, case reports were published on robot-assisted transoral odontoidectomy for decompression of the craniocervical junction [87], on a retroperitoneal transdiaphragmatic robotic-assisted laparoscopic resection of a left thoracolumbar neurofibroma [90], thoracoscopical extirpation of paravertebral mediastinal neurogenic tumors such as schwannomas [92], and in the transperitoneal resection of paravertebral lumbosacral masses [93].

Practical Considerations When Using Image or Robotic Guidance

Image-guidance in spine surgery achieved "maturity" with systems based on cbCT that allowed intraoperative scanning in the "correct" position and registration of several motion segments simultaneously. These systems allow for a check scan before leaving the OR. They reduce occupational exposure for the surgeon and OR staff but result in significant radiation to the patient. An increasing number of surgeons are performing minimally invasive spine surgeries. They are exposed to significant radiation, and there are reports of early revision surgeries in up to 10 % of cases [148]. In response to these issues, the use of some form of guidance seems intuitive. In addition, image or robotic guidance can make a big difference in cases of revision surgery with a posterior fusion mass, abnormal anatomy, or spinal deformity. In all of these instances, the energy spent on lamino-foraminotomy or exposure of other relevant anatomical landmarks for successful screw placement can now be shifted to other important parts of revision surgery, such as osteotomy or decompression of the neural elements. One simple step, using the guidance system software for preplanning, upgrades the surgeon's readiness for the procedure, with preoperative exposure to abnormal bony and neural anatomy, enabling appropriate planning that avoids attempts at screw placement in locations where they cannot be introduced.

The decision by a spine surgeon to use image or robotic guidance is not an easy step. Several obstacles may have to be overcome:

1. The "I do not need it, I can do better than the machine" mindset must be changed. In fact, in most cases the machine will do better than the average surgeon in terms of accuracy with lower radiation exposure. Acknowledging these facts is the first step for a surgeon, before he or she can become interested in looking into guidance systems.

2. There is a learning curve, and it can take some time before a surgeon will benefit from image or robotic guidance. Two-dimensional fluoroscopy image-guidance systems are the most intuitive for spine surgeons. More sophisticated systems will require a longer learning curve; however, after achieving good understanding of the system and the surgical steps, the position of the implants will repeat itself case after case, with very few outliers. Many surgeons lose their patience during the learning curve and stop using the system. It takes motivation and discipline to stay focused on the long-term objective.
3. These systems are expensive and cannot be purchased by every spine surgeon around the world. In the future, their prices will fall as a result of mass production, competition, and device simplification. For now, it is important to work with hospital administration and convey the benefits of guidance for both patients and staff.
4. These systems are cumbersome, they require significant space in the OR, and require trained OR staff to operate them. With most navigation systems, cables run between the sterile area and the navigation system, and the surgeon and the OR staff must keep an open "line of sight" between the infrared camera, the reference arc, and the navigation tools. This requires an appropriate OR set-up. In the future, wireless systems may be available, a line of sight will not be needed, the system will be operated by the surgeon or will run automatically, and systems will become smaller, reducing their footprint in the OR.

Surgeon who choose to use image guidance must remember one simple fact: their eyes are centered on a screen showing virtual anatomy and virtual tools. Navigation errors may occur as a result of:

1. Scanning errors
2. Poor registration between the scan and the patient's anatomy
3. Motion of the relevant anatomy in relation to the reference arc following registration
4. Too great a distance between the reference arc and the relevant anatomy
5. Shift or instability in the reference arc
6. Suboptimal angle of view of the reference arc by the infrared camera
7. Tilted or misshapen tools that create a false trajectory on the screen

Current systems require some form of imaging that involves ionizing radiation. Future systems may be based on registration between preoperative MRI and intra-operative ultrasound, or on EM point-matching to preoperative MRI studies, which would save both the surgeon and the patient from the dangers of ionizing radiation; however, these ideals will not be achieved in the short term.

A surgeon who chooses to use robotic guidance must also remember several simple rules:

1. The platform must not move. No matter whether it is a clamp, Hover T, or a unilateral or bidirectional bed-mount device, the surgeon must make certain to create a stable platform before beginning the procedure.
2. AP and 60° oblique fluoroscopy images must be taken with the target seen clearly at the center of the field. The patient must be still during this step. If the

frame or bed may prevent the patient from remaining motionless, leading to motion during respiration, fluoroscopy images should be taken while respiration has been temporarily stopped by the anesthesiologist.

3. The semi-automatic registration should be visually verified by the surgeon. In case any shift is noted between preop CT and intraoperative fluoroscopy images, the surgeon should verify that the platform is stable and repeat the fluoroscopy study until registration is sufficient for robotic guidance.

4. Ensure that the robot is connected to the right station, and maintain constant and clear communication with the person operating the workstation. Connect the correct arm to the robot, again keeping clear communication with the trajectory plan on the workstation screen. Choose guiding tools and drill of the correct length.

5. Keep the skin incision in line with the point of the trocar. Keeping the trajectory line, cut the fascia. Push the trocar and guiding tube gently through muscle until reaching the pedicle entry point, but do not push the guiding tools too deep. Keep the outer tube floating over the anatomy, thus avoiding skiving (Fig. 14.7). Remove the trocar and tap the toothed working channel to the entry point. This step will have a learning curve, and skiving or slipping on sharp, bony ridges will be identified by the surgeon only after these occur several times. In open surgery, the surgeon must make sure no pressure is applied on the guiding tools by the paravertebral muscles since this may lead to skiving and screw misplacement.

6. Drill in and out, full speed ahead, holding the tip of the working channel to prevent dislodgement.

7. Leave a marker or a KW in each drilled trajectory and move on to the next trajectory. Make sure no force is applied on the robotic arm when disconnecting it, as this may lead to platform motion, especially if a unilateral bed-mount device is used.

Surgeons using robotic guidance should keep in mind an important difference from image guidance. During surgeries performed under image guidance, the surgeon has a sense of "where am I going" from following the virtual trajectory on the screen; however, with robotic guidance there is no control mechanism to alert the surgeon when an incorrect trajectory is drilled. The authors of this chapter consider this the weakest link of the currently available robotic guidance systems, and suggest that efforts should be made to develop a feedback mechanism that will identify any deviation from the planned entry point. With the current system, the entry point should be prepared by a designated tool using a percutaneous approach and by nibbling bone or burring it down in open surgery to create a comfortable "landing area" for the toothed working channel. Moreover, it is of great importance to understand the 3D anatomy of this landing area on the planning software, and to avoid areas with high risk for skiving and slipping. Surgeons in the beginning of their learning curve should be controlling their steps with check fluoroscopy. Later on, when the surgeon has developed the ability to sense skiving and slipping, less fluoroscopy will be required.

Robotic guidance is currently based on a preoperative CT scans. The protocol initially dictated by the company demands thin slices and high energy to allow registration of the CT image to intraoperative fluoroscopy. The radiation dose to the patient from CT scans obtained with this protocol is high, and this has led to an ongoing dialogue between the authors of this chapter and the company. This led to two modifications in the recommended protocol of the preoperative CT. The modified protocol reduced the radiation dose to the patient down to 25 % of the original protocol, a level that is close to a normal CT scan of the relevant area of the spine.

Dedicated tele-surgical systems with haptics will be a big breakthrough, allowing spine surgeons to enjoy the proven benefits of this technology [91]. These benefits include better ergonomics and less fatigue, allowing more procedures per day; compensation for the challenges posed by hand tremor, loss of finger grip power, and visual deterioration in older surgeons; and excellent enlarged 3D visualization of the surgical field. Procedures performed with tele-surgical systems may frequently be less invasive, require less retraction of delicate anatomy, result in less blood loss, lead to less damage to soft tissue surrounding the spine, and a lower tendency to tear the dura while maintaining the feel of the surgical field.

Combining tele-surgical systems with image- and/or robotic guidance will allow the surgeon to perform robotic decompression and spinal instrumentation with guidance, and may assist in complicated tasks such as osteotomy and correction of alignment.

Conclusions

Image guidance systems for spine surgery have greatly advanced. They cover the cervical-to-sacral spine, front and back. They increase accuracy, and reduce radiation exposure for surgeons and operating room staff. Future systems are expected to improve visualization of outlying anatomy, decrease registration errors, and incorporate imaging techniques that are not dependent on ionizing radiation.

Robotic guidance for spine surgery is in its infancy, with many systems at different stages of development. The robotic system that is currently on the market has proven to be accurate and to reduce radiation exposure in the hands of trained surgeons who have advanced down a steep learning curve. This system lacks a mechanism to alert the surgeon and correct skiving and slipping from the correct entry point.

The future of tele-surgical systems used in combination with some form of guidance and haptic capabilities is exciting, and will take spine surgeons far beyond the current state-of-the-art.

Acknowledgment The authors wish to thank Shifra Fraifeld, Research Associate and Senior Medical Writer at the Hadassah-Hebrew University Medical Center, for her editorial contribution to the preparation of this manuscript.

Disclosures The Spine Surgery Unit of the Hadassah-Hebrew University Medical Center is a beta site for MazorRobotics Ltd. Dr. Kaplan and Dr. Barzilay are paid consultants for MazorRobotics, and Prof. Liebergal, Dr. Kaplan, and Dr. Barzilay hold options in the company. The authors have no other disclosures that are relevant to this work.

References

1. Weinstein JN, Lurie JD, Olson PR, Bronner KK, Fisher ES. United States' trends and regional variations in lumbar spine surgery: 1992–2003. Spine (Phila Pa 1976). 2006;31(23):2707–14.
2. Amiot LP, Lang K, Putzier M, Zippel H, Labelle H. Comparative results between conventional and computer-assisted pedicle screw installation in the thoracic, lumbar, and sacral spine. Spine (Phila Pa 1976). 2000;25(5):606–14.
3. Belmont Jr PJ, Klemme WR, Dhawan A, Polly Jr DW. In vivo accuracy of thoracic pedicle screws. Spine (Phila Pa 1976). 2001;26(21):2340–6.
4. Belmont Jr PJ, Klemme WR, Robinson M, Polly Jr DW. Accuracy of thoracic pedicle screws in patients with and without coronal plane spinal deformities. Spine (Phila Pa 1976). 2002;27(14):1558–66.
5. Boachie-Adjei O, Girardi FP, Bansal M, Rawlins BA. Safety and efficacy of pedicle screw placement for adult spinal deformity with a pedicle-probing conventional anatomic technique. J Spinal Disord. 2000;13(6):496–500.
6. Carbone JJ, Tortolani PJ, Quartararo LG. Fluoroscopically assisted pedicle screw fixation for thoracic and thoracolumbar injuries: technique and short-term complications. Spine (Phila Pa 1976). 2003;28(1):91–7.
7. Castro WH, Halm H, Jerosch J, Malms J, Steinbeck J, Blasius S. Accuracy of pedicle screw placement in lumbar vertebrae. Spine (Phila Pa 1976). 1996;21(11):1320–4.
8. Esses SI, Sachs BL, Dreyzin V. Complications associated with the technique of pedicle screw fixation. A selected survey of ABS members. Spine (Phila Pa 1976). 1993;18(15):2231–8; discussion 8–9.
9. Farber GL, Place HM, Mazur RA, Jones DE, Damiano TR. Accuracy of pedicle screw placement in lumbar fusions by plain radiographs and computed tomography. Spine (Phila Pa 1976). 1995;20(13):1494–9.
10. Gertzbein SD, Robbins SE. Accuracy of pedicular screw placement in vivo. Spine (Phila Pa 1976). 1990;15(1):11–4.
11. Laine T, Lund T, Ylikoski M, Lohikoski J, Schlenzka D. Accuracy of pedicle screw insertion with and without computer assistance: a randomised controlled clinical study in 100 consecutive patients. Eur Spine J. 2000;9(3):235–40.
12. Laine T, Makitalo K, Schlenzka D, Tallroth K, Poussa M, Alho A. Accuracy of pedicle screw insertion: a prospective CT study in 30 low back patients. Eur Spine J. 1997;6(6):402–5.
13. Liljenqvist UR, Halm HF, Link TM. Pedicle screw instrumentation of the thoracic spine in idiopathic scoliosis. Spine (Phila Pa 1976). 1997;22(19):2239–45.
14. Lonstein JE, Denis F, Perra JH, Pinto MR, Smith MD, Winter RB. Complications associated with pedicle screws. J Bone Joint Surg Am. 1999;81(11):1519–28.
15. Odgers CJ, Vaccaro AR, Pollack ME, Cotler JM. Accuracy of pedicle screw placement with the assistance of lateral plain radiography. J Spinal Disord. 1996;9(4):334–8.
16. Schulze CJ, Munzinger E, Weber U. Clinical relevance of accuracy of pedicle screw placement. A computed tomographic-supported analysis. Spine (Phila Pa 1976). 1998;23(20):2215–20; discussion 20–1.
17. Ludwig SC, Kramer DL, Balderston RA, Vaccaro AR, Foley KF, Albert TJ. Placement of pedicle screws in the human cadaveric cervical spine: comparative accuracy of three techniques. Spine (Phila Pa 1976). 2000;25(13):1655–67.
18. Yoshimoto H, Sato S, Hyakumachi T, Yanagibashi Y, Masuda T. Spinal reconstruction using a cervical pedicle screw system. Clin Orthop Relat Res. 2005;431:111–9.
19. Gelalis ID, Paschos NK, Pakos EE, Politis AN, Arnaoutoglou CM, Karageorgos AC, et al. Accuracy of pedicle screw placement: a systematic review of prospective in vivo studies comparing free hand, fluoroscopy guidance and navigation techniques. Eur Spine J. 2012;21(2):247–55.
20. Suk SI, Lee CK, Kim WJ, Chung YJ, Park YB. Segmental pedicle screw fixation in the treatment of thoracic idiopathic scoliosis. Spine (Phila Pa 1976). 1995;20(12):1399–405.

21. Tian NF, Huang QS, Zhou P, Zhou Y, Wu RK, Lou Y, et al. Pedicle screw insertion accuracy with different assisted methods: a systematic review and meta-analysis of comparative studies. Eur Spine J. 2011;20(6):846–59.
22. Vaccaro AR, Rizzolo SJ, Allardyce TJ, Ramsey M, Salvo J, Balderston RA, et al. Placement of pedicle screws in the thoracic spine. Part I: morphometric analysis of the thoracic vertebrae. J Bone Joint Surg Am. 1995;77(8):1193–9.
23. Vaccaro AR, Rizzolo SJ, Balderston RA, Allardyce TJ, Garfin SR, Dolinskas C, et al. Placement of pedicle screws in the thoracic spine. Part II: an anatomical and radiographic assessment. J Bone Joint Surg Am. 1995;77(8):1200–6.
24. Weinstein JN, Spratt KF, Spengler D, Brick C, Reid S. Spinal pedicle fixation: reliability and validity of roentgenogram-based assessment and surgical factors on successful screw placement. Spine (Phila Pa 1976). 1988;13(9):1012–8.
25. Xu R, Ebraheim NA, Ou Y, Yeasting RA. Anatomic considerations of pedicle screw placement in the thoracic spine. Roy-Camille technique versus open-lamina technique. Spine (Phila Pa 1976). 1998;23(9):1065–8.
26. Schwarzenbach O, Berlemann U, Jost B, Visarius H, Arm E, Langlotz F, et al. Accuracy of computer-assisted pedicle screw placement. An in vivo computed tomography analysis. Spine (Phila Pa 1976). 1997;22(4):452–8.
27. Welch WC, Subach BR, Pollack IF, Jacobs GB. Frameless stereotactic guidance for surgery of the upper cervical spine. Neurosurgery. 1997;40(5):958–63; discussion 63–4.
28. Boos N, Webb JK. Pedicle screw fixation in spinal disorders: a European view. Eur Spine J. 1997;6(1):2–18.
29. Kakkos SK, Shepard AD. Delayed presentation of aortic injury by pedicle screws: report of two cases and review of the literature. J Vasc Surg. 2008;47(5):1074–82.
30. O'Brien JR, Krushinski E, Zarro CM, Sciadini M, Gelb D, Ludwig S. Esophageal injury from thoracic pedicle screw placement in a polytrauma patient: a case report and literature review. J Orthop Trauma. 2006;20(6):431–4.
31. Tian NF, Xu HZ. Image-guided pedicle screw insertion accuracy: a meta-analysis. Int Orthop. 2009;33(4):895–903.
32. Patel AA, Whang PG, Vaccaro AR. Overview of computer-assisted image-guided surgery of the spine. Semin Spin Surg. 2008;20:186–94.
33. Perisinakis K, Damilakis J, Theocharopoulos N, Papadokostakis G, Hadjipavlou A, Gourtsoyiannis N. Patient exposure and associated radiation risks from fluoroscopically guided vertebroplasty or kyphoplasty. Radiology. 2004;232(3):701–7.
34. Chou LB, Cox CA, Tung JJ, Harris AH, Brooks-Terrell D, Sieh W. Prevalence of cancer in female orthopaedic surgeons in the United States. J Bone Joint Surg Am. 2010;92(1): 240–4.
35. Mastrangelo G, Fedeli U, Fadda E, Giovanazzi A, Scoizzato L, Saia B. Increased cancer risk among surgeons in an orthopaedic hospital. Occup Med (Lond). 2005;55(6):498–500.
36. de Berrington Gonzalez A, Mahesh M, Kim KP, Bhargavan M, Lewis R, Mettler F, et al. Projected cancer risks from computed tomographic scans performed in the United States in 2007. Arch Intern Med. 2009;169(22):2071–7.
37. FDA X-Ray record card. Guidelines. Initiative to reduce unnecessary radiation exposure from medical imaging. 2010. Available from: http://www.fda.gov/downloads/Radiation-EmittingProducts/RadiationSafety/RadiationDoseReduction/UCM200087.pdf. Accessed 23 Jan 2013.
38. Linhardt O, Perlick L, Luring C, Stern U, Plitz W, Grifka J. Extracorporeal single dose and radiographic dosage in image-controlled and fluoroscopic navigated pedicle screw implantation. Z Orthop Ihre Grenzgeb. 2005;143(2):175–9.
39. Perisinakis K, Theocharopoulos N, Damilakis J, Katonis P, Papadokostakis G, Hadjipavlou A, et al. Estimation of patient dose and associated radiogenic risks from fluoroscopically guided pedicle screw insertion. Spine (Phila Pa 1976). 2004;29(14):1555–60.

40. Sagi HC, Manos R, Benz R, Ordway NR, Connolly PJ. Electromagnetic field-based image-guided spine surgery part one: results of a cadaveric study evaluating lumbar pedicle screw placement. Spine (Phila Pa 1976). 2003;28(17):2013–8.
41. Sagi HC, Manos R, Park SC, Von Jako R, Ordway NR, Connolly PJ. Electromagnetic field-based image-guided spine surgery part two: results of a cadaveric study evaluating thoracic pedicle screw placement. Spine (Phila Pa 1976). 2003;28(17):E351–4.
42. Slomczykowski M, Roberto M, Schneeberger P, Ozdoba C, Vock P. Radiation dose for pedicle screw insertion. Fluoroscopic method versus computer-assisted surgery. Spine (Phila Pa 1976). 1999;24(10):975–82; discussion 83.
43. Bindal RK, Glaze S, Ognoskie M, Tunner V, Malone R, Ghosh S. Surgeon and patient radiation exposure in minimally invasive transforaminal lumbar interbody fusion. J Neurosurg Spine. 2008;9(6):570–3.
44. Harstall R, Heini PF, Mini RL, Orler R. Radiation exposure to the surgeon during fluoroscopically assisted percutaneous vertebroplasty: a prospective study. Spine (Phila Pa 1976). 2005;30(16):1893–8.
45. Singer G. Occupational radiation exposure to the surgeon. J Am Acad Orthop Surg. 2005;13(1):69–76.
46. George DC, Krag MH, Johnson CC, Van Hal ME, Haugh LD, Grobler LJ. Hole preparation techniques for transpedicle screws. Effect on pull-out strength from human cadaveric vertebrae. Spine (Phila Pa 1976). 1991;16(2):181–4.
47. Brasiliense LB, Theodore N, Lazaro BC, Sayed ZA, Deniz FE, Sonntag VK, et al. Quantitative analysis of misplaced pedicle screws in the thoracic spine: how much pullout strength is lost? Presented at the 2009 joint spine section meeting. J Neurosurg Spine. 2010;12(5):503–8.
48. Holly LT, Foley KT. Image guidance in spine surgery. Orthop Clin North Am. 2007;38(3):451–61; abstract viii.
49. Quinones-Hinojosa A, Robert Kolen E, Jun P, Rosenberg WS, Weinstein PR. Accuracy over space and time of computer-assisted fluoroscopic navigation in the lumbar spine in vivo. J Spinal Disord Tech. 2006;19(2):109–13.
50. Fitzpatrick JM, West JB, Maurer Jr CR. Predicting error in rigid-body point-based registration. IEEE Trans Med Imaging. 1998;17(5):694–702.
51. Holly LT, Bloch O, Johnson JP. Evaluation of registration techniques for spinal image guidance. J Neurosurg Spine. 2006;4(4):323–8.
52. Nottmeier EW. A review of image-guided spinal surgery. J Neurosurg Sci. 2012;56(1):35–47.
53. Lee TC, Yang LC, Liliang PC, Su TM, Rau CS, Chen HJ. Single versus separate registration for computer-assisted lumbar pedicle screw placement. Spine (Phila Pa 1976). 2004;29(14):1585–9.
54. Nottmeier EW, Crosby TL. Timing of paired points and surface matching registration in three-dimensional (3D) image-guided spinal surgery. J Spinal Disord Tech. 2007;20(4):268–70.
55. Peterson MD, Nelson LM, McManus AC, Jackson RP. The effect of operative position on lumbar lordosis. A radiographic study of patients under anesthesia in the prone and 90–90 positions. Spine (Phila Pa 1976). 1995;20(12):1419–24.
56. Deen HG, Nottmeier EW. Balloon kyphoplasty for treatment of sacral insufficiency fractures. Report of three cases. Neurosurg Focus. 2005;18(3):e7.
57. Florensa R, Munoz J, Cardiel I, Bescos A, Tardaguila M, Plans G, et al. Posterior spinal instrumentation image guided and assisted by neuronavigation. Experience in 120 cases. Neurocirugia (Astur). 2011;22(3):224–34.
58. Sakai Y, Matsuyama Y, Yoshihara H, Nakamura H, Nakashima S, Ishiguro N. Simultaneous registration with ct-fluoro matching for spinal navigation surgery. A case report. Nagoya J Med Sci. 2006;68(1–2):45–52.
59. von Jako R, Finn MA, Yonemura KS, Araghi A, Khoo LT, Carrino JA, et al. Minimally invasive percutaneous transpedicular screw fixation: increased accuracy and reduced radiation exposure by means of a novel electromagnetic navigation system. Acta Neurochir (Wien). 2011;153(3):589–96.

60. von Jako RA, Carrino JA, Yonemura KS, Noda GA, Zhue W, Blaskiewicz D, et al. Electromagnetic navigation for percutaneous guide-wire insertion: accuracy and efficiency compared to conventional fluoroscopic guidance. Neuroimage. 2009;47 Suppl 2: T127–32.

61. Penzkofer T, Isfort P, Bruners P, Wiemann C, Kyriakou Y, Kalender WA, et al. Robot arm based flat panel CT-guided electromagnetic tracked spine interventions: phantom and animal model experiments. Eur Radiol. 2010;20(11):2656–62.

62. Cui G, Wang Y, Kao TH, Zhang Y, Liu Z, Liu B, et al. Application of intraoperative computed tomography with or without navigation system in surgical correction of spinal deformity: a preliminary result of 59 consecutive human cases. Spine (Phila Pa 1976). 2012;37(10):891–900.

63. Nottmeier EW, Crosby T. Timing of vertebral registration in three-dimensional, fluoroscopy-based, image-guided spinal surgery. J Spinal Disord Tech. 2009;22(5):358–60.

64. Scheufler KM, Cyron D, Dohmen H, Eckardt A. Less invasive surgical correction of adult degenerative scoliosis, part I: technique and radiographic results. Neurosurgery. 2010; 67(3):696–710.

65. Scheufler KM, Cyron D, Dohmen H, Eckardt A. Less invasive surgical correction of adult degenerative scoliosis. Part II: complications and clinical outcome. Neurosurgery. 2010;67(6):1609–21; discussion 21.

66. Taylor RH, Stoianovici D. Medical robotics in computer-integrated surgery. IEEE Trans Robot Automat. 2003;19(5):765–81.

67. Barzilay Y, Kaplan L, Liebergall M. Miniature robotic guidance for spine surgery. In: Bozociv V, editor. Medical robotics. Available online: http://www.intechopen.com/books/medical_robotics/miniature_robotic_guidance_for_spine_surgery. Accessed 8 Jan 2013. InTech Open: Rijeka; 2008.

68. Nathoo N, Cavusoglu MC, Vogelbaum MA, Barnett GH. In touch with robotics: neurosurgery for the future. Neurosurgery. 2005;56(3):421–33; discussion –33.

69. Bertelsen A, Melo J, Sánchez E, Borro D. A review of surgical robots for spinal interventions. Int J Med Robot. 2012;1(2):18–34.

70. Devito DP, Kaplan L, Dietl R, Pfeiffer M, Horne D, Silberstein B, et al. Clinical acceptance and accuracy assessment of spinal implants guided with SpineAssist surgical robot: retrospective study. Spine (Phila Pa 1976). 2010;35(24):2109–15.

71. Hu X, Ohnmeiss DD, Lieberman IH. Robotic-assisted pedicle screw placement: lessons learned from the first 102 patients. Eur Spine J. 2013;22:661–6.

72. Kantelhardt SR, Martinez R, Baerwinkel S, Burger R, Giese A, Rohde V. Perioperative course and accuracy of screw positioning in conventional, open robotic-guided and percutaneous robotic-guided, pedicle screw placement. Eur Spine J. 2011;20(6):860–8.

73. Pechlivanis I, Kiriyanthan G, Engelhardt M, Scholz M, Lucke S, Harders A, et al. Percutaneous placement of pedicle screws in the lumbar spine using a bone mounted miniature robotic system: first experiences and accuracy of screw placement. Spine (Phila Pa 1976). 2009;34(4):392–8.

74. Ringel F, Stüer C, Reinke A, Preuss A, Behr M, Auer F, et al. Accuracy of robot-assisted placement of lumbar and sacral pedicle screws: a prospective randomized comparison to conventional freehand screw implantation. Spine (Phila Pa 1976). 2012;37(8):E496–501.

75. Roser F, Tatagiba M, Maier G. Spinal robotics: current applications and future perspectives. Neurosurgery. 2013;72 Suppl 1:A12–8.

76. Sukovich W, Brink-Danan S, Hardenbrook M. Miniature robotic guidance for pedicle screw placement in posterior spinal fusion: early clinical experience with the SpineAssist. Int J Med Robot. 2006;2(2):114–22.

77. Shoham M, Burman J, Zehavi E, Joskowicz L, Batkilin E, Kunicher Y. Bone-mounted miniature robot for surgical procedures: concept and clinical applications. IEEE Trans Robot Automat. 2003;19(5):893–901.

78. Wolf A, Shoham M, Michael S, Moshe R. Feasibility study of a mini, bone-attached, robotic system for spinal operations: analysis and experiments. Spine (Phila Pa 1976). 2004;29(2):220–8.

79. Lieberman IH, Togawa D, Kayanja MM, Reinhardt MK, Friedlander A, Knoller N, et al. Bone-mounted miniature robotic guidance for pedicle screw and translaminar facet screw placement: part I – technical development and a test case result. Neurosurgery. 2006;59(3): 641–50; discussion –50.

80. Togawa D, Kayanja MM, Reinhardt MK, Shoham M, Balter A, Friedlander A, et al. Bone-mounted miniature robotic guidance for pedicle screw and translaminar facet screw placement: part 2 – evaluation of system accuracy. Neurosurgery. 2007;60(2 Suppl 1):ONS129–39; discussion ONS39.

81. Barzilay Y, Liebergall M, Fridlander A, Knoller N. Miniature robotic guidance for spine surgery – introduction of a novel system and analysis of challenges encountered during the clinical development phase at two spine centres. Int J Med Robot. 2006;2(2):146–53.

82. Shoham M, Lieberman IH, Benzel EC, Togawa D, Zehavi E, Zilberstein B, et al. Robotic assisted spinal surgery – from concept to clinical practice. Comput Aided Surg. 2007;12(2):105–15.

83. Kim S, Chung J, Yi BJ, Kim YS. An assistive image-guided surgical robot system using O-arm fluoroscopy for pedicle screw insertion: preliminary and cadaveric study. Neurosurgery. 2010;67(6):1757–67; discussion 67.

84. Kostrzewski S, Duff JM, Baur C, Olszewski M. Robotic system for cervical spine surgery. Int J Med Robot. 2012;8(2):184–90.

85. Ortmaier T, Weiss H, Dobele S, Schreiber U. Experiments on robot-assisted navigated drilling and milling of bones for pedicle screw placement. Int J Med Robot. 2006;2(4):350–63.

86. Lee J, Hwang I, Kim K, Choi S, Chung WK, Kim YS. Cooperative robotic assistant with drill-by-wire end-effector for spinal fusion surgery. Ind Robot: Int J. 2009;36(1):60–72.

87. Lee JY, Lega B, Bhowmick D, Newman JG, O'Malley Jr BW, Weinstein GS, et al. Da Vinci robot-assisted transoral odontoidectomy for basilar invagination. ORL J Otorhinolaryngol Relat Spec. 2010;72(2):91–5.

88. Kim MJ, Ha Y, Yang MS, Yoon do H, Kim KN, Kim H, et al. Robot-assisted anterior lumbar interbody fusion (ALIF) using retroperitoneal approach. Acta Neurochir (Wien). 2010;152(4):675–9.

89. Lee JY, O'Malley BW, Newman JG, Weinstein GS, Lega B, Diaz J, et al. Transoral robotic surgery of craniocervical junction and atlantoaxial spine: a cadaveric study. J Neurosurg Spine. 2010;12(1):13–8.

90. Moskowitz RM, Young JL, Box GN, Pare LS, Clayman RV. Retroperitoneal transdiaphragmatic robotic-assisted laparoscopic resection of a left thoracolumbar neurofibroma. JSLS. 2009;13(1):64–8.

91. Ponnusamy K, Chewning S, Mohr C. Robotic approaches to the posterior spine. Spine (Phila Pa 1976). 2009;34(19):2104–9.

92. Ruurda JP, Hanlo PW, Hennipman A, Broeders IA. Robot-assisted thoracoscopic resection of a benign mediastinal neurogenic tumor: technical note. Neurosurgery. 2003;52(2):462–4; discussion 4.

93. Yang MS, Kim KN, Yoon do H, Pennant W, Ha Y. Robot-assisted resection of paraspinal schwannoma. J Korean Med Sci. 2011;26(1):150–3.

94. Yang MS, Yoon do H, Kim KN, Kim H, Yang JW, Yi S. Robot-assisted anterior lumbar interbody fusion in a swine model in vivo test of the da Vinci surgical-assisted spinal surgery system. Spine (Phila Pa 1976). 2011;36(2):E139–43.

95. Arand M, Hartwig E, Hebold D, Kinzl L, Gebhard F. Precision analysis of navigation-assisted implanted thoracic and lumbar pedicled screws. A prospective clinical study. Unfallchirurg. 2001;104(11):1076–81.

96. Arand M, Schempf M, Fleiter T, Kinzl L, Gebhard F. Qualitative and quantitative accuracy of CAOS in a standardized in vitro spine model. Clin Orthop Relat Res. 2006;450:118–28.

97. Assaker R, Reyns N, Vinchon M, Demondion X, Louis E. Transpedicular screw placement: image-guided versus lateral-view fluoroscopy: in vitro simulation. Spine (Phila Pa 1976). 2001;26(19):2160–4.

98. Austin MS, Vaccaro AR, Brislin B, Nachwalter R, Hilibrand AS, Albert TJ. Image-guided spine surgery: a cadaver study comparing conventional open laminoforaminotomy and two image-guided techniques for pedicle screw placement in posterolateral fusion and nonfusion models. Spine (Phila Pa 1976). 2002;27(22):2503–8.

99. Choi WW, Green BA, Levi AD. Computer-assisted fluoroscopic targeting system for pedicle screw insertion. Neurosurgery. 2000;47(4):872–8.

100. Fu TS, Wong CB, Tsai TT, Liang YC, Chen LH, Chen WJ. Pedicle screw insertion: computed tomography versus fluoroscopic image guidance. Int Orthop. 2008;32(4):517–21.

101. Gruetzner P, Waelti H, Vock B, Axel H, Nolte LP, Wentzensen A. Navitation using fluoro-CT technology: concept and clinical experience in a new method for intraoperative navigation. Eur J Trauma. 2004;30(3):161–70.

102. Hart RA, Hansen BL, Shea M, Hsu F, Anderson GJ. Pedicle screw placement in the thoracic spine: a comparison of image-guided and manual techniques in cadavers. Spine (Phila Pa 1976). 2005;30(12):E326–31.

103. Ito H, Neo M, Yoshida M, Fujibayashi S, Yoshitomi H, Nakamura T. Efficacy of computer-assisted pedicle screw insertion for cervical instability in RA patients. Rheumatol Int. 2007;27(6):567–74.

104. John PS, James C, Antony J, Tessamma T, Ananda R, Dinesh K. A novel computer-assisted technique for pedicle screw insertion. Int J Med Robot. 2007;3:59–63.

105. Kotani Y, Abumi K, Ito M, Takahata M, Sudo H, Ohshima S, et al. Accuracy analysis of pedicle screw placement in posterior scoliosis surgery: comparison between conventional fluoroscopic and computer-assisted technique. Spine (Phila Pa 1976). 2007;32(14):1543–50.

106. Laine T, Schlenzka D, Makitalo K, Tallroth K, Nolte LP, Visarius H. Improved accuracy of pedicle screw insertion with computer-assisted surgery. A prospective clinical trial of 30 patients. Spine (Phila Pa 1976). 1997;22(11):1254–8.

107. Lee GY, Massicotte EM, Rampersaud YR. Clinical accuracy of cervicothoracic pedicle screw placement: a comparison of the "open" lamino-foraminotomy and computer-assisted techniques. J Spinal Disord Tech. 2007;20(1):25–32.

108. Lekovic GP, Potts EA, Karahalios DG, Hall G. A comparison of two techniques in image-guided thoracic pedicle screw placement: a retrospective study of 37 patients and 277 pedicle screws. J Neurosurg Spine. 2007;7(4):393–8.

109. Li SG, Sheng L, Zhao H. Computer-assisted navigation technique in the spinal pedical screw internal fixation. J Clin Rehabil Tissue Eng Res. 2009;13:3365–9.

110. Li Y. The study of clinical anatomy of cervical pedicle with Iso-C arm and clinical application of Iso-C navigation system. Master's thesis, Shandong University; 2007.

111. Liu YJ, Tian W, Liu B, Li Q, Hu L, Li ZY, et al. Accuracy of CT-based navigation of pedicle screws implantation in the cervical spine compared with X-ray fluoroscopy technique. Zhonghua Wai Ke Za Zhi. 2005;43(20):1328–30.

112. Ludwig SC, Kowalski JM, Edwards 2nd CC, Heller JG. Cervical pedicle screws: comparative accuracy of two insertion techniques. Spine (Phila Pa 1976). 2000;25(20):2675–81.

113. Merloz P, Tonetti J, Pittet L, Coulomb M, Lavallee S, Sautot P. Pedicle screw placement using image guided techniques. Clin Orthop Relat Res. 1998;354:39–48.

114. Merloz P, Troccaz J, Vouaillat H, Vasile C, Tonetti J, Eid A, et al. Fluoroscopy-based navigation system in spine surgery. Proc Inst Mech Eng H. 2007;221(7):813–20.

115. Mirza SK, Wiggins GC, Kuntz C, York JE, Bellabarba C, Knonodi MA, et al. Accuracy of thoracic vertebral body screw placement using standard fluoroscopy, fluoroscopic image guidance, and computed tomographic image guidance: a cadaver study. Spine (Phila Pa 1976). 2003;28(4):402–13.

116. Nottmeier EW, Seemer W, Young PM. Placement of thoracolumbar pedicle screws using three-dimensional image guidance: experience in a large patient cohort. J Neurosurg Spine. 2009;10(1):33–9.

117. Rajasekaran S, Vidyadhara S, Ramesh P, Shetty AP. Randomized clinical study to compare the accuracy of navigated and non-navigated thoracic pedicle screws in deformity correction surgeries. Spine (Phila Pa 1976). 2007;32(2):E56–64.

118. Richter M, Cakir B, Schmidt R. Cervical pedicle screws: conventional versus computer-assisted placement of cannulated screws. Spine (Phila Pa 1976). 2005;30(20):2280–7.
119. Sakai Y, Matsuyama Y, Nakamura H, Katayama Y, Imagama S, Ito Z, et al. Segmental pedicle screwing for idiopathic scoliosis using computer-assisted surgery. J Spinal Disord Tech. 2008;21(3):181–6.
120. Schnake KJ, Konig B, Berth U, Schroeder RJ, Kandziora F, Stockle U, et al. Accuracy of CT-based navigation of pedicle screws in the thoracic spine compared with conventional technique. Unfallchirurg. 2004;107(2):104–12.
121. Seller K, Wild A, Urselmann L, Krauspe R. Prospective screw misplacement analysis after conventional and navigated pedicle screw implantation. Biomed Tech (Berl). 2005;50(9):287–92.
122. Tian W, Liu B, Li Q, et al. Experience of pedicle screw fixation in the cervical spine using navigation system. J Spinal Surg. 2003;1:15–8.
123. Xu L, Yu X, Zheng DB, et al. Preliminary application of spinal navigation with the intra-operative 3D-imaging modality in pedicle screw fixation. Orthop J Chin. 2004;12:1895–7.
124. Yan H, Rong K, Shi-yuan F, De-wan Y, Shou-min L, Zhang B, et al. Comparison study between C-arm X-ray and 3D CT in guiding thoracolumbar pedicle screw fixation. Shandong Med J. 2009;49:5–7.
125. Yang LL, Chen HJ, Chen DY. Clinical applications of computer assisted navigation technique in scoliosis surgery. Orthop J Chin. 2007;15:1772–6.
126. Yong-hong YE, Hong Z, Jie Z, Qing Z, Zhang DS. Application of orthopaedic guidance for pedicle screw fixation of spine. Orthop J Chin. 2005;13:75–6.
127. Zhang DS, Yuan JT, Zheng J. Pedical screw placement under the guidance of computer-assisted navigation system. Chin J Min Inv Surg. 2008;8:544–6.
128. Bai YS, Zhang Y, Chen ZQ, Wang CF, Zhao YC, Shi ZC, et al. Learning curve of computer-assisted navigation system in spine surgery. Chin Med J (Engl). 2010;123(21):2989–94.
129. Kim KD, Patrick Johnson J, Bloch BO, Masciopinto JE. Computer-assisted thoracic pedicle screw placement: an in vitro feasibility study. Spine (Phila Pa 1976). 2001;26(4):360–4.
130. Nakanishi K, Tanaka M, Misawa H, Sugimoto Y, Takigawa T, Ozaki T. Usefulness of a navigation system in surgery for scoliosis: segmental pedicle screw fixation in the treatment. Arch Orthop Trauma Surg. 2009;129(9):1211–8.
131. Sasso RC, Garrido BJ. Computer-assisted spinal navigation versus serial radiography and operative time for posterior spinal fusion at L5-S1. J Spinal Disord Tech. 2007;20(2):118–22.
132. Kosmopoulos V, Schizas C. Pedicle screw placement accuracy: a meta-analysis. Spine (Phila Pa 1976). 2007;32(3):E111–20.
133. Shin BJ, James AR, Njoku IU, Hartl R. Pedicle screw navigation: a systematic review and meta-analysis of perforation risk for computer-navigated versus freehand insertion. J Neurosurg Spine. 2012;17(2):113–22.
134. Wu H, Gao ZL, Wang JC, Li YP, Xia P, Jiang R. Pedicle screw placement in the thoracic spine: a randomized comparison study of computer-assisted navigation and conventional techniques. Chin J Traumatol. 2010;13(4):201–5.
135. Yu X, Xu L, Bi LY. Spinal navigation with intra-operative 3D-imaging modality in lumbar pedicle screw fixation. Zhonghua Yi Xue Za Zhi. 2008;88(27):1905–8.
136. Li SG, Sheng L, Zhao H, Zhang JG, Zhai JL, Zhu Y. Clinical applications of computer-assisted navigation technique in spinal pedicle screw internal fixation. Zhonghua Yi Xue Za Zhi. 2009;89(11):736–9.
137. Rampersaud YR, Foley KT, Shen AC, Williams S, Solomito M. Radiation exposure to the spine surgeon during fluoroscopically assisted pedicle screw insertion. Spine (Phila Pa 1976). 2000;25(20):2637–45.
138. Izadpanah K, Konrad G, Sudkamp NP, Oberst M. Computer navigation in balloon kyphoplasty reduces the intraoperative radiation exposure. Spine (Phila Pa 1976). 2009;34(12):1325–9.
139. Mroz TE, Abdullah KG, Steinmetz MP, Klineberg EO, Lieberman IH. Radiation exposure to the surgeon during percutaneous pedicle screw placement. J Spinal Disord Tech. 2011;24(4):264–7.

140. Kim CW, Lee YP, Taylor W, Oygar A, Kim WK. Use of navigation-assisted fluoroscopy to decrease radiation exposure during minimally invasive spine surgery. Spine J. 2008;8(4): 584–90.
141. Smith HE, Welsch MD, Sasso RC, Vaccaro AR. Comparison of radiation exposure in lumbar pedicle screw placement with fluoroscopy vs computer-assisted image guidance with intraoperative three-dimensional imaging. J Spinal Cord Med. 2008;31(5):532–7.
142. Schaeren S, Roth J, Dick W. Effective in vivo radiation dose with image reconstruction controlled pedicle instrumentation vs. CT-based navigation. Orthopade. 2002;31(4):392–6.
143. Zhang J, Weir V, Fajardo L, Lin J, Hsiung H, Ritenour ER. Dosimetric characterization of a cone-beam O-arm imaging system. J Xray Sci Technol. 2009;17(4):305–17.
144. Kim JS, Eun SS, Prada N, Choi G, Lee SH. Modified transcorporeal anterior cervical microforaminotomy assisted by O-arm-based navigation: a technical case report. Eur Spine J. 2011;20 Suppl 2:S147–52.
145. Silbermann J, Riese F, Allam Y, Reichert T, Koeppert H, Gutberlet M. Computer tomography assessment of pedicle screw placement in lumbar and sacral spine: comparison between freehand and O-arm based navigation techniques. Eur Spine J. 2011;20(6):875–81.
146. Johnson JP, Stokes JK, Oskouian RJ, Choi WW, King WA. Image-guided thoracoscopic spinal surgery: a merging of 2 technologies. Spine (Phila Pa 1976). 2005;30(19):E572–8.
147. Lieberman IH, Hardenbrook MA, Wang JC, Guyer RD. Assessment of pedicle screw placement accuracy, procedure time, and radiation exposure using a miniature robotic guidance system. J Spinal Disord Tech. 2012;25(5):241–8.
148. Ringel F, Stoffel M, Stuer C, Meyer B. Minimally invasive transmuscular pedicle screw fixation of the thoracic and lumbar spine. Neurosurgery. 2006;59(4 Suppl 2):ONS361–6; discussion ONS6–7.

Chapter 15
Bone Substitution in Spine Fusion: The Past, the Present, and the Future

Giandomenico Logroscino and Wanda Lattanzi

Introduction

Bone fusion represents a challenge in orthopedics practice, in particular when a pathological condition, such as non-union fractures, osteomyelitis, critical size defects, may imply a reduced biological response. This is why recently basic research has been addressing this issue and new and innovative products have been introduced into clinical practice. Spinal fusion can be defined as the bony union between two vertebral bodies after surgical treatment. Each year in the USA, more than 200,000 spine fusions are performed. From 1993 to 2001, the rate of cervical spine fusion increased to 433 %, while the rate of thoracolumbar fusion increased from 52 to 352 %. Despite the advances in surgical techniques and the increasing use of stabilization systems, the incidence of nonunion for lumbar fusions remains high (10–40 %) [1, 2].

This chapter aims to describe the variety of techniques commonly used for bone fusion in spinal surgery (bone grafts, bone substitutes, growth factors, and stem cells) and the future developments of the research in this field [3, 4].

G. Logroscino, MD (✉)
Department of Orthopaedics and Traumatology,
Università Cattolica del Sacro Cuore,
L.go F. Vito 1, Rome 00168, Italy
e-mail: g.logroscino@fastwebnet.it

W. Lattanzi, MD
Department of Anatomy and Cell Biology,
Università Cattolica del Sacro Cuore,
Rome, Italy

P.P.M. Menchetti (ed.), *Minimally Invasive Surgery of the Lumbar Spine*,
DOI 10.1007/978-1-4471-5280-4_15, © Springer-Verlag London 2014

Fig. 15.1 The "diamond concept"

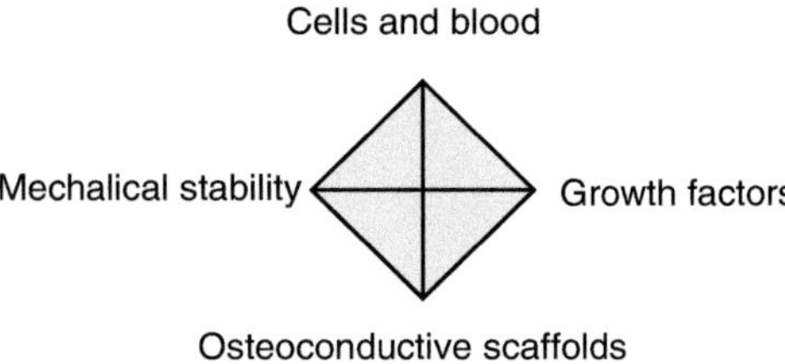

Spine Fusion and Bone Substitutes

The biological principles of bone fusion have been more deeply studied in the past years.

It has been calculated that bone grafting is the second most common tissue transplant in the world, after the blood. In the USA more than 500,000 bone grafts are implanted every year. Of these bone-grafting procedures, the 50 % are spine fusions. The purpose of bone grafts in spinal fusion is to enhance bone healing obtaining a faster biological stability. Spine fusion depends on the availability of adequate osteogenic cells, the presence of osteoconductive matrix within the region in which new bone tissue is desired, osteoinductive signals within the graft, an adequate blood supply to support a local bone healing response, and a local mechanical environment suitable for bone formation.

The basic requirements for bone healing were well described by Giannoudis in 2007 [5] who proposed a more fundamental principle: "the diamond concept."

Bone healing depends on four main factors that interact together. When bone healing is delayed or missing (nonunion), one or more of these factors are lost and bone will never heal. The four factors of "the diamond concept" are the following (Fig. 15.1):

- The osteogenic cells and blood supply
- Mechanical stability
- Growth factors
- Osteoconductive scaffolds (in combination with growth factors)

Theoretically, the ideal bone substitute would be osteoconductive, osteoinductive, resorbable, not immunogenic, free from the risk of disease transmission, and easy to use and, finally, should be mechanically adequate and cost-effective.

The osteogenic properties of a graft is derived from viable stem and progenitor cells that can be transplanted as part of the transplant in conditions where they can survive and directly contribute to the formation of new bone. Osteoinductive activity refers to the ability of certain stimuli, peptide growth factors, to stimulate cellular events that transform an immature cell in a cell that is activated and committed to new bone formation. The prototype of osteoinductive factors is the family of bone morphogenetic proteins (BMP), in particular BMPSs 2, 4, 6, 7, and 9, which are more osteoinductive. Osteoconductive is the result of the structural characteristics

Table 15.1 Bone substitutes resuming

			Osteoinduction	Osteoconduction	Strength	Resorbibility
Biological	Autografts		+	+	+	+
	Allografts		+/−	+	+	+
	Xenografts		+/−	+	+	+
Synthetic	Calcium-based	HA-TCP-HA/TCP	−	+	+/−	+/−
	Polymer-based		−	+/−	+/−	+
Growth factors	BMPs		+	+	−	+
	DBM		+/−	+	−	+
	PDGF		+/−	+	−	+
Cellular based	Bone marrow		+/−	+/−	−	+
	Stem cells		+	+	−	+

+: the material has this property

−: the material does not have this property

+/− : the material has intermediate properties

and the surface of a graft matrix. Osteoconductivity refers to the ability of a matrix graft to improve migration of osteoblastic stem cells and progenitors, as well as other cells that contribute to bone healing response. The osteoconductivity of a matrix is a function of its macrostructure or architecture, the size and the connection between the pores of the material, and its structure and surface chemistry and surface.

Unfortunately, at present, no bone substitutes answer to all of these requirements.

Actually bone replacement can be performed with three main categories of substitutes (Table 15.1):

- Biological bone grafts (autograft, homograft, xenograft)
- Synthetic bone substitutes (calcium-based, polymer-based)
- Growth factors (DBM, BMP, PDGF)
- Bone marrow and stem cells

Each of them has strengths and weaknesses and will be subsequently discussed.

Biological Bone Grafts

Basically three types of bone grafts are available:

- Autografts: the donor is the same as the receiver.
- Allografts: the donor is human but is different from the receiver.
- Xenografts: the donor is from the animal being.

The history of bone grafts was firstly written by the Dutch Job van Meekeren in 1632, which has successfully implanted a bone of a dog in a human. Since the critics of the Catholic Church, the transplant was subsequently explanted. Only in the late nineteenth and early twentieth century, the theory of "creeping substitution" of bone grafts was described by Axhausen [6], Phemister [7], and Barth [8] who described the second integration mechanism of bone grafts.

Autologous bone grafts have an average rate of 77 % fusion (cervical spine) [9]. Autologous bone has all the properties essential for bone formation and is therefore considered the graft material of choice for the fusion of the spine. Autografts achieve osteoconductive and osteoinductive requirements, strength, growth factors, osteogenic cells, no risk of transmission disease, and immune response and are slowly replaced by newly formed bone. The disadvantages include a constant rate of morbidity (30 %) as bleeding or hematoma, infection, neurovascular injury fracture, and cosmetic deformity at the removal site (iliac crest or fibula) and longer operative time [2, 10]. Unfortunately, only limited amounts of autologous bone can be obtained from a patient, and this is a significant limitation.

Allografts are used to avoid the complications of autografts (donor site morbidity and availability). Tissue banks has grown fast in the 1980s, but doubts and concerns arise about the costs and the problems associated with storage. The bone of a human donor is osteoconductive and osteoinductive (growth factors but no cells), but storage is detrimental to the mechanical qualities of the material. The risk of infection was the first critic to allografts. Since 1989 only two documented cases of HIV have been reported with a hazard ratio of 1:1.6 million people. Other infectious risks are most important like HBV (1 case), HCV (2 cases), a fatal infection by Clostridium difficile, and 26 bacterial infections [11, 12].

Xenografts are an alternative and are more documented in the dental surgery than in orthopedic surgery. Xenotransplants are obtained from porcine, bovine, and equine donors. Bovine bone was introduced by Maatz and Bauermeister in 1957 [13, 14]. Heterologous bone (xenograft) fails to induce bone repair because of its high level of antigenicity. Partially deproteinated and partially defatted heterologous bone (Kiel bone or Oswestry bone) exhibits a significantly reduced antigenicity and minimal immune response. The process of denaturation, however, also destroys the proteins matrix, and osteoinductive properties are missed. The impregnation of this material with cells capable of osteogenic activity was studied. Doubts have been argued regarding "zoonoses," diseases transmitted from animals to humans, such as BSE (bovine spongiform encephalopathy) or PERV (porcine endogenous retroviruses) [13]. The results are contradictory with some authors reporting favorable results. However, given the wide availability of allogeneic materials at a similar cost, xenografts are rarely used. In addition [15–19], poor results in hip surgery, with 25 % of pseudo-infection complications, were reported recently. The main advantages are the low cost, the easy availability, the osteoconductivity, and the good mechanical properties [20].

Synthetic Bone Substitutes

The solution for bone replacement has been ideally found in synthetic bone substitutes. A level II and level IV study found less pain, operation time, blood loss, and complications in synthetic substitutes compared to iliac crest grafts [21].

Two categories are known:

- Ceramic bone substitutes
- Polymer bone substitutes

Ceramic-based substitutes are the most often used in the operating theatre. They are osteoconductive but often are rarely good mechanically. They have no osteoinductive capacity and, depending on the degree of the amorphous phase (tricalcium phosphate), are resorbable.

Three categories of ceramic substitutes are mainly present on the market:

- TCP
- HA
- Mix of HA and TCP

Generally the ceramic substitutes are based on calcium. Often a mixture of HA (hydroxyapatite) and the amorphous phase of TCP (tricalcium phosphate) is used. Depending on the concentration, HA is a relatively inert substance that persists in vivo for prolonged periods of time, while the more porous TCP undergoes biodegradation typically within 6 weeks after its introduction in the area of bone formation. TCP with a Ca:P molar ratio of 1.5 is resorbed too quickly, while HA with a Ca:P ratio of 1.67 resorbs too slowly. HA achieves very high mechanical strength, while TCP has poor mechanical qualities. Biphasic calcium phosphates, which combine (40–60 %) TCP with (60–40 %) HA, can produce a more physiological balance between mechanical support and bone resorption [22].

HA is widely known and proven to be safe and effective in bone substitution. HA-TCP are now available in the form of blocks, granules, and injectable kit. Macroporosity of about 100–400 μm and interconnected porosity are necessary for bone growth. Depending on the concentration of HA and TCP, the strength is variable between 10 and 60 MPa that is lower than the compressive strength of cortical bone (150–200 MP), and this is one of the main limitations of ceramic-based biomaterials. A variant of these materials is the coralline HA that is obtained by the hydrothermal conversion of calcium carbonate of the coral skeleton (ProOsteon 200 (50 % porosity) or 500 (65 % porosity)). These materials have been tested on animals for spine fusion [23]. In humans, Dai and Jiang have published a controlled study on interbody cages and concluded that β-TCP is an appropriate treatment for cervical fusion, and good results have been reported by many other authors for HA or HA/TCP [24–26].

Nanometric and Biomimetic Bone Substitutes

In the past, synthetic HA-based substitutes were a mere and simple chemical reproduction of the natural HA (Ca, P). On the contrary, it is well known that bone has a more sophisticated structure and is a nanostructured, precisely organized compound of Ca, P, and collagen [27]. At a nanometric level, bone is structured in crystalline HA units regularly oriented on collagen fibers [28]. New nanotechnologies show that it is possible to assemble materials starting from the primary microscopic units, nano-molecules, by a process called "bottom to the top," producing biologically active and intelligent macromolecules. On this regard, recently, a new class of synthetic HA-based bone substitutes have been proposed, that are both chemically and functionally similar to the bone mineralized matrix. These new synthetic nanotechnology materials have, in their chemical composition, bioactive ions able to interact directly with the environment, to modify the properties of the materials as a function of local stimulus. This is possible by adding to the stoichiometric HA active ions such as Mg_2+ (6–14 % of moles Ca) and CO_3 (3–8 % by weight) and F, Si, Sr, and CO_3 substitutes. These materials are members of a new family of bone substitutes, called "biomimetic," for their capacity to mime human bone. It has been described that these ceramic substitutes achieve biological properties that correspond to those of human bone matrix [28–35]. In fact, Mg-CO_3-substituted hydroxyapatite is highly concentrated in natural bone tissues during the initial phases of osteogenesis, while it tends to disappear when the bone is mature. Magnesium is indeed able to accelerate the kinetics of natural nucleation of HA, while Mg depletion affects negatively bone formation. Furthermore, the Mg replacement adds solubility and faster resorption properties to the material. Consequently, this material has been shown to have a very high kinetics of osseointegration in the biological environment. Newly formed bone matrix synthesis, followed by fast and efficient bone remodeling in structured mature bone, was observed in previous animal studies [34, 35].

Injectable Bone Substitutes

Injectable bone substitutes were recently introduced in the clinical practice to adjuvate minimally invasive procedures (MIS) and tissue-sparing surgery (TSS) in order to reduce morbidity and costs. In spine surgery, two techniques are available for injectable introduction of bone substitutes: vertebroplasty and kyphoplasty (Fig. 15.2).

In these techniques, actually, the most common and the gold standard material used is PMMA (polymethyl methacrylate). This material is not resorbable and it is not indicated in younger patients.

Related to bone response, PMMA is classified as a bio-inert material. An increasing number of young patients with acute traumatic compression and burst fractures

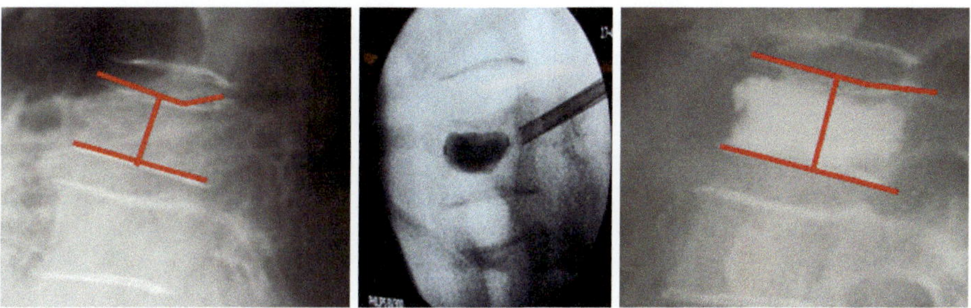

Fig. 15.2 Kyphoplasty restoring the healing of vertebral body fracture

have recently undergone kyphoplasty. For a population of this age, the use of PMMA cement should raise some biocompatibility questions and serious drawbacks. These problems might generate little interest in elderly patients with painful and degenerative spines that are readily and successfully treated by PMMA-based vertebroplasty. However, in a young and active population, the PMMA biocompatibility problems are unacceptable if they have the potential to induce degeneration later in life. Consequently, the selection of a more reliable material is crucial for future spine surgery.

To obviate to these problems and premising that the gold standard, to be compared with, is PMMA, we will try to describe the optimal qualities that will be necessary for an optimal injectable bone substitute to be used in spine surgery:

- Injectable
- Low viscosity (equal to not less than 100 Pa s)
- Mixture time: from 3 to 4.5 min at room temperature (19–22 °C)
- Workability life: from 2 to 2.6 min at room temperature (19–22 °C)
- Early setting time from 4.5 to 10 min at 37 °C
- Delayed hardening time from 12 to 24 h at 37 °C
- Hardening without exothermic reaction (below 56 °C) at 37 °C
- Radiopaque (barium sulfate ($BaSO_4$), zirconium oxide (ZrO_2), or other components)
- Resorbable (in a period variable between 45 days and 6 months)
- Drillable for screw after a few minutes
- Osteoconductive or osteoinductive
- Biomimetic (doped with Mg, CO_3, Sr, F ions)
- Mechanically adequate (60–150 MPa)
- Porosity: macroporosity of 200–500 μ and interconnected microporosity (in total 30–60 %)

Calcium Phosphate Cements

As an alternative, self-hardening synthetic injectable calcium phosphate cements have been developed for this purpose. A milestone study published by Hillmeier et al.

comparing kyphoplasty with PMMA or calcium phosphate in osteoporotic and traumatic fractures either stand-alone or with associated posterior fixation reported comparable results [36, 37]. The suggested biocompatibility problems specifically related to polymethyl methacrylate are not present in calcium phosphate cement. Calcium phosphate cements are biocompatible materials, without local heating or toxic effects on the surrounding bone tissue, and are bioactively degraded over time by creeping substitution and can stimulate the formation of new bone at the bone-material interface (osteoconductivity). Some authors have demonstrated a similar compression strength and stiffness on human cadaveric studies on vertebroplasty with calcium phosphate cement and PMMA but have also shown that calcium phosphate cements are inferior than acrylic cements in withstanding (cyclic) to torque and stress forces. Verlaan et al. [38], in a cadaveric model, found no bone displacement after balloon kyphoplasty with calcium phosphate cements. A biomechanical study on the transpedicular vertebral body reinforcement of thoracolumbar burst fractures with hydroxyapatite cement showed that this augmentation reduced pedicle screw-bending moments and increased significantly initial stiffness in the flexion-extension plane. A recent biomechanical in vitro tests of human osteoporotic lumbar spine after prophylactic kyphoplasty with different materials (PMMA, calcium phosphate, and silicon-based material) showed that the calcium phosphate cements displayed in vitro identical mechanical behavior (similar subsidence) in axial compression to PMMA [39].

Recently, some calcium phosphate biomaterials have been studied in kyphoplasty:

Calcibon (Biomet, Wehrheim, Germany) is a calcium phosphate cement in a radiopaque liquid that hardens quickly. It is a synthetic material which comprises two constituents: powder consisting of (tricalcium phosphate, calcium hydrogen phosphate, calcium carbonate, and hydroxyapatite) and a liquid part (aqueous di-sodium-hydrogen-phosphate solution). The material is available since June 2002 for clinical use. The material is obtained with a time of cohesion of 1 min, a time of initial setting of 3 min, and a final time of 7.5 min at 37 °C without exothermic reaction. A compressive strength of 30 MPa is reached at 6 h and 60 MPa at 3 days. Enhanced capacity of biological osteoconduction after 6 months without cellular toxicity or mutation was confirmed in animal study [37]. Furthermore, the process of rapid hardening of calcium phosphate and the lack of exothermic reaction appear to be advantageous compared to PMMA, in particular in the case of losses in proximity to vital structures [29, 36, 38–50].

KYPHON (ActivOs 10 Bone Cement, Medtronic, Inc.) is a PMMA bone cement containing hydroxyapatite (HA) available on the market since June 2010. ActivOs 10 includes the advantages of HA without sacrificing the reliability of a PMMA cement. The cement has great handling characteristics, is highly radiopaque, and has optimal working time for doctors to complete the procedure kyphoplasty. It is reported that in a nonhuman trial where KYPHON ActivOs 10 Bone Cement with HA was implanted into eight rabbit femurs, new bone was seen to form on the surface of the cement without a layer of fibrous tissue and no foreign body inflammatory reaction was observed. This suggests that the surface of the cement is compatible with bone. Unfortunately, no literature is available on this hybrid procedure.

Although, numerous reports of in vitro and in vivo investigations dealing with calcium phosphate (CaP) cements have been published, there are still some problems to overcome. These mainly concern the setting time, compressive strength, and the rate of degradation of the cement in vivo.

The use of injectable calcium phosphate cements in spine surgery is hampered by two issues: an increased washout trend and a low resistance to mechanical stress (bending, tension, and shear). Actually, PMMA is ten times more resistant to bending forces, tension, and shear, than CaP cements. Experiments are currently underway to investigate the possibility of reducing the effect of washout using different additives (hydroxypropylmethylcellulose, carboxyl methylcellulose, chitosan). Attempts to improve the biomechanical properties of CaP cements are currently following two different paths: on one hand, the possibility of structural stabilization by primary fiber reinforcements (aramide, carbon, bioglass) and, on the other hand, improved bone coverage by osteoinductive substances, resulting in earlier secondary integration [53].

Future Trends in Spine Fusion

All the strenuous research efforts achieved so far, although improving the surgical protocol, did not allow avoiding cortical harvesting or cancellous bone autografts, which are associated with donor site morbidity. The further development of improved strategies for spinal fusion would plausibly benefit from the progress of stem cell biology and applications. In addition, the progressive clarification of the whole molecular scenario that orchestrates osteogenesis and bone healing is regularly providing new osteoinductive genes to be tested as potential therapeutic agents in spine surgery. Diverse studies described possible applications of gene therapy for achieving bone healing and spine fusion in animal models [54–56]. The most convincing results recently obtained from experimental spine fusion strategies are based on the use of cell-based approaches, i.e., engineered cells, which have been appropriately manipulated in vitro to express osteoinductive genes [57]. Genetically engineered cells can therefore maintain physiologic doses of a gene product for a sustained period once inoculated into the selected anatomical site, facilitating an efficient bone healing [58].

Cell-Based Approaches for Spinal Fusion

Cell-based approaches for bone formation and regeneration are widely considered the most effective, as they are able to efficiently produce the physiologic osteogenic process in vivo. In particular, mesenchymal stem cells (MSCs) have been widely used as suitable somatic stem cells to induce bone formation and regeneration [57, 59, 60]. MSCs are pluripotent somatic stem cells, residing in the connective stroma of mesenchymal-derived adult organs and tissues; hence they are also named "stromal stem cells" [61]. They are capable of extensive self-renewal, plasticity, and multilineage potential, being able to differentiate along all mesodermal tissue lineages [62].

Originally, MSCs were isolated from bone marrow aspirates (bone marrow-derived mesenchymal stem cells, BMSCs); thereafter, they have been found in quite any organ endowed with a connective stroma, including adipose tissue, lung, skeletal muscle, synovial, tendons and skin, along with antenatal tissues such as umbilical cord, placenta, and amniotic fluid [63–67]. MSCs are easily isolated through collagenase digestion and adherence selection in vitro; they can be further subcultured for several culture passages, without losing their plasticity and self-renewal potential [68]. Nonetheless, they display a limited plasticity and lifespan in culture compared to embryonic stem cells and induced pluripotent stem cells, lessening the risk of tumorigenicity [69]. Cultured MSCs have proved to be efficient osteoprogenitor cells, as they can easily be induced along the osteogenic lineage, upon appropriate in vitro induction. This property has been exploited for cell-based therapy of congenital bone disorders [70, 71]. In addition, MSCs proved to yield bone formation in vivo, by differentiating into osteoblasts and producing extracellular matrix, increasing ALP activity and the expression of osteo-specific genes in the grafted area [56, 59, 72]. The feasibility of an MSC-based approach to orthopedic surgery comes also from their innate immunomodulatory properties which suggest a potential use in allogeneic transplantation, preventing graft-versus-host disease [73].

Most experimental data on the preclinical use of MSC for bone regeneration purposes were obtained with BMSC. Nevertheless, the main limitation of using BMSC in the clinical setting still derives from the pain and invasiveness of bone marrow collection, the scarcity of this tissue source in adults, and the limited number of bone marrow sample donors available for allogeneic transplantation. In addition, the number of BMSC with osteogenic potential is thought to decrease with old age, when most indications for regenerative medicine approaches arise [74]. At the time of this writing, there is a single active phase I clinical trial testing ex vivo-expanded autologous BMSC for spinal fusion in spine degenerative disease (www. clinicaltrials.gov). Recent findings suggested that MSCs residing in the stromal-vascular fraction of adipose tissue (namely, adipose tissue-derived stromal cells, ATSC) display higher plasticity and extended self-renewal capability, compared to BMSCs. BMSCs and ATSCs share a common immunophenotype and, in part, a gene expression profile that is consistent with their stemness upholding and uncommitted status [75–78]. Not only ATSCs are obtained from a tissue source that is usually abundant in most adults, but also high yield of cell isolation can be easily obtained in primary culture, from limited volume of lipoaspirate. Such features suggest potentially great advantages of ATSC over BMSC, in bridging the bench-to-bed gap in regenerative medicine.

With regard to spinal surgery, distinct preclinical studies have tested the effectiveness of either BMSC or ATSC, in animal model of spinal fusion, combined with alternative scaffold and/or cell engineering strategies, with successful results (Table 15.2). Most studies transplanted allogeneic cells into immunocompetent

Table 15.2 Cell-based gene therapy in animal models of spine fusion

BMSC

Fusion	Species	Type of transplantation	Cell treatment	Graft	Reference
PLF	Rabbit	Autologous	AdBMP2	Collagen sponge	Riew et al. [79]
PLF	Rabbit	Autologous	AdBMP2	None	Cheng et al. [80]
PF	Rat	Xenogenic	None	Matrigel	Cui et al. [81]
PF	Rat	Allogeneic	AdBMP7	Allograft	Hidaka et al. [82]
PLF	Macaque	Autologous	None	Beta-TCP	Orii et al. [83]
PLF	Goat	Autologous	None	Different ceramics	Kruyt et al. [84]
PLF	Rat	Allogeneic	Lenti-BMP2 Adeno-BMP2	Collagen sponge	Miyazaki et al. [85]
PLF	Rat	Allogeneic	Lenti-BMP2	Collagen sponge	Miyazaki et al. [86]
PLF	Rabbit	Xenogeneic	None	CRM	Kim et al. [87]
PLF	Rabbit	Autologous	rhBMP2	Alginate	Fu et al. [88]
PLF	Mouse	Xenogeneic	None	Collagen sponge	Rao et al. [89]
PLF	Rabbit	Autologous	Hyperbaric O_2	Alginate	Fu et al. [90]
PLF	Rabbit	Allogeneic	None	Pro-Osteon 500R	Giannicola et al. [91]
PLF	Rat	Xenogeneic	None	Ceramic	Geuze et al. [92]
PLF	Rabbit	Autologous	AdSmad1C	Gelatin sponge	Douglas et al. [93]
PLF	Rat	Xenogeneic	Oxysterols	Collagen sponge	Johnson et al. [94]
PLF	Rabbit	Allogeneic	None	HA/COL	Huang et al. [72]
AIBF	Pig	Allogeneic	None	mPCL/TCP	Abbah et al. [95]

ATSC

Fusion	Species	Type of transplantation	Cell treatment	Scaffold/graft	Reference
PLF	Rat	Xenogeneic	rhBMP2	Type I collagen	Hsu et al. [96]
PF	Mice	Xenogeneic	rhBMP6	None	Sheyn et al. [97]
PLF	Rat	Xenogeneic	AdenoBMP2	Collagen sponge	Miyazaki et al. [85, 86]
PLF	Rat	Autologous + allogeneic	None	TCP /collagen	Lopez et al. [98]
PLF	Rat	Autologous + allogeneic	None	Beta-TCP/ collagen	McIntosh et al. [99]
PF	Goat	Allogeneic	None	PLCL	Vergroesen et al. [100]
PLF	Rabbit	Autologous	None	nHAC-PLA	Tang et al. [101]

PF posterior fusion, *PLF* posterolateral fusion, *AIBF* anterior interbody fusion, *TCP* tricalcium phosphate, *CRM* compression-resistant matrix, *HA/COL* hydroxyapatite/type 1 collagen, *mPCL* medical grade poly(ε-caprolactone), *PLCL* poly(L-lactide-co-caprolactone), *nHAC-PLA* nano-hydroxyapatite-collagen/polylactic acid recipient animals [72, 86, 91, 95, 98, 100, 102]. In particular, it has been clearly demonstrated that allogeneic ATSCs display a non-immunogenic profile in vitro and evoke neither cell-based immunity when implanted in a rat spinal fusion model [99]. Moreover, ATSC proved to allow bone regeneration in vivo, without the need for ex vivo engineering and/or induction [59]. Taken together, this data could provide quite convincing proof-of-principle on the potential safeness and efficacy of banked MSC from healthy donors. Though, the required standards for clinical-grade cell manufacturing (i.e., the current good manufacturing practices, cGMP, guidelines) would be quite hardly to be met by currently experimental protocol for ATSC isolation and culture [103].

Besides MSCs, fibroblasts have been proposed as suitable cell types for bone regenerative purposes. In particular, dermal fibroblasts (DF) can be easily isolated from small skin biopsies, with reduced local morbidity, and rapidly expanded in culture. Dermal fibroblasts share significant similarities with MSC, being considered the skin-derived MSC, and can be induced rapidly towards the osteogenic lineage [58, 104, 105]. Such features render DF a potentially promising tool for bone formation and regeneration.

Cell Engineering Strategies

In order to increase the osteogenic potential of bone-forming cells and obtain a faster bone formation in vivo, diverse genetic engineering strategies have been proposed and tested as promising tool in spinal surgery.

Bone morphogenetic proteins (BMP), being the best characterized molecules implicated in the osteogenic cascade, have been widely employed to induce bone formation in spinal fusion models [106].

The BMP family comprises over 20 distinct highly conserved secreted proteins, further categorized into multiple subgroups according to functional and/or structural features [107, 108]. BMPs play a pivotal role in skeletogenesis during all processes associated with limb development; in particular, they induce the osteoblastic commitment of mesenchymal cells, while inhibiting their differentiation along the myoblastic and adipogenic lineage and increase osteoclastogenesis [108–111]. The osteogenic BMPs, namely, BMP2, BMP4, and BMP7 (also known as osteogenic protein-1, OP-1), can induce the differentiation of multipotent mesenchymal cells into both osteochondrogenic lineage cells and osteoblast precursor cells, suggesting their essential contribution to both direct and indirect ossification mechanisms occurring in vertebrates [112–114]. A wide number of preclinical studies have been demonstrating that these small molecules are capable of inducing ectopic bone formation upon intramuscular implantation and efficient bone healing/regeneration, when delivered in the appropriate concentration and on the appropriate scaffold into a bone defect site [57, 115]. In addition, the use of recombinant human BMP2 (rhBMP2) and BMP7 (rhBMP7) has been approved in both Europe and the United States for selected clinical applications, including anterior interbody spinal fusion. However, despite significant evidence of their potential benefit to bone repair, there is, to date, a dearth of convincing clinical trials [116]. Various genetic engineering approaches are being considered to produce second-generation BMPs, aimed at improving binding affinity to specific target cells, reducing sensitivity to natural inhibitors, reducing immunogenicity, and increasing solubility and stability [117].

On this regard, the main limitation of using recombinant proteins for inducing bone formation in clinical applications is the need for delivery systems that provide a sustained, biologically appropriate concentration of the osteogenic factor at the site of the defect [58, 59]. To this aim, gene delivery vectors based on defective human adenovirus are well suited, as they are able to mediate high-level and short-term gene expression. Although their use implies several disadvantages in view of a potential clinical application [57], adenoviral vectors carrying osteoinductive genes have been successfully used in preclinical spinal fusion models (Table 15.2). In particular, most studies employed defective adenoviral vectors carrying the BMP2 gene (AdBMP2), either for ex vivo cell transduction [79, 80, 86, 96, 104] or for direct percutaneous injection [118]. With regard to the cell type, Mayazaki and colleagues recently demonstrated that the efficacy of AdBMP2-transduced MSC treatment is not related to the tissue source of MSC, as ATSC and BMSC proved to exert comparable results in a rat spinal fusion model [102]. Adenoviral vectors carrying BMP4 [119], BMP6 [120], and BMP9 [121] were also used for direct injection into the paraspinal musculature, which proved to be effective. Also BMP7 has been tested as a suitable molecule delivered ex vivo in BMSC to induce spine fusion [82].

Several contraindications hinder the use of adenoviral vectors in humans, including systemic toxicity, immunization (over 95 % adults have neutralizing antibodies against adenovirus serotype 5), and low cell selectivity [57].

A BMP2 vector based on lentivirus (lenti-BMP2) that is a specialized retrovirus capable of random integration in the host cell genome has been also tested as a feasible tool to induce stable osteogenic commitment of BMSC, to be used in a rat spinal fusion model [85]. Although, enabling sufficient bone formation, this strategy proved to be more effective than AdBMP2-based cell transduction [86], the possible risks of insertional mutagenesis should be carefully considered when using lentiviral vectors [57].

A nonviral approach was attempted using nucleofection, i.e., the intranuclear transfection by electroporation, of rhBMP6 in ATSC [122]. The results obtained through this virus-free technology sound encouraging, although the plasmid DNA used in the procedure still retains some inherent bacterial-related toxicity.

Besides BMPs, other molecules have been tested for their osteogenic potential in gene therapy approaches for spinal fusion. These included the Nel-like molecule (NELL1) [123], the LIM mineralization protein (LMP) [58, 124], and the mothers against decapentaplegic homolog 1 (Smad1) [93]. NELL1 is a heterotrimeric secretory protein thought to be involved in cell growth regulation and differentiation, acting specifically in osteoblasts. NELL1 is overexpressed in synostotic calvaria of patients affected by sporadic plagiocephaly [125] and is able to induce bone regeneration in rat calvarial defects [126]. Based on the evidence that this gene is more osteoblast specific than BMPs, the efficacy of AdNell-1 injection in a rat posterolateral spinal fusion model has been tested, with successful results [123].

LMP is an intracellular LIM-domain protein acting as a potent positive regulator of the osteoblast differentiation program, being able to induce the activation of BMPs and downstream signaling pathway [127, 128]. In humans, three different splice variants are transcribed from the LMP-coding gene (PDZ and LIM domain-7, PDLIM7), named LMP1, LMP2, and LMP3. Both LMP1 and LMP3 induce osteogenic differentiation of mesenchymal progenitors and pre-osteoblasts in vitro and bone formation in diverse animal models [58, 59, 116, 82, 119–122, 124, 128–133]. Similarly to NELL1, in humans LMPs are overexpressed in calvarial tissues and cells isolated from synostosis of patients affected by sporadic synostosis, where it possibly plays a pathogenetic role [134]. LMP1 has been used successfully to induce spine fusion in rats and rabbits, upon plasmid transfection and adenoviral vector-mediated delivery, respectively [124, 127]. Adenoviral-mediated ex vivo transduction was also used to overexpress LMP3 in dermal fibroblast, in a mouse model of paravertebral ectopic bone formation, resulting in the formation of an overwhelming new bony mass [58].

Finally, another gene therapy approach to spine fusion has been recently performed in a rabbit model, using the Hoxc-8-interacting domain of Smad1. In this case, ex vivo transduction was performed using an adenoviral vector, modified to target specifically BMSC, in order to improve the efficiency of gene transfer [93].

Overall the genetic engineering strategies proposed so far in spinal orthopedics surgery proved to be extremely effective, although much effort should be further spent in improving the safety of the gene delivery strategies, by limiting the toxicity and avoiding modification that could lead to genomic instability.

References

1. Etminan M, Girardi FP, Khan SN, et al. Revision strategies for lumbar pseudarthrosis. Orthop Clin North Am. 2002;33:381–92.
2. Boden SD. Overview of the biology of lumbar spine fusion and principles for selecting a bone graft substitute. Spine (Phila Pa 1976). 2002;27(16 Suppl 1):S26–31.
3. Cowan JA, Dimick JB, Wainess R, Upchurch GR, Chandler WF, La Marca F. Changes in the utilization of spinal fusion in the United States. Neurosurgery. 2006;59:15–20.
4. Reid JJ, Johnson JS, Wang JC. Challenges to bone formation in spinal fusion. J Biomech. 2011;44(2):213–20.
5. Giannoudis PV, Einhorn TA, Marsh D. Fracture healing: the diamond concept. Injury. 2007;38 Suppl 4:S3–6.
6. Axhausen G. Arch k1in Chir. 1909;88:23–28.
7. Phemister DB. Surg Gynecol Obstet. 1914;19:303–307.
8. Barth A. Die entstehung und das wachstum der freien gelenkkorper. Eine histologisch-klinische studie. Arch f Klin Chir. 1898;56:507–73.
9. Wigfield CC, Nelson RJ. Nonautologous interbody fusion materials in cervical spine surgery: how strong is the evidence to justify their use? Spine. 2001;26:687–94.
10. Rawlinson JN. Morbidity after anterior cervical decompression and fusion. The influence of the donor site on recovery, and the results of a trial of surgibone compared to autologous bone. Acta Neurochir (Wien). 1994;131:106–18.

11. Khan SN, Cammisa Jr FP, Sandhu HS, Diwan AD, Girardi FP, Lane JM. The biology of bone grafting. J Am Acad Orthop Surg. 2005;13(1):77–86.
12. Tomford WW. Transmission of disease through transplantation of musculoskeletal allografts. J Bone Joint Surg Am. 1995;77:1742–54.
13. Laurencin CT, El-Amin SF. Xenotransplantation in orthopaedic surgery. J Am Acad Orthop Surg. 2008;16(1):4–8.
14. Maatz R, Bauermeister A. A method of bone maceration. Results of animal experiments. J Bone Joint Surg Am. 1957;39:153–66.
15. Lofgren H, Johannsson V, Olsson T, Ryd L, Levander B. Rigid fusion after cloward operation for cervical disc disease using autograft, allograft, or xenograft: a randomized study with radiostereometric and clinical follow-up assessment. Spine. 2000;25:1908–16.
16. Malca SA, Roche PH, Rosset E, Pellet W. Cervical interbody xenograft with plate fixation: evaluation of fusion after 7 years of use in post-traumatic discoligamentous instability. Spine. 1996;21:685–90.
17. Ramani PS, Kalbag RM, Sengupta RP. Cervical spinal interbody fusion with Kiel bone. Br J Surg. 1975;62:147–50.
18. Savolainen S, Usenius JP, Hernesniemi J. Iliac crest versus artificial bone grafts in 250 cervical fusions. Acta Neurochir (Wien). 1994;129:54–7.
19. Siqueira EB, Kranzler LI. Cervical interbody fusion using calf bone. Surg Neurol. 1982;18:37–9.
20. Beer M, Charalambides C, Cobb AG. Poor results after augmenting autograft with xenograft (surgibone) in hip revision surgery: a report of 27 cases. Acta Orthop. 2005;76(4):544–9.
21. Lerner T, Bullmann V, Schulte TL, Schneider M, Liljenqvist U. A level-1 pilot study to evaluate of ultraporous beta-tricalcium phosphate as a graft extender in the posterior correction of adolescent idiopathic scoliosis. Eur Spine J. 2009;18(2):170–9.
22. Boyan BD, McMillan J, Lohmann CH, Ranly DM, Schwartz Z. Bone graft substitutes: basic information for successful clinical use with special focus on synthetic graft substitutes. In: Laurencin CT, editor. Bone graft substitutes. West Conshohocken: ASTM International; 2003. p. 231–59.
23. Yamamuro T, Shikata J, Okumura H, et al. Replacement of lumbar vertebrae of sheep with ceramic prostheses. J Bone Joint Surg Br. 1990;72:889–93.
24. Dai L, Jiang L. Anterior cervical fusion with interbody cage containing beta-tricalcium phosphate augmented with plate fixation: a prospective randomized study with 2-year follow-up. Eur Spine J. 2008;17:698–705.
25. Kim P, Wakai S, Matsuo S, Moriyama T, Kirino T. Bisegmental cervical interbody fusion using hydroxyapatite implants: surgical results and long-term observation in 70 cases. J Neurosurg. 1998;88:21–7.
26. Suetsuna F, Yokoyama T, Kenuka E, Harata S. Anterior cervical fusion using porous hydroxyapatite ceramics for cervical disc herniation. A two-year follow-up. Spine J. 2001;1:348–57.
27. Lowenstam HA, Weiner S. On biomineralization. New York: Oxford University Press; 1989.
28. Le Geros RZ. Calcium phosphates in oral biology and medicine. In: Myers KH, editor. Monographs in oral science, vol. 15. Basel: AG Publishers; 1991. p. 82–107.
29. Korovessis P, Repantis T, Petsinis G, Iliopoulos P, Hadjipavlou A. Direct reduction of thoracolumbar burst fractures by means of balloon kyphoplasty with calcium phosphate and stabilization with pedicle-screw instrumentation and fusion. Spine (Phila Pa 1976). 2008;33(4):E100–8.
30. Bigi A, Foresti E, Gregoriani R, Ripamonti A, Roveri N, Shah JS. The role of magnesium on the structure of biological apatite. Calcif Tissue Int. 1992;50:439–44.
31. Bigi A, Falini G, Foresti E, Gazzano M, Ripamonti A, Roveri N. Magnesium influence on hydroxyapatite crystallization. J Inorg Biochem. 1993;49:69–78.
32. TenHuisen KS, Brown PW. Effects of magnesium on the formation of calcium deficient hydroxyapatite from $CaHPO_4 \cdot 2H_2O$ and $Ca_4(PO_4)_2O$. J Biomed Mater Res. 1997;36:306–14.

33. Rey C, Renugopalakrishnan V, Collins B, Glimcher M. Fourier transform infrared spectroscopic study of the carbonate ions in bone mineral during aging. Calcif Tissue Int. 1991;49:251–8.
34. Landi E, Tampieri A, Mattioli-Belmonte M, Celotti G. Biomimetic Mg- and Mg, CO3-substituted hydroxyapatites: synthesis characterization and in vitro behaviour. J Eur Ceramic Soc. 2006;26:2593–601.
35. Landi E, Logroscino G, Proietti L, Tampieri A, Sandri M, Sprio S. Biomimetic Mg-substituted hydroxyapatite: from synthesis to in vivo behaviour. J Mater Sci Mater Med. 2008;19:239–47.
36. Hillmeier J, et al. Augmentation von Wirbelkörperfrakturen mit einem neuen Calciumphosphate-Zement nach Ballon-Kphoplastie. Orthopade. 2004;33(1):31–9.
37. Maestretti G, Cremer C, Otten P, Jakob RP. Prospective study of standalone balloon kyphoplasty with calcium phosphate cement augmentation in traumatic fractures. Eur Spine J. 2007;16(5):601–10.
38. Verlaan JJ, Oner FC, Slootweg PJ, Verbout AJ, Dhert WJ. Histologic changes after vertebroplasty. J Bone Joint Surg Am. 2004;86:1230–8.
39. Chow LC, Takagi S, Constantino PD. Self-setting calcium phosphate cements. Mat Res Soc Symp Proc. 1991;179:1–24.
40. Driessens FC, Planell JA, Gil FJ. Calcium phosphate bone cements. In: Wise DL et al., editors. Encyclopedic handbook of biomaterials and bioengineering part B, applications, vol. 2. New York: Marcel Dekker; 1995. p. 855–77.
41. Toyone T, Tanaka T, Kato D, Kaneyama R, Otsuka M. The treatment of acute thoracolumbar burst fractures with transpedicular intracorporeal hydroxyapatite grafting following indirect reduction and pedicle screw fixation: a prospective study. Spine. 2006;31:E208–14.
42. Lim TH, Brebach GT, Renner SM, Kim WJ, Kim JG, Lee RE, et al. Biomechanical evaluation of an injectable calcium phosphate treatment of acute thoracolumbar burst fractures with kyphoplasty an intracorporeal grafting with calcium phosphate: a prospective study. Spine. 2002;27:1297–302.
43. Tomita S, Molloy S, Jasper LE, Abe M, Belkoff SM. Biomechanical comparison of kyphoplasty with different bone cements. Spine. 2004;29:1203–7.
44. Cho DY, Lee WY, Sheu PC. Treatment of thoracolumbar burst fractures with polymethyl methacrylate vertebroplasty and short segment pedicle screw fixation. Neurosurgery. 2003;53:1354–61.
45. Gelb H, Schumacher HR, Cuckler J, Ducheyne P, Baker DG. In vivo inflammatory response to polymethylmethacrylate particulate debris: effect of size, morphology and surface area. J Orthop Res. 1994;12:83–92.
46. San Millán Ruíz D, Burkhardt K, Jean B, Muster M, Martin JB, Bouvier J, et al. Pathology findings with acrylic implants. Bone. 1999;25:85S–90.
47. Bai B, Jazrawi LM, Kummer FJ, Spivak JM. The use of an injectable, biodegradable calcium phosphate bone substitute for the prophylactic augmentation of osteoporotic vertebrae and the management of vertebral compression fractures. Spine. 1999;24:1521–6.
48. Dujovny M, Aviles A, Agner C. An innovative approach for cranioplasty using hydroxyapatite cement. Surg Neurol. 1997;48:294–7.
49. LeGeros RZ. Properties of osteoconductive biomaterials: calcium phosphates. Clin Orthop Relat Res. 2002;395:81–98.
50. Ooms EM, Wolke JG, van der Waerden JP, Jansen JA. Trabecular bone response to injectable calcium phosphate (Ca-P) cement. J Biomed Mater Res. 2002;61:9–18.
51. Verlaan JJ, van Helden WH, Oner FC, Verbout AJ, Dhert WJ. Balloon vertebroplasty with calcium phosphate cement augmentation for direct restoration of traumatic thoracolumbar vertebral fractures. Spine. 2002;27:543–8.
52. Korovessis P, Repantis T, George P. Treatment of acute thoracolumbar burst fractures with kyphoplasty and short pedicle screw fixation: transpedicular intracorporeal grafting with calcium phosphate: a prospective study. Indian J Orthop. 2007;41(4):354–61.

53. Blattert TR, Jestaedt L, Weckbach A. Suitability of a calcium phosphate cement in osteoporotic vertebral body fracture augmentation: a controlled, randomized, clinical trial of balloon kyphoplasty comparing calcium phosphate versus polymethylmethacrylate. Spine (Phila Pa 1976). 2009;34(2):108–14.
54. Yoon ST, Boden SD. Spine fusion by gene therapy. Gene Ther. 2004;11(4):360–7.
55. Baltzer AW, Lieberman JR. Regional gene therapy to enhance bone repair. Gene Ther. 2004;11(4):344–50.
56. Pneumaticos SG, Triantafyllopoulos GK, Chatziioannou S, Basdra EK, Papavassiliou AG. Biomolecular strategies of bone augmentation in spinal surgery. Trends Mol Med. 2011;17(4):215–22.
57. Lattanzi W, Pola E, Pecorini G, Logroscino CA, Robbins PD. Gene therapy for in vivo bone formation: recent advances. Eur Rev Med Pharmacol Sci. 2005;9(3):167–74.
58. Lattanzi W, Parrilla C, Fetoni A, Logroscino G, Straface G, Pecorini G, Stigliano E, Tampieri A, Bedini R, Pecci R, Michetti F, Gambotto A, Robbins PD, Pola E. Ex vivo-transduced autologous skin fibroblasts expressing human Lim mineralization protein-3 efficiently form new bone in animal models. Gene Ther. 2008;15(19):1330–43. PubMed PMID: 18633445.
59. Parrilla C, Saulnier N, Bernardini C, Patti R, Tartaglione T, Fetoni AR, Pola E, Paludetti G, Michetti F, Lattanzi W. Undifferentiated human adipose tissue-derived stromal cells induce mandibular bone healing in rats. Arch Otolaryngol Head Neck Surg. 2011;137(5):463–70.
60. Gómez-Barrena E, Rosset P, Müller I, Giordano R, Bunu C, Layrolle P, Konttinen YT, Luyten FP. Bone regeneration: stem cell therapies and clinical studies in orthopaedics and traumatology. J Cell Mol Med. 2011;15(6):1266–86.
61. Horwitz EM, Le Blanc K, Dominici M, Mueller I, Slaper-Cortenbach I, Marini FC, Deans RJ, Krause DS, Keating A, International Society for Cellular Therapy. Clarification of the nomenclature for MSC: The International Society for Cellular Therapy position statement. Cytotherapy. 2005;7(5):393–5.
62. Pittenger MF, Mackay AM, Beck SC, Jaiswal RK, Douglas R, Mosca JD, Moorman MA, Simonetti DW, Craig S, Marshak DR. Multilineage potential of adult human mesenchymal stem cells. Science. 1999;284(5411):143–7.
63. De Bari C, Dell'Accio F, Tylzanowski P, Luyten FP. Multipotent mesenchymal stem cells from adult human synovial membrane. Arthritis Rheum. 2001;44(8):1928–42.
64. Asakura A, Komaki M, Rudnicki M. Muscle satellite cells are multipotential stem cells that exhibit myogenic, osteogenic, and adipogenic differentiation. Differentiation. 2001;68(4–5):245–53.
65. Zuk PA, Zhu M, Mizuno H, Huang J, Futrell JW, Katz AJ, Benhaim P, Lorenz HP, Hedrick MH. Multilineage cells from human adipose tissue: implications for cell-based therapies. Tissue Eng. 2001;7(2):211–28.
66. Erices A, Conget P, Minguell JJ. Mesenchymal progenitor cells in human umbilical cord blood. Br J Haematol. 2000;109(1):235–42.
67. Saulnier N, Lattanzi W, Puglisi MA, Pani G, Barba M, Piscaglia AC, Giachelia M, Alfieri S, Neri G, Gasbarrini G, Gasbarrini A. Mesenchymal stromal cells multipotency and plasticity: induction toward the hepatic lineage. Eur Rev Med Pharmacol Sci. 2009;13 Suppl 1:71–8.
68. Prockop DJ, Oh JY. Medical therapies with adult stem/progenitor cells (MSCs): a backward journey from dramatic results in vivo to the cellular and molecular explanations. J Cell Biochem. 2012;113(5):1460–9.
69. Prockop DJ, Kota DJ, Bazhanov N, Reger RL. Evolving paradigms for repair of tissues by adult stem/progenitor cells (MSCs). J Cell Mol Med. 2010;14(9):2190–9.
70. Horwitz EM, Gordon PL, Koo WK, Marx JC, Neel MD, McNall RY, Muul L, Hofmann T. Isolated allogeneic bone marrow-derived mesenchymal cells engraft and stimulate growth in children with osteogenesis imperfecta: implications for cell therapy of bone. Proc Natl Acad Sci USA. 2002;99(13):8932–7.
71. Chamberlain JR, Schwarze U, Wang PR, Hirata RK, Hankenson KD, Pace JM, Underwood RA, Song KM, Sussman M, Byers PH, Russell DW. Gene targeting in stem cells from individuals with osteogenesis imperfecta. Science. 2004;303(5661):1198–201.

72. Huang JW, Lin SS, Chen LH, Liu SJ, Niu CC, Yuan LJ, Wu CC, Chen WJ. The use of fluorescence-labeled mesenchymal stem cells in poly(lactide-co-glycolide)/hydroxyapatite/collagen hybrid graft as a bone substitute for posterolateral spinal fusion. J Trauma. 2011;70(6):1495–502.

73. Uccelli A, Moretta L, Pistoia V. Mesenchymal stem cells in health and disease. Nat Rev Immunol. 2008;8(9):726–36.

74. Zaim M, Karaman S, Cetin G, Isik S. Donor age and long-term culture affect differentiation and proliferation of human bone marrow mesenchymal stem cells. Ann Hematol. 2012;91(8):1175–86.

75. Zuk PA, Zhu M, Ashjian P, De Ugarte DA, Huang JI, Mizuno H, Alfonso ZC, Fraser JK, Benhaim P, Hedrick MH. Human adipose tissue is a source of multipotent stem cells. Mol Biol Cell. 2002;13(12):4279–95.

76. Katz AJ, Tholpady A, Tholpady SS, Shang H, Ogle RC. Cell surface and transcriptional characterization of human adipose-derived adherent stromal (hADAS) cells. Stem Cells. 2005;23(3):412–23.

77. Saulnier N, Puglisi MA, Lattanzi W, Castellini L, Pani G, Leone G, Alfieri S, Michetti F, Piscaglia AC, Gasbarrini A. Gene profiling of bone marrow- and adipose tissue-derived stromal cells: a key role of Kruppel-like factor 4 in cell fate regulation. Cytotherapy. 2011;13(3):329–40.

78. Gimble JM, Bunnell BA, Chiu ES, Guilak F. Concise review: adipose-derived stromal vascular fraction cells and stem cells: let's not get lost in translation. Stem Cells. 2011;29(5):749–54.

79. Riew KD, Wright NM, Cheng S, Avioli LV, Lou J. Induction of bone formation using a recombinant adenoviral vector carrying the human BMP-2 gene in a rabbit spinal fusion model. Calcif Tissue Int. 1998;63(4):357–60.

80. Cheng SL, Lou J, Wright NM, Lai CF, Avioli LV, Riew KD. In vitro and in vivo induction of bone formation using a recombinant adenoviral vector carrying the human BMP-2 gene. Calcif Tissue Int. 2001;68(2):87–94.

81. Cui Q, Ming Xiao Z, Balian G, Wang GJ. Comparison of lumbar spine fusion using mixed and cloned marrow cells. Spine (Phila Pa 1976). 2001;26(21):2305–10.

82. Hidaka C, Goshi K, Rawlins B, Boachie-Adjei O, Crystal RG. Enhancement of spine fusion using combined gene therapy and tissue engineering BMP-7-expressing bone marrow cells and allograft bone. Spine (Phila Pa 1976). 2003;28(18):2049–57.

83. Orii H, Sotome S, Chen J, Wang J, Shinomiya K. Beta-tricalcium phosphate (beta-TCP) graft combined with bone marrow stromal cells (MSCs) for posterolateral spine fusion. J Med Dent Sci. 2005;52(1):51–7.

84. Kruyt MC, Wilson CE, de Bruijn JD, van Blitterswijk CA, Oner CF, Verbout AJ, Dhert WJ. The effect of cell-based bone tissue engineering in a goat transverse process model. Biomaterials. 2006;27(29):5099–106.

85. Miyazaki M, Sugiyama O, Tow B, Zou J, Morishita Y, Wei F, Napoli A, Sintuu C, Lieberman JR, Wang JC. The effects of lentiviral gene therapy with bone morphogenetic protein-2-producing bone marrow cells on spinal fusion in rats. J Spinal Disord Tech. 2008;21(5):372–9.

86. Miyazaki M, Sugiyama O, Zou J, Yoon SH, Wei F, Morishita Y, Sintuu C, Virk MS, Lieberman JR, Wang JC. Comparison of lentiviral and adenoviral gene therapy for spinal fusion in rats. Spine (Phila Pa 1976). 2008;33(13):1410–7.

87. Kim HJ, Park JB, Lee JK, Park EY, Park EA, Riew KD, Rhee SK. Transplanted xenogenic bone marrow stem cells survive and generate new bone formation in the posterolateral lumbar spine of non-immunosuppressed rabbits. Eur Spine J. 2008;17(11):1515–21.

88. Fu TS, Chen WJ, Chen LH, Lin SS, Liu SJ, Ueng SW. Enhancement of posterolateral lumbar spine fusion using low-dose rhBMP-2 and cultured marrow stromal cells. J Orthop Res. 2009;27(3):380–4.

89. Rao RD, Gourab K, Bagaria VB, Shidham VB, Metkar U, Cooley BC. The effect of platelet-rich plasma and bone marrow on murine posterolateral lumbar spine arthrodesis with bone morphogenetic protein. J Bone Joint Surg Am. 2009;91(5):1199–206.

90. Fu TS, Ueng SW, Tsai TT, Chen LH, Lin SS, Chen WJ. Effect of hyperbaric oxygen on mesenchymal stem cells for lumbar fusion in vivo. BMC Musculoskelet Disord. 2010;11:52.

91. Giannicola G, Ferrari E, Citro G, Sacchetti B, Corsi A, Riminucci M, Cinotti G, Bianco P. Graft vascularization is a critical rate-limiting step in skeletal stem cell-mediated posterolateral spinal fusion. J Tissue Eng Regen Med. 2010;4(4):273–83.

92. Geuze RE, Prins HJ, Öner FC, van der Helm YJ, Schuijff LS, Martens AC, Kruyt MC, Alblas J, Dhert WJ. Luciferase labeling for multipotent stromal cell tracking in spinal fusion versus ectopic bone tissue engineering in mice and rats. Tissue Eng Part A. 2010;16(11):3343–51.

93. Douglas JT, Rivera AA, Lyons GR, Lott PF, Wang D, Zayzafoon M, Siegal GP, Cao X, Theiss SM. Ex vivo transfer of the Hoxc-8-interacting domain of Smad1 by a tropism-modified adenoviral vector results in efficient bone formation in a rabbit model of spinal fusion. J Spinal Disord Tech. 2010;23(1):63–73.

94. Johnson JS, Meliton V, Kim WK, Lee KB, Wang JC, Nguyen K, Yoo D, Jung ME, Atti E, Tetradis S, Pereira RC, Magyar C, Nargizyan T, Hahn TJ, Farouz F, Thies S, Parhami F. Novel oxysterols have pro-osteogenic and anti-adipogenic effects in vitro and induce spinal fusion in vivo. J Cell Biochem. 2011;112(6):1673–84.

95. Abbah SA, Lam CX, Ramruttun AK, Goh JC, Wong HK. Fusion performance of low-dose recombinant human bone morphogenetic protein 2 and bone marrow-derived multipotent stromal cells in biodegradable scaffolds: a comparative study in a large animal model of anterior lumbar interbody fusion. Spine (Phila Pa 1976). 2011;36(21):1752–9.

96. Hsu WK, Wang JC, Liu NQ, Krenek L, Zuk PA, Hedrick MH, Benhaim P, Lieberman JR. Stem cells from human fat as cellular delivery vehicles in an athymic rat posterolateral spine fusion model. J Bone Joint Surg Am. 2008;90(5):1043–52.

97. Sheyn D, Pelled G, Zilberman Y, Talasazan F, Frank JM, Gazit D, Gazit Z. Nonvirally engineered porcine adipose tissue-derived stem cells: use in posterior spinal fusion. Stem Cells. 2008;26(4):1056–64.

98. Lopez MJ, McIntosh KR, Spencer ND, Borneman JN, Horswell R, Anderson P, Yu G, Gaschen L, Gimble JM. Acceleration of spinal fusion using syngeneic and allogeneic adult adipose derived stem cells in a rat model. J Orthop Res. 2009;27(3):366–73.

99. McIntosh KR, Lopez MJ, Borneman JN, Spencer ND, Anderson PA, Gimble JM. Immunogenicity of allogeneic adipose-derived stem cells in a rat spinal fusion model. Tissue Eng Part A. 2009;15(9):2677–86.

100. Vergroesen PP, Kroeze RJ, Helder MN, Smit TH. The use of poly(L-lactide-co-caprolactone) as a scaffold for adipose stem cells in bone tissue engineering: application in a spinal fusion model. Macromol Biosci. 2011;11(6):722–30.

101. Tang ZB, Cao JK, Wen N, Wang HB, Zhang ZW, Liu ZQ, Zhou J, Duan CM, Cui FZ, Wang CY. Posterolateral spinal fusion with nano-hydroxyapatite-collagen/PLA composite and autologous adipose-derived mesenchymal stem cells in a rabbit model. J Tissue Eng Regen Med. 2012;6(4):325–36.

102. Miyazaki M, Zuk PA, Zou J, Yoon SH, Wei F, Morishita Y, Sintuu C, Wang JC. Comparison of human mesenchymal stem cells derived from adipose tissue and bone marrow for ex vivo gene therapy in rat spinal fusion model. Spine (Phila Pa 1976). 2008;33(8):863–9.

103. Gimble JM, Bunnell BA, Chiu ES, Guilak F. Taking stem cells beyond discovery: a milestone in the reporting of regulatory requirements for cell therapy. Stem Cells Dev. 2011;20(8):1295–6.

104. Olabisi RM, Lazard Z, Heggeness MH, Moran KM, Hipp JA, Dewan AK, Davis AR, West JL, Olmsted-Davis EA. An injectable method for noninvasive spine fusion. Spine J. 2011;11(6):545–56.

105. Parrilla C, Lattanzi W, Rita Fetoni A, Bussu F, Pola E, Paludetti G. Ex vivo gene therapy using autologous dermal fibroblasts expressing hLMP3 for rat mandibular bone regeneration. Head Neck. 2010;32(3):310–8.

106. Lattanzi W, Bernardini C. Genes and molecular pathways of the osteogenic process. In: Yunfeng Lin, editor. Osteogenesis. InTech; 2012. ISBN:978-953-51-0030-0. Available from: http://www.intechopen.com/books/osteogenesis/genes-and-molecular-pathways-of-the-osteogenic-process.

107. Miyazono K, Maeda S, Imamura T. BMP receptor signaling: transcriptional targets, regulation of signals, and signaling cross-talk. Cytokine Growth Factor Rev. 2005;16(3):251–63.
108. Wu X, Shi W, Cao X. Multiplicity of BMP signaling in skeletal development. Ann N Y Acad Sci. 2007;1116:29–49.
109. Katagiri T, Yamaguchi A, Komaki M, Abe E, Takahashi N, Ikeda T, Rosen V, Wozney JM, Fujisawa-Sehara A, Suda T. Bone morphogenetic protein-2 converts the differentiation pathway of C2C12 myoblasts into the osteoblast lineage. J Cell Biol. 1994;127(6 Pt 1):1755–66.
110. Okamoto M, Murai J, Yoshikawa H, Tsumaki N. Bone morphogenetic proteins in bone stimulate osteoclasts and osteoblasts during bone development. J Bone Miner Res. 2006;21(7):1022–33.
111. Pham L, Beyer K, Jensen ED, Rodriguez JS, Davydova J, Yamamoto M, Petryk A, Gopalakrishnan R, Mansky KC. Bone morphogenetic protein 2 signaling in osteoclasts is negatively regulated by the BMP antagonist, twisted gastrulation. J Cell Biochem. 2011;112(3):793–803.
112. Bahamonde ME, Lyons KM. BMP3: to be or not to be a BMP. J Bone Joint Surg Am. 2001;83-A(Suppl 1(Pt 1)):S56–62.
113. Balint E, Lapointe D, Drissi H, van der Meijden C, Young DW, van Wijnen AJ, Stein JL, Stein GS, Lian JB. Phenotype discovery by gene expression profiling: mapping of biological processes linked to BMP-2-mediated osteoblast differentiation. J Cell Biochem. 2003;89(2):401–26.
114. Canalis E, Economides AN, Gazzerro E. Bone morphogenetic proteins, their antagonists, and the skeleton. Endocr Rev. 2003;24(2):218–35.
115. Evans C. Gene therapy for the regeneration of bone. Injury. 2011;42(6):599–604.
116. Hwang CJ, Vaccaro AR, Lawrence JP, Hong J, Schellekens H, Alaoui-Ismaili MH, Falb D. Immunogenicity of bone morphogenetic proteins. J Neurosurg Spine. 2009;10(5):443–51.
117. Alaoui-Ismaili MH, Falb D. Design of second generation therapeutic recombinant bone morphogenetic proteins. Cytokine Growth Factor Rev. 2009;20(5–6):501–7.
118. Alden TD, Pittman DD, Beres EJ, Hankins GR, Kallmes DF, Wisotsky BM, Kerns KM, Helm GA. Percutaneous spinal fusion using bone morphogenetic protein-2 gene therapy. J Neurosurg. 1999;90(1 Suppl):109–14.
119. Zhao J, Zhao DY, Shen AG, Liu F, Zhang F, Sun Y, Wu HF, Lu CF, Shi HG. Promoting lumbar spinal fusion by adenovirus-mediated bone morphogenetic protein-4 gene therapy. Chin J Traumatol. 2007;10(2):72–6.
120. Laurent JJ, Webb KM, Beres EJ, McGee K, Li J, van Rietbergen B, Helm GA. The use of bone morphogenetic protein-6 gene therapy for percutaneous spinal fusion in rabbits. J Neurosurg Spine. 2004;1(1):90–4.
121. Helm GA, Alden TD, Beres EJ, Hudson SB, Das S, Engh JA, Pittman DD, Kerns KM, Kallmes DF. Use of bone morphogenetic protein-9 gene therapy to induce spinal arthrodesis in the rodent. J Neurosurg. 2000;92(2 Suppl):191–6.
122. Sheyn D, Kallai I, Tawackoli W, Cohn Yakubovich D, Oh A, Su S, Da X, Lavi A, Kimelman-Bleich N, Zilberman Y, Li N, Bae H, Gazit Z, Pelled G, Gazit D. Gene-modified adult stem cells regenerate vertebral bone defect in a rat model. Mol Pharm. 2011;8(5):1592–601.
123. Lu SS, Zhang X, Soo C, Hsu T, Napoli A, Aghaloo T, Wu BM, Tsou P, Ting K, Wang JC. The osteoinductive properties of nell-1 in a rat spinal fusion model. Spine J. 2007;7(1):50–60.
124. Kim HS, Viggeswarapu M, Boden SD, Liu Y, Hair GA, Louis-Ugbo J, Murakami H, Minamide A, Suh DY, Titus L. Overcoming the immune response to permit ex vivo gene therapy for spine fusion with human type 5 adenoviral delivery of the LIM mineralization protein-1 cDNA. Spine (Phila Pa 1976). 2003;28(3):219–26.
125. Ting K, Vastardis H, Mulliken JB, Soo C, Tieu A, Do H, Kwong E, Bertolami CN, Kawamoto H, Kuroda S, Longaker MT. Human NELL-1 expressed in unilateral coronal synostosis. J Bone Miner Res. 1999;14(1):80–9.

126. Aghaloo T, Cowan CM, Chou YF, Zhang X, Lee H, Miao S, Hong N, Kuroda S, Wu B, Ting K, Soo C. Nell-1-induced bone regeneration in calvarial defects. Am J Pathol. 2006;169(3):903–15.

127. Boden SD, Titus L, Hair G, Liu Y, Viggeswarapu M, Nanes MS, Baranowski C. Lumbar spine fusion by local gene therapy with a cDNA encoding a novel osteoinductive protein (LMP-1). Spine (Phila Pa 1976). 1998;23(23):2486–92.

128. Bernardini C, Saulnier N, Parrilla C, Pola E, Gambotto A, Michetti F, Robbins PD, Lattanzi W. Early transcriptional events during osteogenic differentiation of human bone marrow stromal cells induced by Lim mineralization protein 3. Gene Expr. 2010;15(1):27–42.

129. Minamide A, Boden SD, Viggeswarapu M, Hair GA, Oliver C, Titus L. Mechanism of bone formation with gene transfer of the cDNA encoding for the intracellular protein LMP-1. J Bone Joint Surg Am. 2003;85-A(6):1030–9.

130. Strohbach CA, Rundle CH, Wergedal JE, Chen ST, Linkhart TA, Lau KH, Strong DD. LMP-1 retroviral gene therapy influences osteoblast differentiation and fracture repair: a preliminary study. Calcif Tissue Int. 2008;83(3):202–11. PubMed PMID: 18709396.

131. Wang X, Cui F, Madhu V, Dighe AS, Balian G, Cui Q. Combined VEGF and LMP-1 delivery enhances osteoprogenitor cell differentiation and ectopic bone formation. Growth Factors. 2011;29(1):36–48. PubMed PMID: 21222516.

132. Yoon ST, Park JS, Kim KS, Li J, Attallah-Wasif ES, Hutton WC, Boden SD. ISSLS prize winner: LMP-1 upregulates intervertebral disc cell production of proteoglycans and BMPs in vitro and in vivo. Spine (Phila Pa 1976). 2004;29(23):2603–11. PubMed PMID: 15564908.

133. Viggeswarapu M, Boden SD, Liu Y, Hair GA, Louis-Ugbo J, Murakami H, Kim HS, Mayr MT, Hutton WC, Titus L. Adenoviral delivery of LIM mineralization protein-1 induces new-bone formation in vitro and in vivo. J Bone Joint Surg Am. 2001;83-A(3):364–76. PubMed PMID: 11263640.

134. Lattanzi W, Barba M, Novegno F, Massimi L, Tesori V, Tamburrini G, Galgano S, Bernardini C, Caldarelli M, Michetti F, Di Rocco C. Lim mineralization protein is involved in the premature calvarial ossification in sporadic craniosynostoses. Bone. 2013;52(1):474–84. doi:10.1016/j.bone.2012.09.004.

Chapter 16
Microsurgical Approach for the Treatment of Juxtafacet Synovial Cysts of the Lumbar Spine

Giuseppe Costanzo, Alessandro Ramieri, Alessandro Landi, Maurizio Domenicucci, and Roberto Delfini

Introduction

Synovial cysts and ganglia can arise from any synovial-lined articulation or tendon sheath, affected by osteoarthritis or rheumatoid arthritis. They are encountered predominantly in the extremities, especially at the wrist and knee. However, they can be associated with any diarthrodial joint in the body. The disease is caused by cystic dilatation of the synovial membrane of the joints. Compared with the number of lesions involving the extremities, spinal localization is considered a rare finding. Nevertheless, over the last few years, synovial cysts of the spine have been increasingly reported, probably due to the availability of high-quality CT and MRI [1]. Intraspinal development of this kind of cystic lesion may be asymptomatic or responsible for back pain and neurological disorders. Classically, there is a predilection for these cysts to develop at the L4–L5 facet joint, which is known to be the most mobile segment and the point of maximum axial loading of the spine. This particular predilection for cysts to occur adjacent to the L4–L5 facet joints has also been attributed to the amount of degenerative spondylosis at that level of the spine. Synovial cysts can also be detected in the presence of L4–L5 degenerative spondylolisthesis [2].

G. Costanzo, MD (✉)
Department of Orthopedic Surgery, Polo Pontino,
University of Rome Sapienza, Rome, Italy
e-mail: g.costanzo@giomi.com

A. Ramieri, MD, PhD
Division of Orthopedic, Don Gnocchi Foundation, Milan, Italy

A. Landi, MD, PhD • M. Domenicucci, MD • R. Delfini, MD
Division of Neurosurgery, Department of Neurology and Psychiatry,
University of Rome Sapienza, Rome, Italy

P.P.M. Menchetti (ed.), *Minimally Invasive Surgery of the Lumbar Spine,*
DOI 10.1007/978-1-4471-5280-4_16, © Springer-Verlag London 2014

History and Nomenclature

In 1877, Baker originally described synovial cysts as being secondary to processes occurring within an adjacent degenerated joint. He reported a cyst in a patient with osteoarthritis of the knee, a condition since named for him. Soon after Baker published his description, in 1880 Von Gruker reported an intraspinal cyst found at autopsy. Subsequently, many cases of these lesions that arise from the facet joints of the spine have been reported in the neurosurgical, orthopedic, rheumatological, and radiological literature. In 1950, Vosschulte and Borger were the first to report associated nerve root compression secondary to a cyst adjacent to the facet joint [3].

Regarding the nomenclature of synovial cysts arising from (or adjacent to) the lumbar zygapophyseal joint, the literature presents a broad range of variation. Historically, the term *juxtafacet cyst* was first introduced by Kao et al. in 1974 to characterize two types of periarticular cystic alterations, synovial and ganglion, that can occur in the paraspinal region. It often is not possible to distinguish clearly between these two forms of periarticular cysts. Also, synovial or ganglion cysts have been described in the ligamentum flavum, interspinous ligament, and lumbar annulus. In 1992, Goffin et al. used the term *spinal degenerative articular cysts* to identify such lesions arising specifically from the facets [4].

Therefore, some confusion still exists today over the terms *synovial cyst* and *ganglion cyst*, used interchangeably with respect to cysts found within the spine.

Histological Pictures

In 1997, Rosenberg and Schiller pointed out that the distinction between synovial and ganglion cysts is of pathological interest only. With respect to clinical presentation and treatment, the two lesions share identical characteristics and responses.

It is thought that, over time, microtrauma associated with the degeneration process leads to weak areas in a joint's capsule. A herniation of synovium occurs and the newly formed cavity is filled by the synovial fluid, until the formation of a cyst directly communicating with the joint. When the cyst loses its connection with the adjacent joint, mixoid degeneration, typical of ganglion, may begin.

A synovial cyst is filled with clear or xantochromic fluid, has a synovial-like epithelial lining, and, as indicated earlier, a demonstrable communication to a synovial sheath or joint capsule. In most instances, such operation to remove the cystic formation takes place a shorter or longer time after a synovial cyst has formed and produced clinical symptoms. During that time period, secondary changes due to mechanical pressure, inflammation, and hemorrhage into the cyst lumen can alter the delicate synovial villi originally lining the cystic wall.

In the preserved cysts, there are synovial villi with well-vascularized stalks covered by multiple layers of normal-appearing synovial cells and, generally, the formation of a precipitated fibrin layer on their luminal side. In the more advanced stage, the synovial lining cells completely disappear and are replaced by layers of fibrin. Sometimes, the stroma contains hemosiderin-laden macrophages or, in other cases, chondroid metaplasia takes place. In the final stage, the cyst wall is transformed into dense, acellular hyalinized scar tissue with moderate to severe calcification.

Ganglion cysts have a collagenous capsule without a mesothelial cell lining, are filled with a mixoid material, and do not communicate with the joint cavity. For these characteristics, it has been proposed that a synovial cyst may evolve into a ganglion cyst by losing its communication to the facet joint and subsequently may undergo mucinous degeneration. Unfortunately, to add further confusion, it has been reported that, within a ganglion cyst, the synovial-like lining can reproduce [5].

Hemorrhagic Variant

The hemorrhagic variant is a rare occurrence: few cases of acute intracystic bleeding have been described in the literature. It is likely that intracystic bleeding leads to severe compression of the nerve roots and/or the spinal cord, thus justifying the patients' acute symptomatology [6–9]. The hemorrhagic nature of these cysts is attributable to neoangiogenesis due to chronic inflammation. In our report, we distinguished blood or hemosiderin deposits that indicate bleeding; the former were observed when there had been recent massive hemorrhages, while the latter were associated with smaller hemorrhages. The presence of vascular neoendothelium was observed within the cystic formation. Tatter and Cosgrove [10], on the basis of that demonstrated by Koch et al. [11] and by others [12, 13] regarding the release of angiogenic factors during inflammation, suggested a correlation between the production of the vascular neoendothelium, proliferation of new vessels into the synovial structures, and the chronic inflammatory processes that accompany the evolution of a synovial cyst. We endorse the etiological hypothesis that attributes repeated hemorrhage to the rupture of these neo-formed vessels. Furthermore, the neoangiogenetic nature of these vessels justifies their fragility and consequent tendency to rupture, even in the absence of a significant traumatic event [14].

Classification

From a morphological point of view, cysts are generally classified into:

- Juxtafacet cysts

  - Synovial cyst: in continuity with the capsule of the facet joints
  - Ganglion cyst: the cyst loses continuity with the capsule of the facet joints and it is free inside and/or outside the spinal canal

- Cysts of the ligamentum flavum
- Cysts of the posterior longitudinal ligament

As outlined above, true synovial cysts have a synovial lining membrane that communicates with the facet joint. Ganglion cysts, in opposition, have no synovial lining and develop from mucinous degeneration of the periarticular tissue and usually contain proteinaceous fluid.

True synovial juxtafacet cysts are thought to be more commonly located on the dorsal aspect of the facet joint and, therefore, they are asymptomatic. Other cysts are dumbbell shaped or purely ventral. In a large series reported by Sachdev et al. in 1991, 31 of 42 cysts (73 %) were incidental dorsal nodules and only 11 (27 %) were ventral and symptomatic [15].

Ligamentum flavum and posterior longitudinal ligament cysts usually contain clear or xanthochromic fluid and also present no real communication with the facet joint.

Although some authors have previously defended that such morphological differentiation does not bear any clinical significance, as one cyst type could evolve into the other and, ultimately, all of them would receive the same surgical treatment based on cystectomy, it is possible to distinguish such entities after a careful preoperative evaluation of the neuroradiological investigations. In our opinion, this is essential for the decision-making process and useful to apply the best surgical procedure to correctly remove the real cause of pain.

Etiology

The etiology of synovial cyst is still unclear. Possibilities include extrusion of synovial fluid from a defect in the joint capsule, myxoid degeneration of cyst formation in collagenous connective tissue, increased production of hyaluronic acid by fibrobrast, and nonspecific proliferation of mesenchimal cells [16, 17].

Abnormal or increased motion appear to have some role in many synovial cysts. The relationship to increased motion is strong, as most cysts arise at L4–L5 level, in presence of spondylolistesis or scoliosis, as reported by Sabo et al. in 1996 [15].

The role of trauma has been frequently questioned. The hemosiderin in many of the pathological specimens seems to be one of the stronger arguments for the role of trauma [18].

Ultimately, the most likely hypothesis attributes these cysts to a natural process of degeneration of the facet joints, although a less plausible correlation with injury at the same level has been proposed. In particular, we believe that synovial cyst is an epiphenomenon of spinal motor unit degeneration. It can be configured in a more complex picture of metameric degeneration. In fact, the articular processes represent only one of the multiple components of the motor unit that may be degenerated: many other components of active and passive movement control may be involved in the pathological degenerative process, such as intervertebral disk, LLA, LLP, ligamentum flavum, inter- and supraspinous ligaments and paravertebral muscles, particularly longissimus dorsi and multifidus. Clearly, a more complex picture of degeneration, involving more than two elements, may define a condition of "suspect instability." In the advanced stages of metameric degeneration, true synovial cysts can be considered the last involvement of the zygapophysial joint, which, after becoming loose and widened, presents partial herniation of the synovial content to the periarticular space. In such cases, even if part of the facet joint is preserved, the long-term risk of instability is high, and various grades of spondylolisthesis may accompany cyst formation [19].

The association between juxtafacet synovial cysts and instability has been discussed in literature. Onofrio and Mih [20] reported that, in a series of 13 patients, two of five patients who had postoperative radiographic control had signs of instability. Eight of twelve lumbar cysts examined by these authors were associated with spondylolisthesis. However, they performed no fusions and a number of their patients continued to have chronic back pain. Freidberg et al. described only 1 patient with late instability out of 26 patients, following surgical cyst excision. Feldman and McCulloch reported 6 cases of juxtafacet cyst requiring surgery. Of their 4 patients with spondylolisthesis, 2 required fusion, 1 at the original cyst resection and the other at 2-year follow-up for backache. Kurz and colleagues described 4 patients with symptomatic synovial cyst and found 3 with spondylolisthesis. They performed no fusion and the patients did well. In contrast, Yarde et al. reported [21] that 2 patients from a series of 8 who had spondylolisthesis underwent lumbar fusion in addition to cyst excision. Finally, Sabo et al. [15] performed 7 fusions in 15 spondylolistheses, concluding that fusion should be considered at the time of first operation if the patient is deemed unstable or at high risk of becoming unstable following mesial facetectomy.

Clinical Presentation

Most of the patients with lumbar synovial cyst tend to be in their sixth decade of life with a slight female predominance. The incidence of lumbar synovial cyst is thought to be less than 0.5 % of the general population with back pain. It may be asymptomatic and found incidentally [22].

Epidural expansion of lumbar synovial cyst into the spinal canal can cause, more or less rapidly, compression of neural structures. Most of the symptomatic patients present with radicular pain and neurological deficits (claudicatory pain), located more often at L4–L5 level. More frequently, symptoms are unilateral and monoradicular, though some authors report bilateral and/or multilevel disturbances [23]. Rapid enlargement of the cyst may be responsible for cauda equina syndrome [24].

The onset of symptoms is usually progressive, according to the slow degeneration of the spinal motor unit. But, in particular cases, onset may be sudden, due to a rapid increase in volume or as a result of massive bleeding within the cyst. In fact, the hemorrhagic variant of lumbar synovial cyst usually differs from the nonhemorrhagic one in terms of onset, pain intensity, and response to pharmacological treatment.

The cause of the acute onset of symptoms in case of sudden bleeding is still a matter of debate. It is not clear whether pain is due to the rapid expansion of the cyst or to nerve root irritation subsequent to an inflammatory reaction to the hemorrhage. In our opinion, expansion of the cyst after bleeding is the cause of symptoms because this occurs even in rare cases of rapid growth of the cyst without hemorrhage [25].

As stated by Roessaux et al. [26], when there is internal bleeding, a massive hemorrhage (macro-hemorrhage) might occur, producing a sudden increase in size and, consequently, a mass effect responsible for an acute and severe compression of the nervous structures. It is likely that in cases of micro-hemorrhage that might occur repeatedly, the compressive mass effect is usually moderate, producing a persistent subacute symptomatology.

Radiological Investigation

Sophisticated and newer imaging capabilities have resulted in increased reporting and treatment options of lumbar synovial cyst.

Diagnosis is currently made easier by MRI, which is the gold standard [27, 28]. The imaging signal can be variable, depending on the type of fluid within the cyst. When there is a serous fluid, as in case of simple synovial cyst, there is a low-intensity T1 signal and a hyperintensity on T2-weighted images. With the proteinaceous content of the ganglion cyst, there is hyperintensity in comparison to cerebrospinal fluid on all sequences. Usually, a low-intensity rim surrounds the cyst on T2-weighted images of both ganglion and synovial cyst. After gadolinium administration, ring enhancement, associated with inflammatory processes, is visible.

In presence of intracystic bleeding, the MRI signal is extremely variable owing to the hematic content of the cyst that differs according to the amount of time that has passed since hemorrhage. Intracystic hemorrhage, generally referred to as subacute, typically appears as heterogenous hyperintensity on all sequences due to the metahemoglobin it contains. However, when there are blood products older than 7 days, there may be areas of hypointensity on T2-weighted sequences. The hypointense rim reflects a combination of hemosiderin deposits, fibrous capsule, and calcification in the cystic wall. After gadolinium, ring enhancement is detected.

MRI is also important for a correct differential diagnosis from other pathologies that may have a similar clinical presentation. The differential diagnosis of synovial cyst includes a herniated nucleus pulposus, especially a free extruded fragment. With the accuracy of MRI, signal characteristics can often distinguish a cyst from a disk fragment. Neurofibroma, hematoma, meningioma, abscess, lipoma, and metastatic disease also may be included in differential diagnosis. The use of gadolinium, as well as the signal change, should assist in an accurate diagnosis. One other rare but important process that needs to be considered in the differential diagnosis is pigmented villonodular synovitis. In 1996, Giannini et al. described a series of 12 patients with pigmented villonodular synovitis of the spine. This is a benign neoplasm of histiocytic origin that is noted histopatholocically and a hypercellular area with hemosiderin and multinucleated giant cells. Pigmented villonodualr synovitis located at other joints has undergone malignant transformation and, therefore, requires synoviectomy [15].

Juxtafacet cysts also require differentiation from perineural and arachnoid cysts. The perineural cyst arises from the posterior root ganglion. It is usually quite small and its cyst wall contains nerve fibers. The arachnoid cyst has a pedicle attachment to the spinal dura near the nerve root. It is usually single and may be longitudinally elongated over several spinal levels. The arachnoid cyst has a connective tissue capsule and may fill with contrast material approximately 50 % of the time.

Although MRI is indicated as the best instrument for diagnosing of juxtafacet lumbar synovial cyst, CT scan also provides abundant information regarding the nature, type, and evolution of the lesion [29]. The cyst often has a calcified rim and there may be gas in association with the facet joint space. Bone erosion has been described, but is uncommon. Hemorrhage increases the density of the soft tissue mass that originates from the articular processes, which are generally severely arthrotic. Peripheral and internal calcification may be present at the chronic stage after hemorrhage. Moreover, CT may be useful to evaluate the inclination of the facet joints, which can be a predisposing factor for instability. Finally, dynamic X-rays are important preoperatively to exclude instability and indication for spinal fusion [15, 30].

Treatment Options

Treatment options are various, ranging from conservative to standard open surgical procedures. Conservative treatment modalities include no treatment, bed rest, oral analgesics, physical therapy, brace, chiropractic care, CT-guided needle aspiration, or intraarticular injection of corticosteroid drugs. Surgical procedures are different, from minimally invasive technique to standard open procedures, with or without instrumentation and fusion. The literature describes simple laminotomy with cystectomy, laminectomy, foraminotomy, mesial facetectomy, and/or fusion when necessary.

There are some considerations regarding treatment:

1. Nonsurgical treatment can achieve unsafe and nondurable results (aspiration of the cyst, instillation of steroids, physiokinesitherapy, and more)
2. Surgical treatment can obtain a complete resolution of symptoms in a high percentage of patients with a low incidence of complications.
3. Identification of the best surgical option requires knowledge of the biomechanics of each individual patient's spine.

Microsurgical Approach

Operative Technique

Under general anesthesia, the patient is positioned prone and intraabdominal pressure is minimized. After surgical preparation, draping, and level control by means of fluoroscopy, a 2 cm midline incision is made. We perform a monolateral lamina exposure without using a monopolar device to prevent muscle damage and with the aid of a dedicated bivalve retractor. Exposing the bone more laterally, we can completely identify the articular process. Using curets, rongeurs, Kerrison punches, and/or high-speed drill, laminotomy is performed. After removal of the ligamentum flavum, the intraspinal cyst is identified. With microscope, as for microdiscectomy, the lesion is dissected off the adjacent dura and nerve root to the level of its attachment to the facet joint. The associated capsule is sharply removed along with the cyst. The laminotomy is then safely widened, with preservation at least of two-thirds of the medial facet. The root is retracted medially and the canal is explored to exclude disk herniation (no disk tissue was discovered to be causing of radicular pain in any of our patients). Nerve root mobility is tested to exclude any residual stenosis. A free fat graft or anti-adhesions gel is placed over the exposed dura and closure is routine.

The patient may be allowed out of the bed on the following day. The remaining postoperative management and rehabilitation are the same as after disk surgery.

Personal Experience

In our experience, the surgical approach has always been microsurgical [30]. Laminotomy with preservation of the medial articular facet is our preferred technique to expose the cyst, so that it can be entirely removed. This particular attention in bone resection is extremely useful in order not to jeopardize vertebral stability and to avoid the need for fusion. In fact, correlation between total removal of the facets and the onset of symptomatic spondylolisthesis is reported in literature.

Bone exposure, performed without using the monopolar device, is useful to prevent muscle atrophy. By using operative microscope, performing a light removal of the one-third of the medial facet of the articular mass, we can identify the capsular origin of the cyst and excise it completely. Resection of the joint capsule ensures prevention of any recurrence.

Another microsurgical option is a decompression and removal of the cysts through a contralateral laminectomy approach [31]. A comparison between the angle of approach, provided by the contralateral laminectomy, and the ipsilateral one shows that the contralateral laminectomy achieves additional access to the lateral recess, which is not obtainable through an ipsilateral approach without resection of the facet. We have never used this approach; however, this approach is described as useful in case of extension of the cyst through the lateral recess.

Recently, minimally invasive techniques for removal of the synovial cyst have been described [32]. The technique most widely used is performed by an 18-mm incision approximately 15 mm lateral to the midline. A K-wire under fluoroscopic control is used to penetrate fascia and muscles. Serial dilators are passed over the wire and docked at the junction of the lamina and facet. Lateral fluoroscopy is again used, this time to confirm proper positioning of the tubular retractor. With visualization provided by the operative microscope, the thin layer of soft tissue over the lamina and medial facet is removed using monopolar cautery. A curette is used to expose the inferior edge of the lamina. A Kerrison instrument and/or high-speed drill is then used to perform the laminotomy and medial facetectomy. If a complete hemilaminectomy is required, the tubular retractor can be angled more medially and the patient tilted away from the surgeon to provide a more contralateral view. The pedicle frequently serves as an excellent landmark from which to determine the extent of necessary lateral bone removal and to maintain anatomical orientation. The ligamentum flavum is opened either cephalad or caudal to the cyst. At this point, the cyst should be carefully separated from the dura mater by using curved curettes as well as sharp dissection. The traversing nerve root should be identified. In some cases, the cyst can be resected en bloc, but commonly it requires piecemeal removal, particularly with larger cysts. Careful dissection and establishment of the proper anatomical planes can minimize the risk of cerebrospinal fluid leakage, but, in some cases, dural tearing is unavoidable.

In 2010, Bydon et al. [31] carried out a wide review of all possible treatment options, including minimally invasive and open procedures, comparing decompression alone with decompression plus instrumented fusion. They concluded that it is fundamental to include an appraisal of any micro-instability in preoperative planning in order to decide when to perform fusion and emphasize that fusion must be planned whenever there are signs of instability. These authors also compared open and minimally invasive techniques for decompression alone and did not find any substantial differences in terms of outcomes: these results support our hypothesis according to which the presence of active instability makes fusion mandatory.

In the light of the evidence reported in the literature, we believe that the microsurgical technique has some advantages in comparison to minimally invasive procedures:

1. Duration of the procedure: the open microsurgical technique requires about 90 min compared to 156 min for minimally invasive techniques.
2. Risk of postoperative instability: the technique we adopted preserves the medial two-thirds of the articular facet, whereas the minimally invasive technique requires a total medial arthrectomy, which, in our opinion, can increases the risk of long-term instability in a spinal segment that already displays degeneration.
3. Minimization of the risk of cerebrospinal fistula: exposure of the lesion via microsurgical technique makes it easy to identify and repair any dural tears. This is far more difficult in mini-invasive techniques, also in view of the fact that synovial cyst may be the cause of dural adherences.

Outcomes

It is universally accepted that cystectomy is succesful. About 80–90 % of patients reported improvement or disappearance of their radicular pain immediately after surgery. Less satisfactory seems to be the improvement of back pain.

Recurrence and complication rates after surgical treatment are completely acceptable. There is a recurrence rate of 6 % at a mean 2-year follow-up. The most frequent complication is dural tear. Some patients develop spinal instability and require later fusion. In fact, the treatment of cyst does not end with this surgical excision, and follow-up is important to detect any possible late complications. Generally, the reappearance of symptoms could indicate a recurrence or the onset of instability. Dynamic X-rays, performed at 2-year follow-up, seem to be effective for recognizing an unstable spondylolisthesis, after a time interval sufficient to develop this late complication. Moreover, a questionnaire issued for assessing outcome was useful for finding out how patients perceive their disease and their prognosis. It also represents a possible means for the assessment of outcome. Recently, we administered a questionnaire for assessing patient outcome and satisfaction at 2-year follow-up. It was based on eight questions:

1. Is your overall pain better since surgery?
2. Any numbness or tingling in legs or feet?
3. Any problems with control of bladder and bowels?
4. Any leg or foot pain?
5. Any back pain?
6. Any walking difficulties?
7. List specific areas of pain since your operation.
8. Satisfaction of surgical outcome: yes, could repeat procedure or no, would have avoided surgery.

Our results, in a series of 18 synovial cysts, all treated by microsurgical procedure (laminotomy, light removal of medial facet, and radical cystectomy), were good or excellent in 80 % of cases and fair in 20 %. We observed one case of spondylolisthesis, clinically asymptomatic, and no recurrence [30] (Figs. 16.1, 16.2, and 16.3).

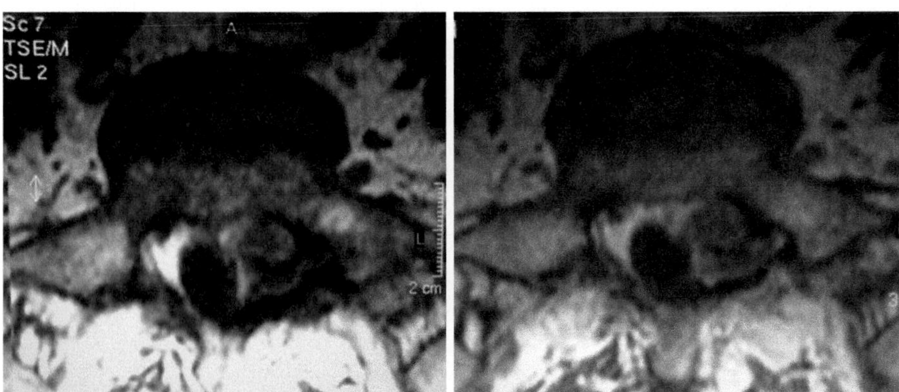

Fig. 16.1 Preoperative MRI. Comparison of axial T1-weighted images before (**a**) and after (**b**) gadolinium injection. The left L5–S1 heterogeneously hyperintense cystic lesion, compressing the cauda, shows a moderate increase of the signal after the contrast injection, particularly around the edges of the lesion. Diagnosis was lumbar hemorrhagic synovial cyst

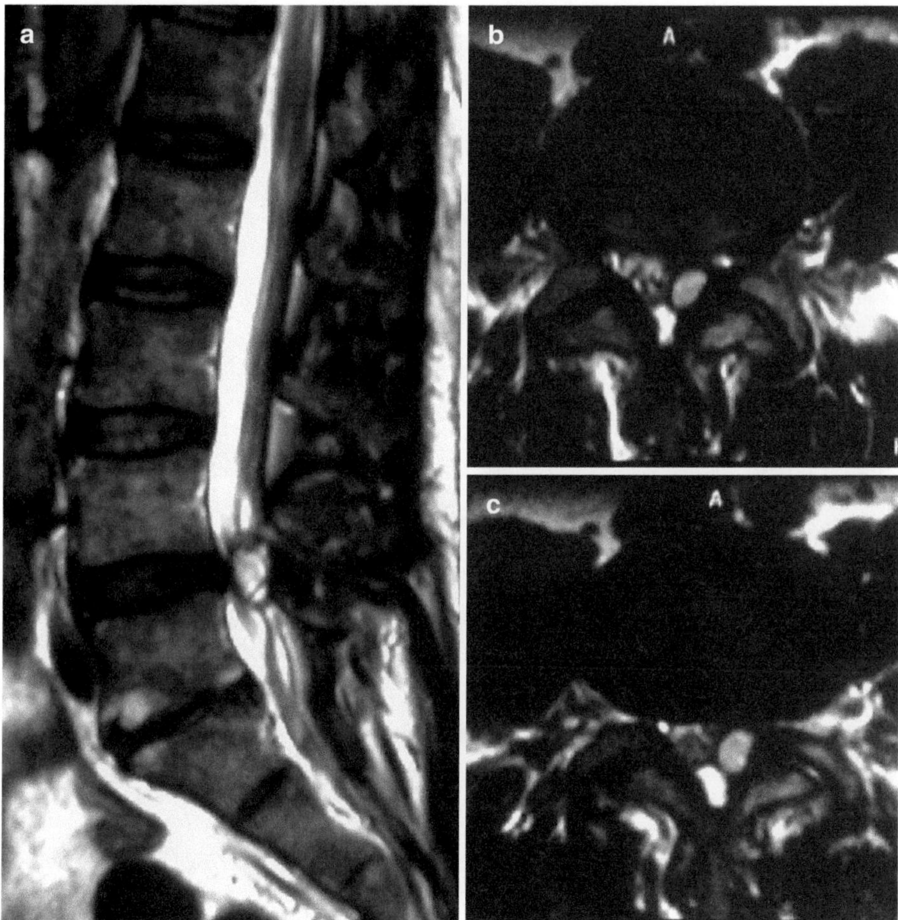

Fig. 16.2 Preoperative MRI. Sagittal (**a**) and axial (**b**, **c**) T2-weighted images that show an L4–L5 true synovial cyst arises from the left L4–L5 facet joint

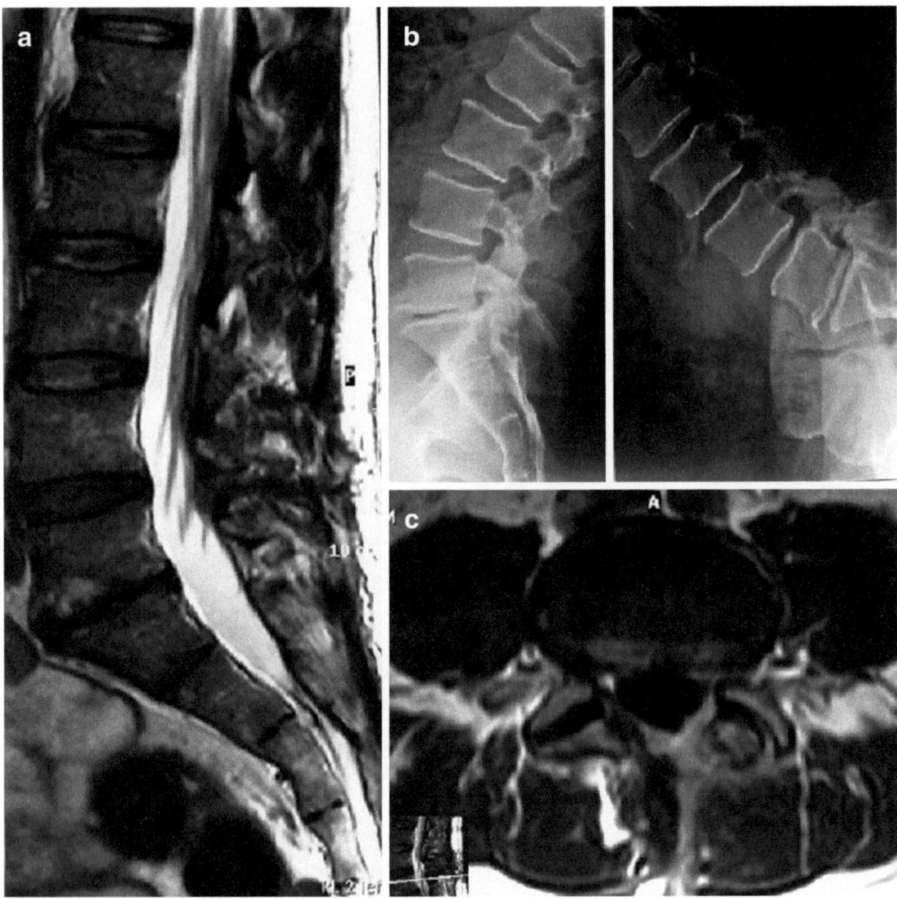

Fig. 16.3 Same case as Fig. 16.2. Postoperative MRI. Sagittal (**a**) and axial (**c**) T2-weighted images that show complete excision of the cyst and preservation of the facet joint. Maintenance of vertebral stability is demonstrated by dynamic X-rays at 2-year follow-up (**b**)

Conclusion

Juxtafacet intraspinal synovial cysts are unusual lesions of the spine associated with facet arthropathy. Advances in neuroimaging have aided in improved preoperative recognition of this pathology. Debate continues regarding the cause of synovial cysts, with arthritis, trauma, or segmental instability being the most often reported.

In the lumbar spine, cysts can cause radicular symptoms. Rapid exacerbation of pain or cauda equina syndrome are possible if sudden enlargement or massive bleeding occur.

Although conservative procedures have been proposed, the gold standard for their treatment remains complete surgical excision. Resection and nerve root or cauda equina decompression can be performed with low risk and an expectation of good to excellent surgery-related outcomes. Sound surgical judgment combined with pre- and intraoperative findings should be used to determine the indication for concomitant fusion in each patient. When preoperative radiological instability, detected by dynamic X-rays, is absent and bone demolition is minimal, no fusion is required.

A minimally invasive microsurgical approach, consisting of laminotomy and partial arthrectomy with preservation of the two-thirds of the medial facet, seems to be a viable treatment option with a low risk of complications and low rate of recurrence.

References

1. Artico M, Cervoni L, Carloia S, et al. Synovial cysts: clinical and neuroradiological aspects. Acta Neurochir (Wien). 1997;139:1176–81.
2. Howington JU, Connolly ES, Voorhies RM. Intraspinal synovial cysts: 10-year experience at the Ochsner Clinic. J Neurosurg Spine. 1999;91:193–9.
3. Savitz M. Synovial cysts of the lumbar spine: a review. Br J Neurosurg. 1998;12:465–6.
4. Lyons MK, Atkinson JL, Wharen RE, et al. Surgical evaluation and management of lumbar synovial cysts: the Mayo Clinic experience. J Neurosurg Spine. 2000;93:53–7.
5. Kjerulf TD, Terry WD, Boubelik RJ. Lumbar synovial or ganglion cysts. Neurosurgery. 1986;19:415–20.
6. Henriet M, Nubourgh Y. Hemorragie dans un kyste synovial lombaire avec compression polyradiculaire aigue. Rachis. 1998;10:89–90.
7. Howling SJ, Kessel D. Case report: acute radiculopathy due to haemorrhagic lumbar synovial cyst. Clin Radiol. 1997;52:73–4.
8. Kaneko K, Inoue Y. Haemorrhagic lumbar synovial cyst. A cause of acute radiculopathy. J Bone Joint Surg Br. 2000;82:583–4.
9. Summers RM, Quint DJ. Case report 712. Hemorrhagic synovial cyst arising from right L2-3 facet joint. Skeletal Radiol. 1992;21:72–5.
10. Tatter SB, Cosgrove GR. Hemorrhage into a lumbar synovial cyst causing an acute cauda equina syndrome. Case report. J Neurosurg. 1994;81:449–52.
11. Kock AE, Polverini PJ, Kunkel SL, et al. Interleukin-8 as a macrophage-derived mediator of angiogenesis. Science. 1992;258:1798–801.
12. Brown RA, Weiss JB, Tomlinson IW, et al. Angiogenic factors from synovial fluid resembling that from tumors. Lancet. 1980;1:682–5.
13. Fritz P, Klein C, Mischlinski A, et al. Morphometric analysis of the angioarchitecture of the synovial membrane in rheumatoid arthritis and osteoarthritis. Zentralbl Pathol. 1992;138:128–35.
14. Ramieri A, Domenicucci TM, Seferi A, Paolini S, Petrozza V, Delfini R. Lumbar hemorrhagic synovial cysts: diagnosis, pathogenesis, and treatment. Report of 3 cases. Surg Neurol. 2006;65:385–90.
15. Sabo RA, Tracy PT, Weinger JM. A series of 60 juxtafacet cysts: clinical presentation, the role of spinal instability and treatment. J Neurosurg. 1996;85:560–5.
16. Brisch A, Payan HM. Lumbar intraspinal extradural ganglion cyst. J Neurol Neurosurg Psychiatry. 1972;35:771–5.
17. Radatz M, Jakubowski J, Cooper J, et al. Synovial cysts of the lumbar spine: a review. Br J Neurosurg. 1997;11:520–4.
18. Franck JI, King RB, Petro GR, et al. A posttraumatic lumbar synovial cyst. Case report. J Neurosurg. 1987;66:293–6.

19. Reust P, Wendling D, Lagier R, et al. Degenerative spondylolisthesis, synovial cyst of the zigapophyseal joints, and sciatic syndrome: report of two cases and review of the literature. Arthritis Rheum. 1988;31:288–94.
20. Onofrio BM, Mih AD. Synovial cysts of the spine. Neurosurgery. 1988;22:642–7.
21. Yarde WL, Arnold PM, Kepes JJ, et al. Synovial cysts of the lumbar spine: diagnosis, surgical management and pathogenesis. Report of eight cases. Surg Neurol. 1995;43:459–65.
22. Eyster EF, Scott WR. Lumbar synovial cysts: report of eleven cases. Neurosurgery. 1989;24:112–5.
23. Pendleton B, Carl B, Pollay M. Spinal extradural benign synovial or ganglion cyst: case report and review of the literature. Neurosurgery. 1983;13:322–6.
24. Cameron SE, Hanscom DA. Rapid development of a spinal synovial cyst. Spine. 1992;17:1528–30.
25. Paolini S, Ciappetta P, Santoro A, Ramieri A. Rapid, symptomatic enlargement of a lumbar juxtafacet cyst: case report. Spine. 2002;27(11):E281–3.
26. Rosseaux P, Durot JF, Pluot M. Kystes synoviaux et synovialomes du rachis lombaire. Aspects histo-pathologiques et neuro-chirurgicaux à propos de 8 observations. Neurochirurgie. 1989;35:31–9.
27. Jackson DE, Atlas SW, Mani JR, et al. Intraspinal synovial cysts: MR imaging. Radiology. 1989;170:527–30.
28. Yuh WT, Drew JM, Weinstein JN, et al. Intraspinal synovial cysts. Magnetic resonance evaluation. Spine. 1991;16:740–5.
29. Lemish W, Apsimon T, Chakera T. Lumbar intraspinal synovial cysts: recognition and CT diagnosis. Spine. 1989;14:1378–83.
30. Landi A, Marotta N, Tarantino R, Ruggeri AG, Cappelletti M, Ramieri A, Domenicucci M, Delfini R. Microsurgical excision without fusion as a safe option for resection of synovial cyst of the lumbar spine: long-term follow-up in mono-institutional experience. Neurosurg Rev. 2012;35:245–53.
31. Bydon A, Xu R, Parker SL, McGirt MJ, Bydon M, Gokaslan ZL, Witham TF. Recurrent back and leg pain and cyst reformation after surgical resection of spinal synovial cysts: systematic review of reported postoperative outcomes. Spine J. 2010;10:820–6.
32. Nouzhan S, Khoo LT. Holly LT treatment of lumbar synovial cysts using minimally invasive surgical techniques. Neurosurg Focus. 2006;20(3):E2.

Index